Radiologic Examination of the Orohypopharynx and Esophagus

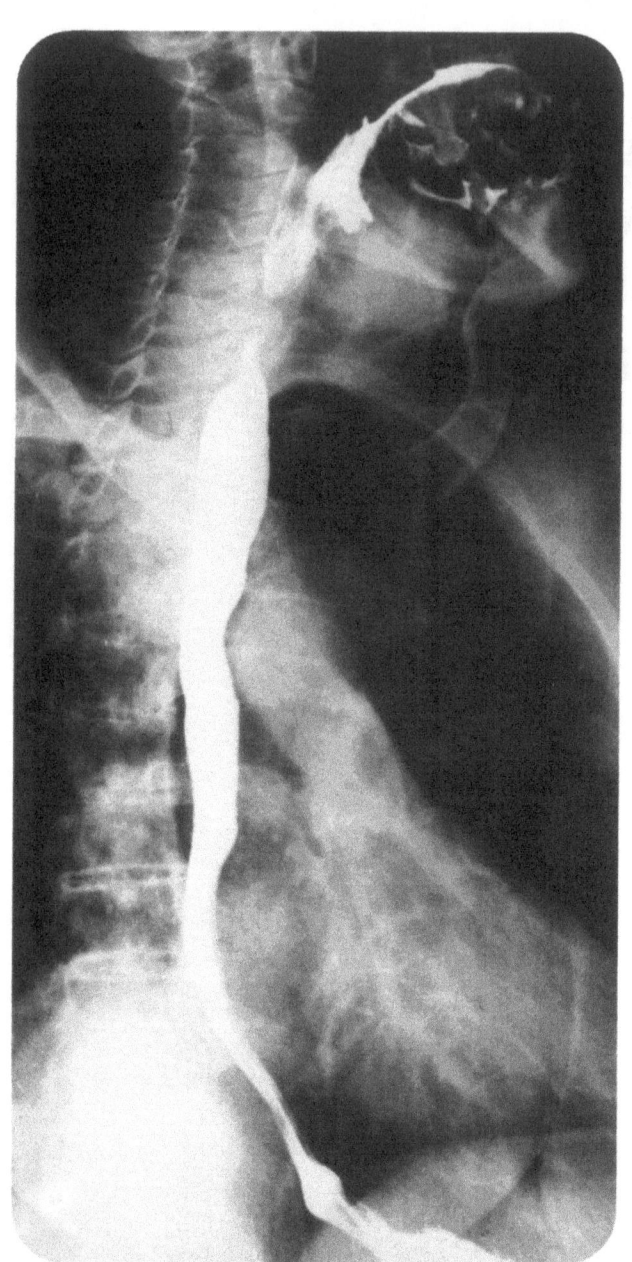

Costantino Zaino

Thomas C. Beneventano

Radiologic Examination of the Orohypopharynx and Esophagus

THE BARIUM SWALLOW

WITH 450 ILLUSTRATIONS

SPRINGER-VERLAG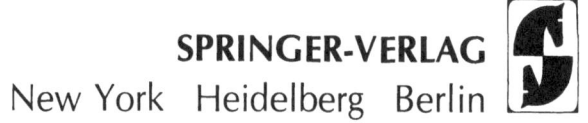
New York Heidelberg Berlin

Dr. Costantino Zaino
Associate Research Fellow
Department of Diagnostic Radiology
Montefiore Hospital and Medical Center

Send correspondence to:
Dr. Costantino Zaino
18 Warren Avenue
Tuckahoe, New York 10707

Dr. Thomas C. Beneventano
Department of Radiology
Montefiore Hospital and Medical Center
111 East 210 Street
Bronx, New York 10467

Library of Congress Cataloging in Publication Data

Zaino, Costantino.
   Radiologic examination of the orohypopharynx and esophagus.

   Bibliography: p.
   Includes index.
   1. Esophagus—Radiography.   2. Pharynx—Radiography.   I. Beneventano,
Thomas C., joint author.   II. Title
RC815.7.Z34   616.3′2′07572   77-21426

Softcover reprint of the hardcover 1st edition 1977

9 8 7 6 5 4 3 2 1

ISBN-13: 978-1-4612-6346-3   e-ISBN-13: 978-1-4612-6344-9
DOI: 10.1007/978-1-4612-6344-9

Designer: Natasha Sylvester

Dedicated to our wives

Yole Zaino
Marilyn L. Beneventano

Basic anatomic differences between infants and adults may affect the technique in radiologic studies. For example, infants have less esophageal muscular tone than adults and the sphincters may not be fully functional, so that the esophagus appears dilated. Also, as a result, there is frequent regurgitation and air is often present in the infants' esophagus. True pharyngeal and/or lower esophageal incoordination may be evaluated by means of special cine studies (see Chapter 3).

The larynx in infants is at a higher level than in adults and the sphincter is located in the area of C-3 (94a) (Fig. 4). The paravertebral soft tissue zone is wider and varies with the respiratory phase and phonation. Buckling and compression of the trachea may also be noted. The retropharyngeal and nasal airway can best be observed in the lateral position while the infant is asleep or during quiet breathing through the nose (neonatal period). After the first month, infants become mouth breathers (6).

The average adult patient

The technique used in the average adult is generally standardized. The rate of swallowing is usually rapid and forceful and is studied by using a standard barium meal mixture or by the use of any standard commercial preparation. Normally forceful expulsion of the bolus from the oropharynx and hypopharynx occurs with almost complete obliteration of the barium lining the esophagus. Residual air in the food channels or the esoph-

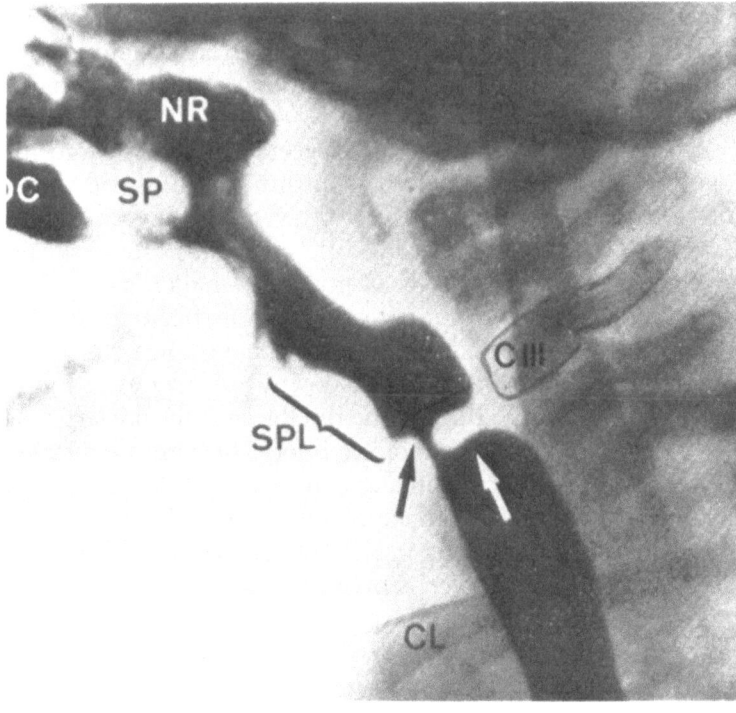

FIGURE 4
Barium swallow in an infant. Upper sphincter at arrows. OC, oral cavity; SP, soft palate; NR, nasal regurgitation; SPL, cricoid impression, CL, clavicle. From Giedion, A. The non-obstructive pharyngoesophageal cross roll. Ann. Radio. *16*-3/4, 129-125, 1973. Paris, France.

agus is usually absent. The routine films and standard positions are described in Chapter 2.

The elderly patient

The elderly population is rapidly increasing with a corresponding increase in the number of patients with swallowing disorders and symptoms of dysphagia. With advancing age, a number of anatomic involutional and degenerative changes ordinarily appear, which may be considered part of the aging process. For example, thinning and atrophy of muscular and ligamentous structures as well as atrophy of body organs occur. A general laxity and loss of muscular tone (reverting back to infant and childhood patterns in the esophagus) also occurs. Functional changes also become more apparent. A slower rate of swallowing, loss of the normal smooth peristaltic waves, and a more segmental type of propulsive action with some degree of incoordination are frequently observed.

With advancing years, impaired mastication becomes an important factor. Because of dental caries, missing teeth, or poorly fitting dental plates, the normal chewing process becomes impaired, causing the patient to select a soft or even liquid diet. This alteration in diet often delays the detection of early esophageal lesions that may obstruct the passage of more solid foods.

Because the bolus is normally reduced in size by the tongue and swallowed in stages, the effectiveness of the tongue in this process partly determines the rate of clearance of a bolus. Increasing age impairs the ability of the tongue to function in this capacity. The lateral food channels, e.g., valleculae and pyriform sinuses, become dilated because of loss of muscle tone. Food is therefore retained longer in these structures. Retained air may also be noted in the lateral channels at rest in the elderly.

A thick barium paste requires exaggerated and more forceful repetitive swallowing motions than thin mixtures and therefore serves as an excellent test of the swallowing mechanism in the aged. The epiglottis is less likely to bend posteriorly and appears radiographically to be sharper and smaller in size than in the younger adult. Air swallowing is more frequent and the upper esophagus can be delineated by trapped air.

As a part of the aging process, a downward and forward shift of the larynx occurs, affecting the thickness of the prevertebral soft tissue area above the thoracic inlet. This shift produces a forward arching of the sphincter zone segment. Relaxation of the phrenoesophageal membrane causes a more frequent demonstration of hiatal hernia in the elderly. Because of the upward shift of the lower esophagus, redundancy is more common, with resultant sluggish passage of the bolus, increased stasis, and dilatation. Because of the redundancy of the esophagus, variations in its position or location in different degrees of obliquity and in various respiratory phases occur.

TYPES OF EXAMINATIONS

The roentgenologic examination of the orohypopharynx and esophagus requires visualization both in motion and at rest. The initial examination is performed during the active process of swallowing a standard barium meal when this area is dilated, followed by reexamination immediately after the patient has swallowed the barium with the esophagus contracted. It is essential to examine this area in action in order to analyze the motor function and to identify any abnormal area of protrusion, compression, deviation, or obstruction. Examining the esophagus in its contracted state aids in the visualization of abnormalities of the mucosal pattern.

The hypopharynx and esophagus, in action, can be examined in a number of ways. Standard fluoroscopy with conventional spot filming remains in use. Image intensification has greatly improved visibility and markedly reduced the exposure to the patient.

Cinefluorography is replacing cineradiography, which requires a greater exposure dose to the patient. Cinefluorography consists of photographing on cine films, the image transmitted by the image intensifier. Cinefluorography with 16 mm or 35 mm films has added a greater dimension to this examination, especially of the hypopharyngeal area. By increasing the number of frames per second, motion can be slowed down considerably so that the normal and abnormal functioning of this area can now be studied at leisure.

Photofluorography instead of cinefluorography may also be used. For example, spot films in which the image is transmitted through the intensifier with either 70 mm, 90 mm, or 105 mm rolled film are excellent in general in the entire GI tract. The use of a stationary grid improves the contrast of the photographed image, being especially useful in sequential filming in children, while further reducing the radiation dose associated with conventional films.

Videotapes used in conjunction with TV monitors are now replacing cinefluorography. These also reduce the exposure to the patient and permit instant replay.

Many newer, more sophisticated radiologic units are now employed, including remote-control equipment and various preprogrammed radiographic techniques which, to a degree, have mechanized barium meal examinations. Although such innovations are desirable in mass screenings, detailed and successful study still requires the personal attention of the radiologist. Also, whereas cineradiography and tapes constitute excellent tools in the examination of the pharyngoesophagus, the images are not as sharp as those obtained with high-quality radiographs, employing optimally functioning screens, grids, and standard films. Whereas functional disturbances are best analyzed by the fluoroscopic image and cineradiographic studies, early structural changes are best evaluated with standard film techniques, including, of course, multiple spot films.

Computerized tomographic x-ray scanning equipment is the

latest innovation and may offer, in the near future, additional aid in the differential diagnosis between mediastinal masses involving the esophagus and esophageal tumors.

FLUOROSCOPIC AND FILMING TECHNIQUE

Fluoroscopic screening in asymptomatic patients is best performed in the prone right anterior oblique position, while the patient drinks a standard barium meal through a flexible straw (dentures should be removed). The detailed observations to be noted in the various segments of the oropharynx and esophagus are presented in Chapter 2. The gastroesophageal junction should also be studied with full sustained inspiration and expiration. The patient is then rotated and examined in other appropriate positions, specifically to exclude the presence of a small lesion which may have been overlooked or to clarify any abnormal areas of compression or deviation. If any abnormality has been detected, the examination should then be repeated immediately using a standard, commercial thick barium paste to determine the rate of travel of the bolus and to better visualize the mucosal pattern. Self-prepared barium paste of a uniform consistency can also be used, but because the rate of transit changes with the viscosity of the bolus it is considered preferable to use a standard commercial preparation instead of a self-prepared barium paste mixture material. Each bolus is followed from the oral cavity to the stomach. After the esophagus has passed the greater part of the bolus, enough barium clings to the mucosal surface to detect any gross abnormality of the mucosal pattern. Mucosal detail, however, is best evaluated on films. The transport time may be measured by means of a stopwatch during fluoroscopy, which helps detect abnormal motor function. The normal emptying time (complete emptying of the barium) following the ingestion of a 15 ml bolus of a standard barium meal has been estimated at 180 seconds (152).

In any routine upper gastrointestinal tract examination with a normal fluoroscopic examination and in the absence of specific symptoms referrable to the hypopharynx and esophagus, at least one roentgenogram, and preferably more, of the entire hypopharynx and esophagus should be obtained in the prone right anterior oblique position while the patient is swallowing continuously through a straw. The upper edge of the 14 × 17 cassette should be at the level of the nose in order to include the oral cavity. In short-statured individuals the oropharynx, esophagus, and gastroesophageal junction can be visualized on one film (see frontispiece). In tall patients, two films, positioned at different levels to include the entire esophagus for a composite evaluation, are obtained.

The filming of the oropharynx, especially if a lesion is suspected, requires a special technique. A preliminary lateral view of the cervical region, including the oral cavity, is obtained before the barium mixture is given (Fig. 5). The patient is examined standing at a distance of 6 feet from the x-ray tube with shoulders down and retracted. The head is held forward with the right or left side resting against a 10 × 12 inch screen cassette. The central ray is aligned with the angle of the jaw to the center of the cassette. An average technique of 85 KV and 100 MA at $1/20$ second achieves good bone and soft tissue contrast. If a lesion high in the hypopharynx and oropharynx is suspected two additional films are obtained, one with the patient breathing through the nose with the mouth closed (which better visualizes the nasopharynx) and the other with the patient breathing through the mouth (which better visualizes the oropharynx). Films are then exposed while the patient swallows a barium mixture with momentary cessation of respiration. In addition, when desirable, other films may be obtained during the Valsalva or Müller maneuver (see Special Maneuvers and Positions). Anteroposterior and oblique films may also be included.

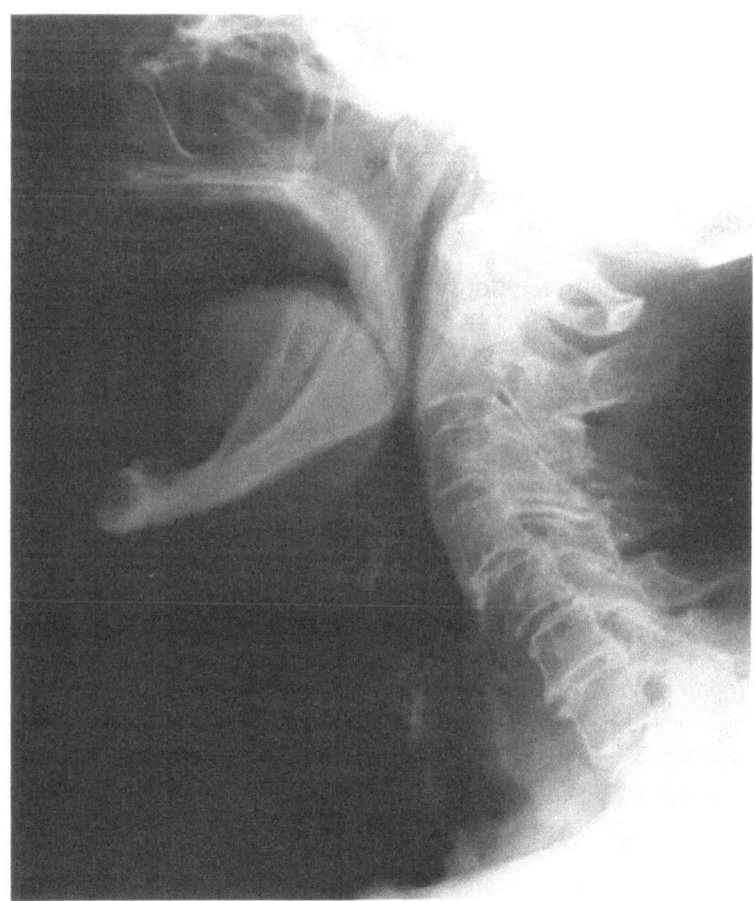

FIGURE 5

Normal lateral film of the neck with dental plates removed and mouth open.

In filming the esophagus even after a normal fluoroscopic examination, a minimum of four films should be used, in the prone PA (posterior-anterior) and RAO (right anterior oblique) positions and the supine AP (anterior posterior) and LPO (left posterior oblique) positions (left side against the table and the right side elevated). These films are obtained while the patient is drinking the barium mixture through a straw or following the ingestion of barium paste. Additional films in the right anterior oblique position in full inspiration and expiration are included if the patient has been referred for the detection of an hiatal hernia. Films of the partially dilated esophagus generally will show the mucosal pattern. If the latter is not evident, additional delayed films following the ingestion of the barium mixture with the esophagus nearly empty usually demonstrate a satisfactory mucosal pattern. Films in the Trendelenburg, Müller, Valsalva bending-over position, or during coughing, sneezing, and bearing down (as in defecation) may also be needed. Films exposed with the patient standing are usually unnecessary but may be helpful in instances where gravity effects certain changes.

SPECIAL EXAMINATIONS

Several special examinations exist which may be used to confirm the presence of a lesion and to clarify the differential possibilities. Tomography is important in differentiating laryngeal from hypopharyngeal lesions. In the hypopharynx, naso or laryngopharyngography can be used to localize a lesion. Cervical pneumography has been employed to delineate lesions of the thyroid gland. Pneumodiastinography may be helpful in differentiating a mediastinal mass from an intrinsic esophageal lesion. Pneumoperitoneum or retropneumoperitoneum is useful in delineating lesions of the lower esophagus and gastroesophageal junction. These are used infrequently. Angiography is now commonly performed to detect the site of bleeding and to determine the vascularity of a tumor.

Double exposure films of the hypopharynx and esophagus following ingestion of a thick barium bolus can be used to determine the degree of mobility of the esophagus. Double contrast studies are most useful in optimally visualizing the mucosal pattern.

Biplane rapid serialograms, e.g., Schonander, have been used on an investigative basis, in both the hypopharyngeal and the lower esophageal regions in a small number of cases. However, because of the excessive radiation involved, their use should be restricted to exceptional instances where rapid exposures are considered essential.

The techniques for these various specialized examinations follow:

Nasopharyngography

Barium nasopharyngography (44) is performed with the patient seated and the neck hyperextended. Water is first sprayed into each nostril as a mist. Then a dry collodial barium powder is insufflated through each nostril with a power blower, the nozzle being directed toward the inferior meatus. Roentgenograms are then obtained. No anesthesia is required so that the procedure may be repeated until the examination is considered satisfactory.

Contrast nasopharyngography

A more complicated method of contrast nasopharyngography requires proper local anesthesia of the nasopharynx (125). A barium sulfate mixture in the form of a paste is injected through a rubber catheter inserted into the right or left naris, so that its tip reaches the posterior wall of the pharynx. Under fluoroscopic control, this paste is injected several cubic centimeters at a time and the patient is instructed to swallow. The scope of this study can be extended to include opaque visualization of the oropharynx and hypopharynx. It is an excellent method for the experimental study of the dynamics of the nasopharynx and the demonstration of the roentgen anatomy of this area, but it is of only limited use for practical purposes.

Tomography

Tomography, especially in the AP views of the region of the neck with and without the ingestion of a contrast medium, is valuable in demonstrating lesions of the pyriform fossa. Lateral tomograms are useful in demonstrating more clearly a previously detected lesion and in the examination of the retropharyngeal area. The levels of the tomographic "cuts" can be determined by the location of the suspected lesion (Fig. 6).

Tomographic studies of the opacified esophagus following the ingestion of a thick barium or tantalum paste can be used in the detection of esophageal varices or early mucosal changes associated with other abnormalities. Pneumoesophagotomography has also been advocated (190) to determine the thickness of the esophageal wall.

Contrast laryngopharyngography

Contrast laryngopharyngography can yield a high degree of accuracy in the diagnosis of laryngeal and hypopharyngeal le-

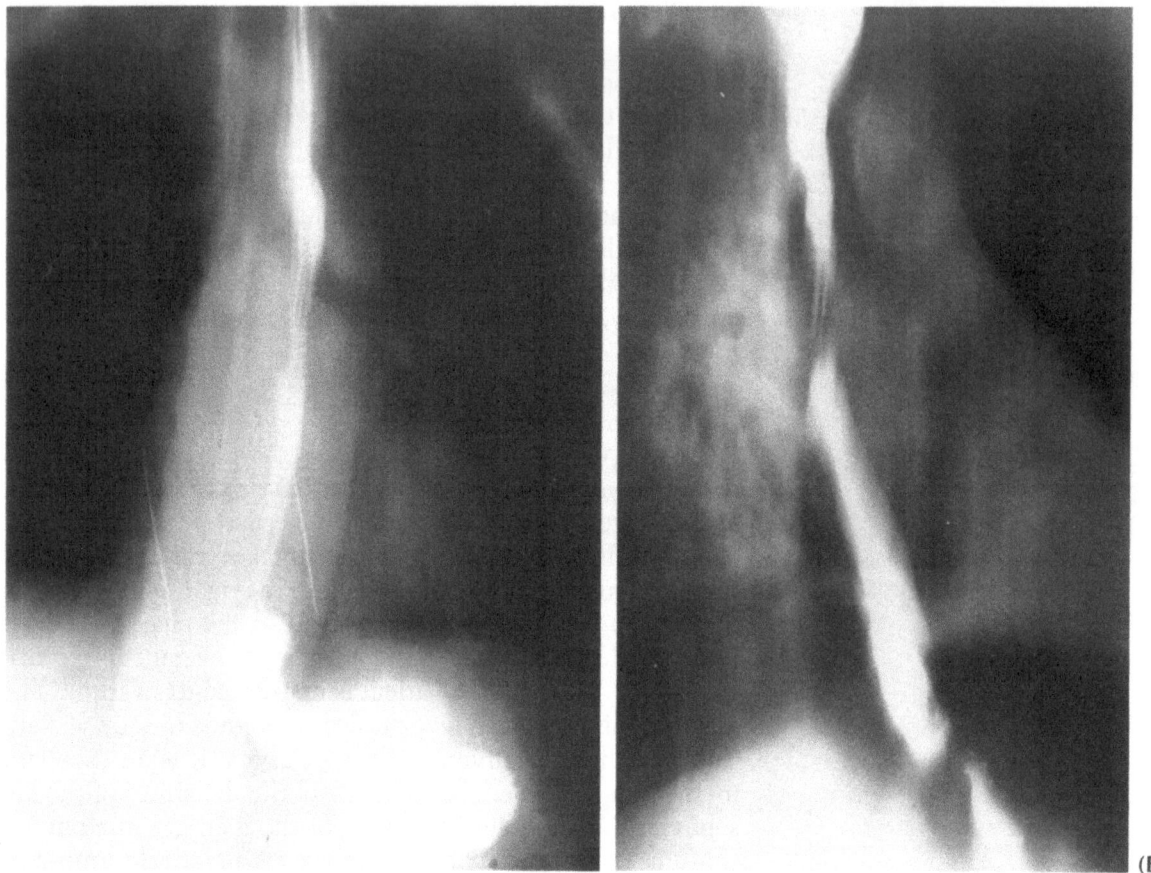

(A)   (B)

FIGURE 6

Normal esophagus: *Tomography* following ingestion of thick barium paste. (A) Anteroposterior (AP) view, (B) Right anterooblique (RAO) view. From Zaino, C., et al. *The Lower Esophageal Vestibular Complex,* 1963. Courtesy Charles C Thomas, Publisher, Springfield, Illinois.

sions (10). The patient is prepared with nembutal and atropine. Xylocaine (1%) is sprayed into the pharynx and larynx. Dionosil is then dripped slowly over the base of the tongue during quiet inspiration. Films in the modified Valsalva maneuver are helpful in demonstrating lesions of the pyriform sinuses, especially in the oblique views. However, difficulty may be encountered in demonstrating postcricoid lesions.

Cervical pneumography

In cervical pneumography 200 ml of oxygen is injected into the midline area of the neck in the subthyroid region. This procedure is used chiefly by some European investigators (136) to study the thyroid gland but can be employed to distinguish intrinsic lesions of the cervical esophagus from surrounding structures. Lateral tomograms after injection of the oxygen and opacification of the esophagus are particularly helpful. (Fig. 7).

Pneumomediastinography

Pneumomediastinography is comparable to cervical pneumography, except that oxygen is injected downward into the mediastinal region. This procedure is helpful in differentiating intrinsic from extrinsic lesions of the esophagus.

Pneumoperitoneum

Pneumoperitoneum is useful in demonstrating and differentiating lesions of the abdominal segment of the esophagus and cardia (270). The patient is placed supine and, using sterile surgical technique and local anesthesia, 300–500 cc of air is injected through a 19 gage needle into the abdominal cavity midway between the costal margin and the umbilicus in the midline (Fig. 8; also see Chapter 2).

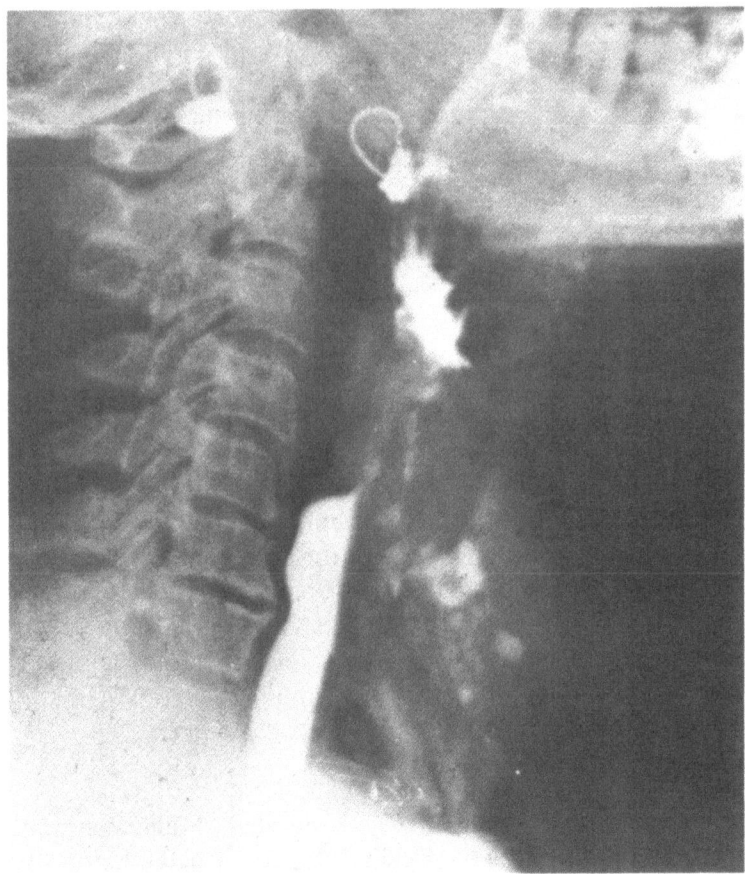

FIGURE 7
Cervical pneumography showing presence of a thyroid gland carcinoma. From La Croix, L., Sulla visualizzione Radiologica Della Tiroide. Minerva Med. *48*:50, 1957. Torino, Italy.

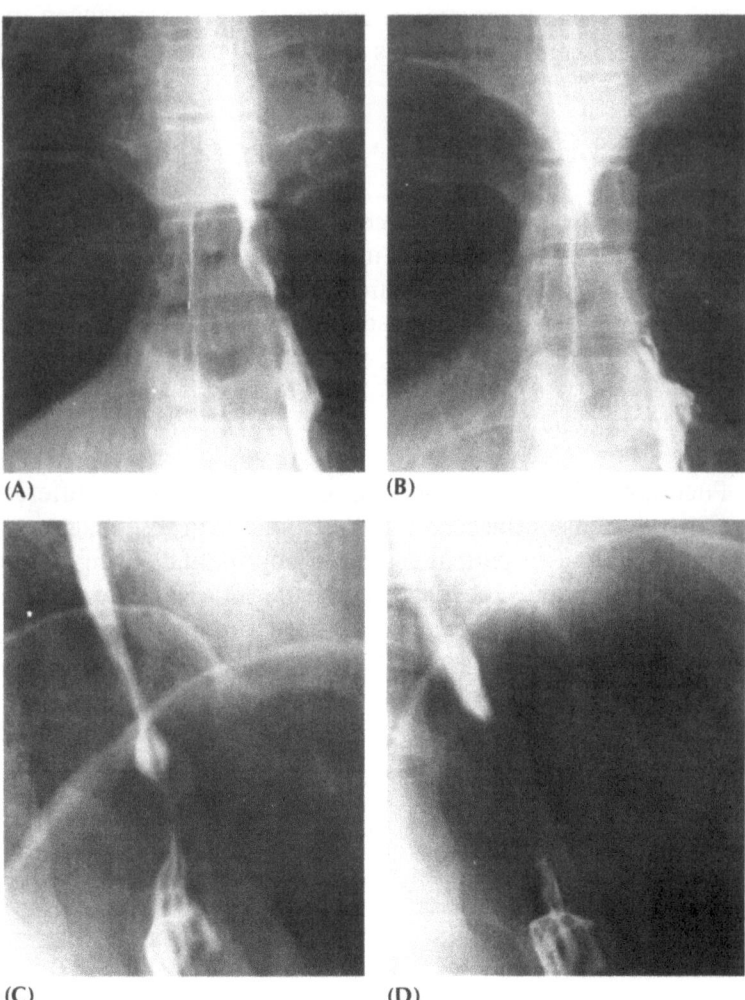

(A)   (B)

(C)   (D)

FIGURE 8
Normal pneumoperitoneum.
(A) Upright PA in inspiration,
(B) upright PA in expiration,
(C) upright RAO in inspiration,
(D) upright RAO in expiration.

Retropneumoperitoneum

Retropneumoperitoneum, performed by injected air through the coccygeal area, can be used to visualize the abdominal segment of the esophagus. Following local anesthesia in the precoccygeal area, a puncture is made with a needle directed to the left of the midline retroperitoneally with the patient on his right side. One thousand cubic centimeters of air are injected slowly. When the air has reached the subdiaphragmatic region, barium is given orally and films are obtained. This procedure is rarely used and generally has been discarded. Unexplained deaths have occurred.

Angiography

Angiography (167) encompasses a number of approaches, depending on the site of the lesion. Selective catheterization with a flexible guided catheter is the keystone to the procedure with the femoral artery a favorite site of entry. Substraction techniques are often helpful.

As examples, selective arteriography via the celiac artery may be useful in detecting the site of a bleeding esophageal varix, or the site of the gastroesophageal tear in the Mallory–Weiss syndrome. Azygography has also been advocated in the study of malignant tumors of the mid-esophagus (94b).

Double exposure films

Double exposure films of the entire esophagus and/or hypopharynx are valuable in determining the degree of mobility of the larnyx or the diaphragm, as well as in visualizing the sphincter zones. Films are obtained in the right anterior oblique prone position after the ingestion of a barium paste. The patient is first instructed to take a deep breath and to hold it (full inspiration) with one-half of the exposure time being used on this first exposure. The patient is then instructed to immediately exhale without changing his or her position and the remaining one-half of the exposure time is now used on the same film. A double exposure is thus produced (Fig. 9).

FIGURE 9
Normal double exposure films, (A) Neck region, (B) esophagus.

(A)　　　　　　　　　　　(B)

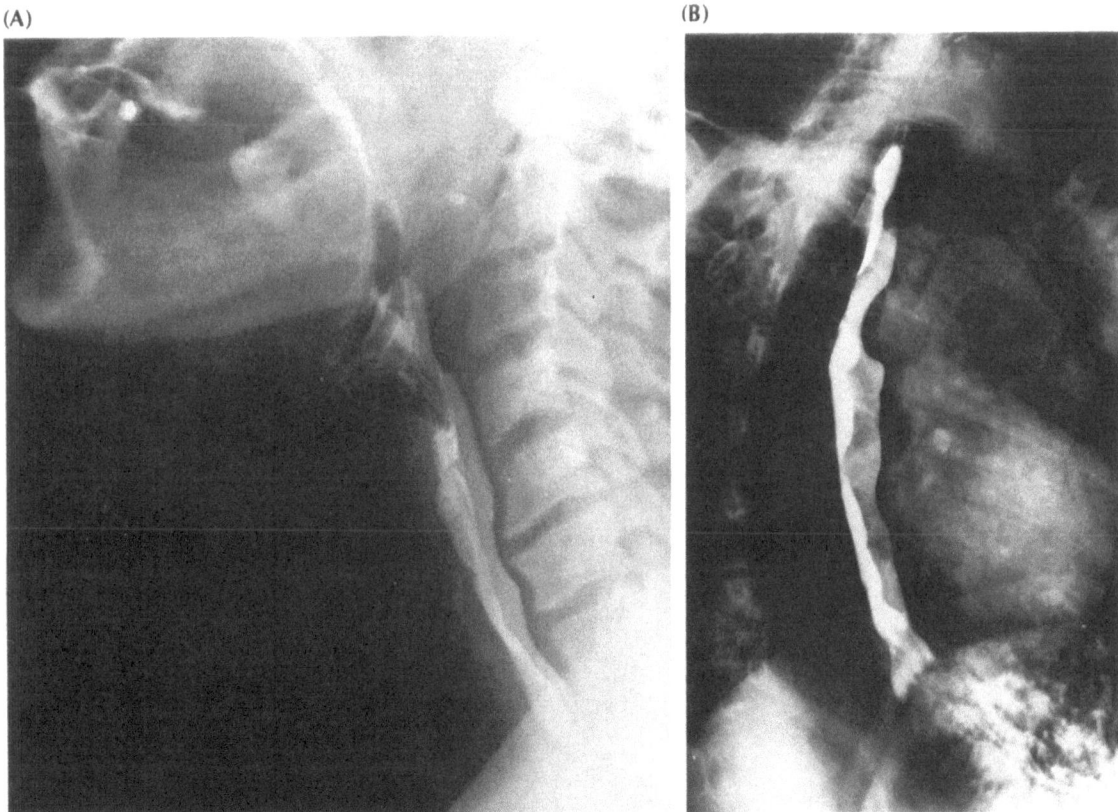

Biplane rapid film serialography

Biplane rapid film serialography (e.g., Schonander) can be carried out for evaluating the hypopharyngeal and the lower esophageal regions. Fourteen by 14 inch films are used; these are exposed simultaneously in the AP and lateral positions at 1-second intervals, after the ingestion of several heaping teaspoonsful of thick barium. In the hypopharyngeal area the series is started, at rest, followed immediately by a swallowing motion and the Valsalva maneuver. An alternative method consists of the patient holding the bolus in his or her mouth and beginning the series immediately on swallowing (Fig. 10). In the lower esophageal regions, films are exposed on full inspiration and expiration after the ingestion of the barium (Fig. 11).

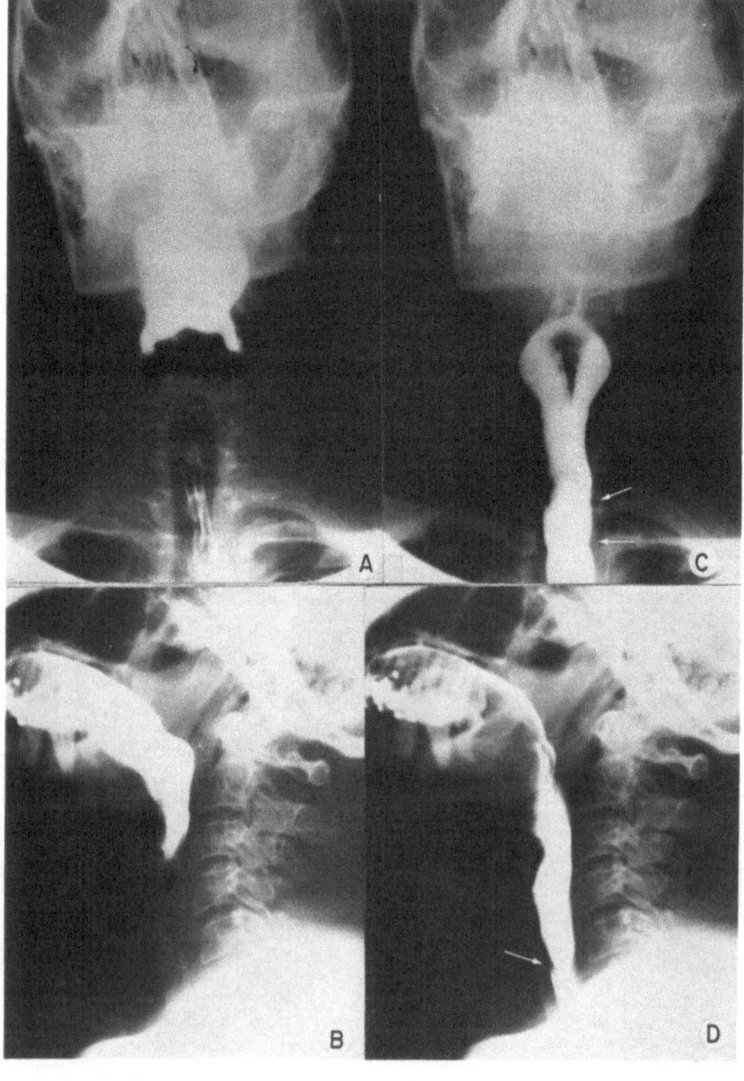

FIGURE 10
Normal Schonander biplane serialography, prone position, neck region. (A) AP views, beginning of a barium swallow; (B) lateral view, beginning of a barium swallow; (C) AP view, immediately following the barium swallow; (D) lateral view, immediately following the barium swallow. Arrows in (C) delineate the dilated upper sphincter. The arrow at (D) is at the pharyngoesophageal junction. From Zaino, C., et al. *The Pharyngoesophageal Sphincter*, 1970. Courtesy Charles C Thomas, Publisher, Springfield, Illinois.

FIGURE 11

Normal Schonander biplane serialography prone position, lower esophagus (A) AP view on expiration; (B) lateral view expiration; (C) AP view on inspiration; (D) lateral view on inspiration. From Zaino, C., et al. *The Lower Esophageal Vestibular Complex,* 1963. Courtesy Charles C Thomas, Publisher, Springfield, Illinois.

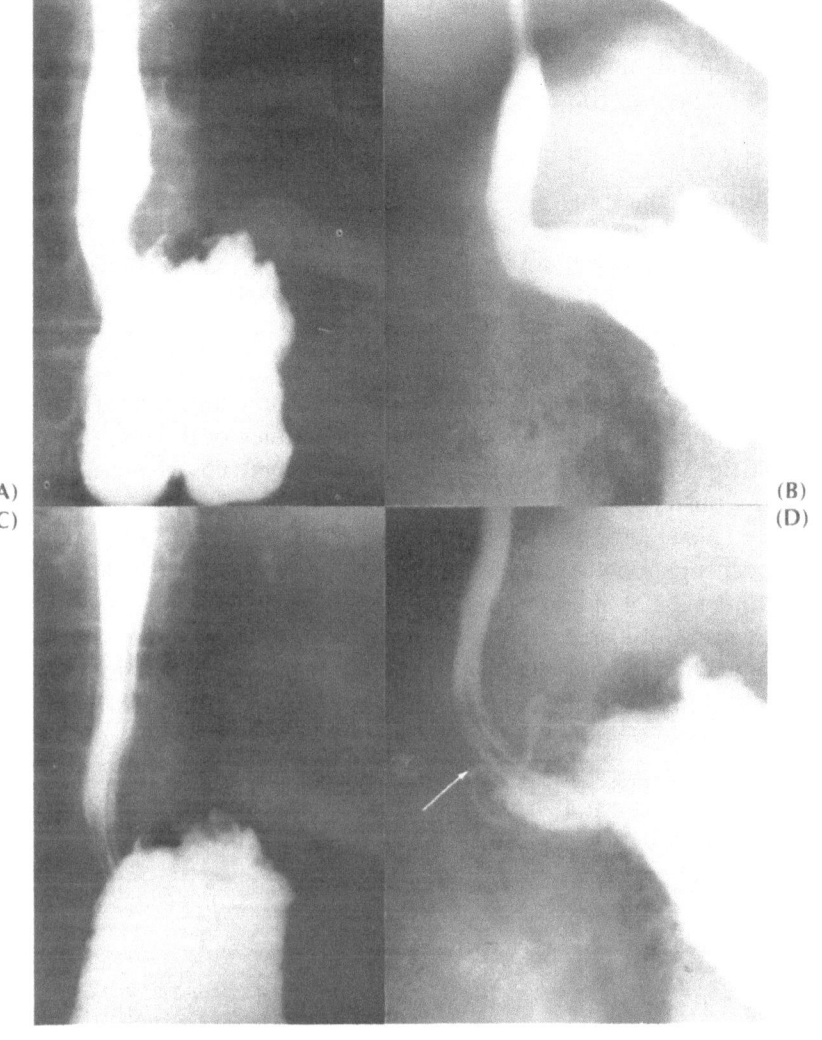

(A)
(B)
(C)
(D)

One-plane serialography may also be performed, using the Schonander or Fairchild roll film and Odelca camera. However, the exposure dose to the patient is often excessive. This method of examination has now been replaced by the 70 mm or 105 mm "spot" filming camera in conjunction with the image intensifier. These newer "spot" films have virtually eliminated the need for polygraph views of the hypopharynx and lower esophagus used previously (271).

Surgical insertion of metal clips

Roentgenologic examination after the surgical insertion of metal clips during thoracic or abdominal surgery, or placed through the esophagoscope at certain designated locations, has also been used by a number of investigators (179). In the study of the gastroesophageal junction it has provided useful information about the localization of the esophageal hiatus in its relationship to the projected dome of the diaphragm (Fig. 12).

Xeroradiography

Xeroradiography is a method of obtaining images that relies upon a positively charged electric plate. This plate is then exposed to radiation in a similar fashion as a radiographic film. The uniform charge distribution on the plate is modified during exposure, depending on the radiation incident on it. The charge distribution remaining on the surface of the plate constitutes a latent electrostatic image which is a charge picture of the object being delineated.

This electrostatic image may be revealed by a process of depositing a powder in proportion to the charge density, surface potential, or field strength. The resolution of the image depends on the size of powder particles used, because the charge plate itself has no grain. The powdered image itself may be transferred to adhesive paper or photographic film (178).

Xeroradiography is particularly suitable for examining soft tissues, especially in the neck (Fig. 13). The radiation dose, however, is usually considerably in excess of films obtained with standard radiography.

Trendelenburg

The Trendelenburg position, as originally described, consisted of the patient lying on his or her back (supine) with the plane of the table inclined cephalad 30 to 40°. For radiographic purposes it has been modified so that the patient is, in addition, rotated to the right (right side against the table) to separate the lower portion of the esophagus from the spine. In addition, during the study, the patient may be rotated from side to side in order to facilitate the localization of a lesion. The original modification and a more extensively used variation consists in rotating the patient to the left while he or she lies supine and is usually combined with the application of abdominal manual pressure.

Wolf

Wolf's position (263a) is used to increase the intraabdominal pressure, to facilitate demonstration of a hiatal hernia or reflux. The patient is placed prone with his or her left side slightly elevated while lying on a radiolucent bolster. The central ray is tilted cephalad and at right angles to the spine. Expo-

SPECIAL MANEUVERS AND POSITIONS

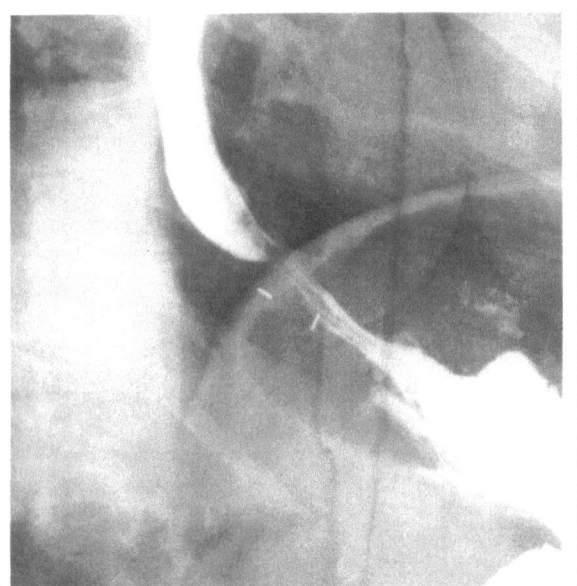 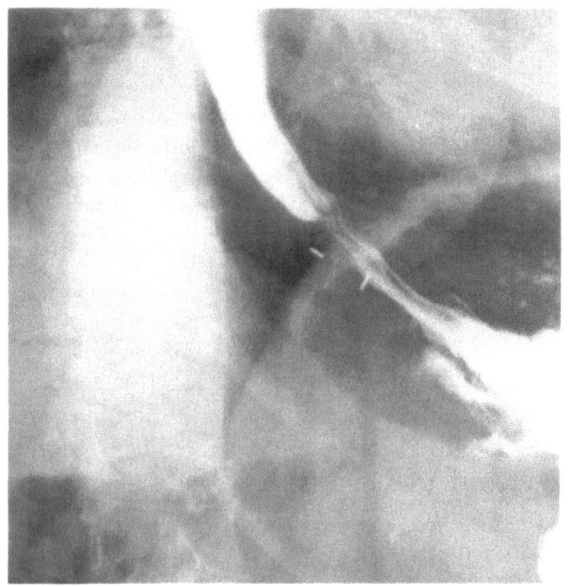

(A)

(B)

FIGURE 12
Normal view following surgical implantation of metal clips placed on posterior and anterior lips of the esophageal hiatus. (A) On inspiration; (B) on expiration. From Zaino, C., et al. *The Lower Esophageal Vestibular Complex*, 1963. Courtesy Charles C Thomas, Publisher, Springfield, Illinois.

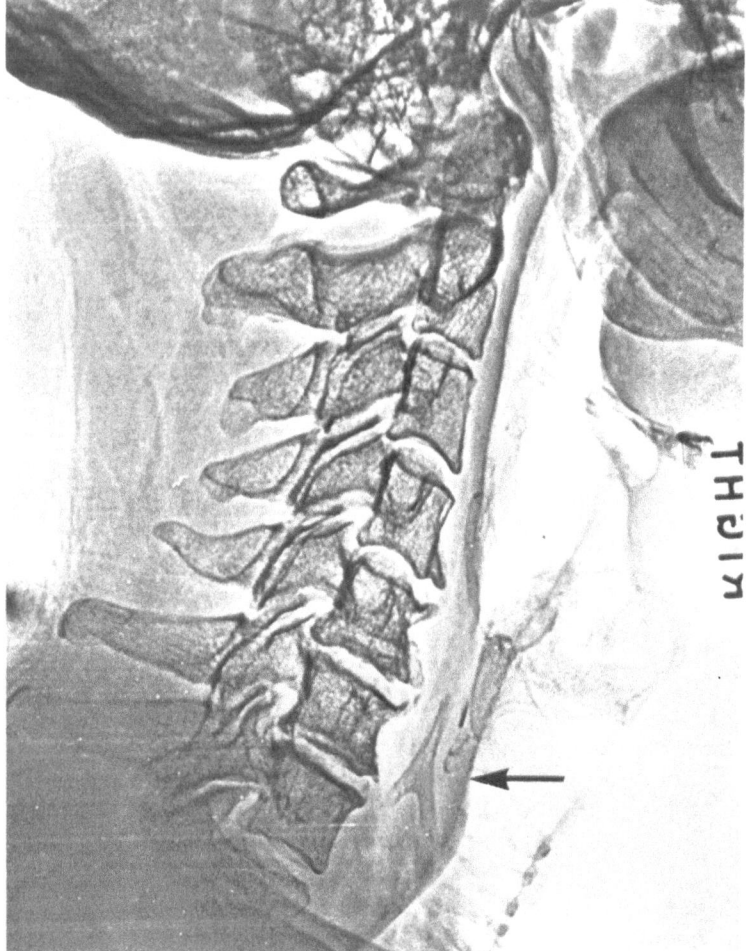

FIGURE 13
Xeroradiography of the neck showing a *foreign body* (chicken bone) in the sphincter zone (at arrow).

sures are made while the patient is swallowing (to demonstrate a hiatal hernia) or after swallowing to visualize reflux. Wolf's position also may be combined with a modified Trendelenburg technique. A straight leg raising test can also be used to increase the intraabdominal pressure during which the patient is placed supine, while raising both heels off the table with legs fully extended during normal breathing.

Johnston

Johnston's bending-over position (toe-touch position) may be helpful in demonstrating a hiatal hernia or reflux. The patient stands lateral to the table and bends forward as much as possible with the arms hanging down and the knees straight (119). This position is also used in conjunction with the Valsalva or Müller maneuvers.

Valsalva

The Valsalva maneuver consists of having a patient strain against a closed glottis. The modified Valsalva maneuver consists of forceful blowing against the cheeks with the lips closed tightly (Fig. 14A).

Müller

The Müller maneuver consists of inhaling forcefully against a

FIGURE 14
Normal (A) Valsalva maneuver, (B) Müller maneuver in same patient.

(A)

(B)

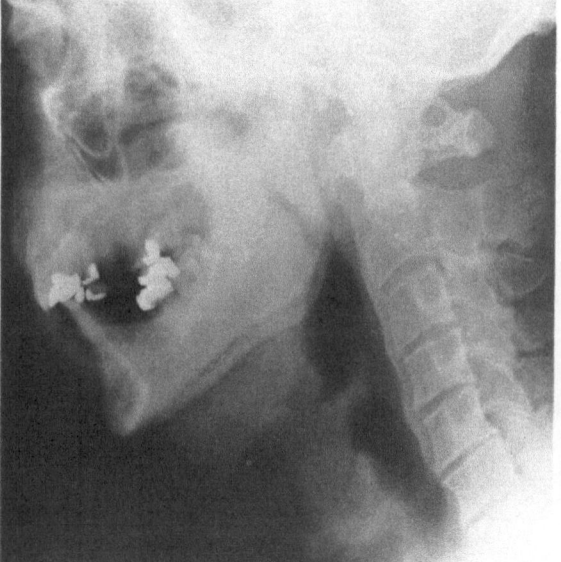
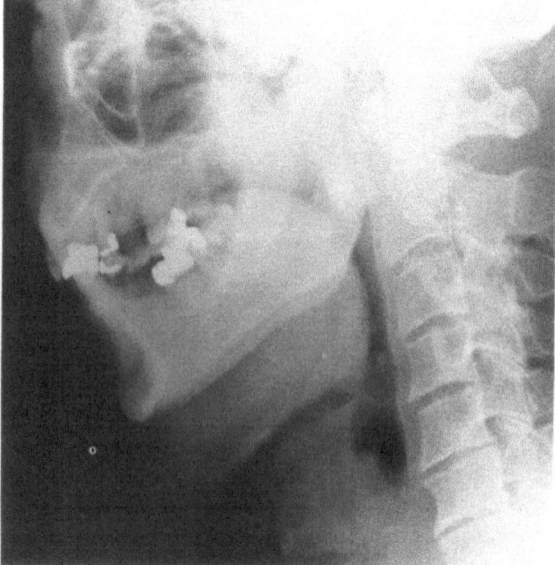

closed glottis, thus increasing the intraabdominal pressure (Fig. 14B).

SPECIAL TESTS

Water siphonage

The water siphonage test (146) is used primarily to demonstrate gastroesophageal reflux. After the ingestion of barium, the patient is placed on his or her back (supine) and turned to the right about 45° (left side elevated). The patient holds a container of cold water with his or her right hand, with the left arm flexed over his or her head out of the way of the examining field. During fluoroscopic observation, the patient drinks the water as rapidly as possible through a tube or straw. Reflux is demonstrated when barium leaves the stomach and passes into the esophagus.

Captured bolus

The captured bolus test (234) is used in the detection of a hiatal hernia. The patient is placed prone in the RAO position. Immediately after taking a swallow of barium, the patient inhales deeply and, while holding his or her breath, performs a sustained straining effort (modified Valsalva maneuver) as films are obtained. Normally, some "tenting" or "funneling" takes place at the esophageal hiatus. In the presence of a hernia, the bolus is trapped between the distal end of the sphincter and the diaphragm (the "captured bolus").

Double lumen tube–balloon

The double lumen tube with an inflatable distal balloon test is used to visualize esophageal varices (184). The test is performed by passing the tube down the esophagus to a level slightly above the junction of its middle and lower third. Inflation of the lower balloon to a pressure of 650 mm of water compresses the veins in this area, causing venous dilatation distal to this area. The injection of barium through the second lumen of the tube opening below the balloon aids in the demonstration of varices, if present in the lower esophagus.

Acid barium

The use of acid barium is a simple test to elicit substernal pain related to the sensitivity of the lower esophagus to acid perfusion. Acid barium is prepared by mixing 10 ml of standard barium sulfate suspension with 1 ml of concentrated hydrochloric acid, producing a mixture with a pH of 1.7 (62). The esophagus is first examined fluoroscopically with a nonacidic barium mixture. Acid barium is then ingested. The appearance of abnormal esophageal contraction and reflux represents a positive test and usually indicates the presence of a peptic esophagitis. After the ingestion of an alkali medication to counteract the effects of the acid, the esophageal motility returns to normal. Bernstein's test (20) was originally used, but this required intubation and perfusion with a hydrochloric acid solution for periods up to 15 minutes. A negative test implies angina or other cardiac abnormality, rather than esophagitis, as a cause of the patient's pain.

Mecholyl

Mecholyl (73) is used in the differential diagnosis of early achalasia from carcinoma, benign stricture, and scleroderma. Mecholyl, a synthetic choline derative, is a parasympathetic drug that increases the tone and peristalsis of the esophagus. A subcutaneous injection of 2.5 mg of mecholyl is given after the esophagus has been filled with a barium paste. Within 2–3 minutes, a positive response is indicated by the appearance of increased, disordered esophageal contractions. If there is no response, another dose is given 5 minutes later, with the total maximum dose not to exceed 10 mg. The greater the degree of esophageal dilatation, the greater will be the dosage needed. One milligram of atropine sulfate injected subcutaneously counteracts the effect of the stimulating dose.

USE OF OTHER DRUGS. A number of drugs may be used in the differential diagnosis of various motor disturbances. Probanthine, and more recently buscopan, temporarily relieves sphincteric or local spasm and relaxes the esophagus sufficiently to permit engorgement of esophageal varices when present. Thirty milligrams of probanthine given intramuscularly 15 minutes before examination (92) usually relieves any spasm, facilitating the diagnosis of esophageal neoplasms, esophagitis, or other disorders.

Amyl nitrate pearls, benzedrine, atropine, or tincture of belladonna can produce temporary disappearance of "curling." A nitroglycerine tablet under the tongue may temporarily relieve diffuse spasm. Alkalinization of the gastric contents produces relaxation of the lower esophageal sphincter and therefore is used to relieve spasm particularly secondary to gastric hyperacidity.

Esophageal varices

SPECIAL STUDIES

The radiologic demonstration of esophageal varices requires careful technique and the knowledge of certain fundamental physical factors that influence their appearance (145). It may not always be possible to demonstrate esophageal varices, even when present. The dimension of the varices may vary at times because of varying conditions, such as a fluctuating portal venous pressure, changing blood volume (i.e., after a hemorrhage or phlebotomy), and variable collateral circulations.

The patient is usually fluoroscoped in the horizontal, Trendelenburg, and both right and left anterior oblique positions. In this way the rate of passage of barium is slowed, permitting a longer period of observation. A thin mixture of barium should be used initially. Overfilling of the esophagus should be avoided because it can efface and obscure varices. Because it is preferable that the varices be engorged for optimal visualization, all possible methods of producing engorgement should be attempted during the examination (192).

Relaxation of the esophagus can be obtained by giving the patient one small swallow of thin barium and insuring that the patient does not take additional swallows. If this fails, the Valsalva maneuver immediately following the ingestion of barium may be attempted. A good mucosal study is imperative; therefore, double contrast techniques should be tried (e.g., the use of mineral oil, oxygen insufflation, carbonated drinks, or air sucked through a perforated straw with barium). At any rate, multiple filming is essential. For this reason, cineradiography is an ideal method of demonstrating varices (2,172). The Müller maneuver of forceful expiration also leads to good results. A special double lumen tube with an inflatable balloon can be used to produce engorgement of the varices by mechanical blockage of venous drainage. The balloon is positioned in the lower esophagus and inflated enough to compress the esophageal wall. Then a thin barium mixture is injected through the second lumen below the level of the compressing balloon, producing visualization of the engorged varices.

A number of drugs have been used to enhance variceal visualization. Probanthine diminishes smooth muscle peristalsis, causing a decrease in motor activity and thus allowing the varices to remain engorged (53,92). Thirty milligrams of probanthine administered intramuscularly or 8 mg intravenously, after the patient has voided, to prevent urinary retention. Several minutes after the intravenous injection or about 15 minutes after the intramuscular injection, a barium swallow is given and the esophagus is examined. The administration of this drug is contraindicated in the presence of glaucoma, advanced heart disease, or prostatic hypertrophy.

Buscopan is now replacing probanthine (46) because of fewer contraindications and complications. Twenty milligrams of buscopan are given intravenously, immediately after the ingestion of a barium paste. Within several minutes, the esophagus dilates and peristalsis is diminished or stopped, with subsequent esophageal relaxation and engorgement of varices. Improved radiologic visualization results.

In cirrhotic patients, an infusion of 1 liter or 6% dextran has been recommended preceding radiologic examination to produce engorgement of esophageal varices. Dextran should not be used in the presence of ascites.

Atropine sulfate (1 mg) injected subcutaneously 30 minutes before the examination will allow the barium to cling to the mucosal surface for a longer time. Pitressin (10 units subcutaneously or by intramuscular injection) facilitates disappearance of esophageal varices because of a fall in portal pressure and may be used in the differential diagnosis from carcinoma.

The presence of varices may be confirmed by splenic portography, which visualizes gastric as well as esophageal varices. The radiologic technique for this procedure is as follows. The patient is supine. Films are centered to the xyphoid process. Under local anesthesia and sterile technique an 18 gauge flexible Teflon needle and obturator is inserted into the spleen at the ninth intercostal space and midaxillary line. The needle is connected to flexible tubing and 20 to 50 ml of 75% aqueous contrast material are injected. Serial filming is started near the end of the injection.

Celiac arteriography is another method of investigating the presence of varices and collateral venous drainage. With catheterization of the celiac artery and occasionally subselective catheterization of the splenic artery itself, detailed study of vascular flow patterns through the abdominal viscera with opacification of arterial as well as venous channels is feasible. By concentrating on the venous phase of timed vascular contrast injections, varices, where present, can be demonstrated to a satisfactory degree. Also, in the postsplenectomy patient, where splenoportography is impossible or following certain splenorenal shunts, the celiac study is most useful in demonstrating altered flow dynamics and the results of the surgical correction of varices. High-dose left gastric angiography (198) and portal venography (173) have been used for visualization of esophageal varices.

Hiatal hernia

The radiologic demonstration of an esophageal hiatal hernia may at times require meticulous technique. Increased abdominal pressure on a filled gastric cardia and fundus in the Trendelenburg position usually reveals the hernia if it is not observed on previous more standard studies. However, the Johnston position, the Wolf position, films after the Valsalva or Müller's maneuvers, films on sustained inspiration, films with straight leg raising, and the captured bolus test may all be tried. During fluoroscopic examination, while the patient is continuously drinking the standard barium mixture or during the ingestion of a thick barium bolus, a hiatal hernia or insufficiency, if present, can be seen without too much difficulty. However, here again cineradiography, taking the place of multiple filming or serial "spot filming," is helpful in detecting a hiatal hernia not previously apparent. A small hiatal hernia may be inconstantly demonstrated because of variable dynamic causes related to muscular tone and abdominal pressure. In infants and children, hiatal hernia is best visualized in the right anterior oblique position, with the esophagus well filled and during active swallowing (see Chapter 3).

Gastroesophageal reflux

Gastroesophageal reflux may be difficult to demonstrate radiologically. In infants, regurgitation is frequent and can be seen by adding barium to the formula and examining the infant fluoroscopically in the prone right anterior oblique position while the infant is sucking from the bottle. The demonstration of abnormal regurgitation, however, usually requires the use of abdominal palpation, with pressure applied to the full stomach after the ingestion of the barium meal. This is done in various supine positions, including the Trendelenburg. The water siphon test may also be tried, particularly in adults. Dry swallows are tried at first, followed by sips of water, while using normal pressure over the filled stomach. Reflux is diagnosed if the barium is observed to regurgitate and refill the lower esophagus. The ease with which this regurgitation and its extent occurs is an indication of the degree of lower sphincter incompetence.

Foreign bodies

The accidental ingestion of foreign bodies is not uncommon, particularly in infants and children. If the object is not opaque, however, other alternatives exist.

Ordinarily, a lateral film of the cervical region and films of the chest and abdomen are obtained as a start. The lateral cervical film should be exposed at the height of a dry swallow to include the sphincter zone. If no opaque foreign body is identified and symptoms are present, or if the history of ingestion is initially unchallenged, the hypopharynx and esophagus should be examined with the ingestion of a thin barium mixture. If no foreign body is noted, barium-filled capsules or tablets should be administered to determine the presence of obstruction of the esophagus at the site of a nonopaque foreign body.

In the instance of a fish bone adherent to the "back of the throat" (usually in the oropharynx), a pledget of cotton soaked in an aqueous contrast medium can be ingested, with the hope that the descent of the cotton pledget can be impeded by the foreign body. Some danger exists in inducing hyperperistalsis, which could facilitate perforation. If the obstruction is more distal in the esophagus, a solid marshmallow can be swallowed with the aid of a barium mixture, under fluoroscopic observation, and the site of obstruction may be identified. The marshmallow gradually dissolves, thus offering no additional problems. A barium-impregnated marshmallow may also be used.

Webs

Webs, strictures, and rings are best observed in a fully distended esophagus during fluoroscopic examination. They can also be visualized during the Valsalva maneuver. The presence of lower esophageal rings is also confirmed by the ingestion of barium-filled capsules, tablets, or a barium-impregnated marshmallow.

Atresia

The detection of atresia and/or tracheoesophageal fistulae in infants requires a specialized technique. Where atresia with or without tracheoesophageal fistula is suspected, a small polyethylene catheter is passed through the nose down to the site of the obstruction. A thin barium mixture is ingested under fluoroscopic control. The patient is placed in the prone position to prevent aspiration of the contrast. Fistulae, when present, are usually located in the anterior wall of the esophagus. Examination in the Trendelenburg (prone) position should also be done to detect proximally located fistulae. In the absence of obstruction, the tip of the catheter should be placed in the mid-esophagus and the contrast injected during fluoroscopy. Aspiration of the contrast into the larynx because of overflow may interfere with the examination. A technique to obviate this difficulty has been described recently (see Chapter 3).

Acute esophagitis

Acute esophagitis is usually suspected on clinical grounds. The radiologic findings usually lag behind the acute inflammatory changes. However, the acid barium test can be used to detect esophagitis, which ordinarily may be missed on a routine study of the esophagus.

2

NORMAL ANATOMICOROENTGEN STUDIES AND CORRELATIONS

GROSS ANATOMY
Introductory remarks

Before the normal radiologic anatomy of the orohypopharynx and esophagus is reviewed, a brief presentation of the relevant gross and histologic anatomy of this area is considered, with special reference to the upper and lower sphincters of the esophagus. Following extensive gross anatomic dissections, histologic sectioning, and anatomicoroentgen studies, both the upper and lower sphincters have been shown to be anatomic transitional zones rather than isolated specific muscles (267,271). Some pertinent aspects of the general gross anatomy of the oral cavity, including the tongue, soft palate, and uvula, are presented. The epiglottis, nasopharynx, oropharynx, hypopharynx and upper sphincter zone, cervical esophagus, thoracic esophagus, lower esophageal sphincter, esophageal hiatus, gastroesophageal junction, and gastric cardia are reviewed in sequence. The musculature and other related structures of the orohypopharynx and esophagus are then considered in greater detail in order to correlate the radiologic and anatomic findings (Figs. 15 and 16).

The oral cavity is the beginning of the alimentary tract, extending from the lips anteriorly to the soft palate and uvula posteriorly. The tongue lies between the floor of the mouth inferiorly and the hard palate superiorly. The gums and teeth form the anterior lateral border. This zone is divided into the main oral cavity enclosed by the palate and teeth as well as the vestibular area or space between the closed teeth and cheeks. The entire oral and pharyngeal surfaces are lined with squamous epithelium.

The tongue is a very mobile mass of striated muscle arising

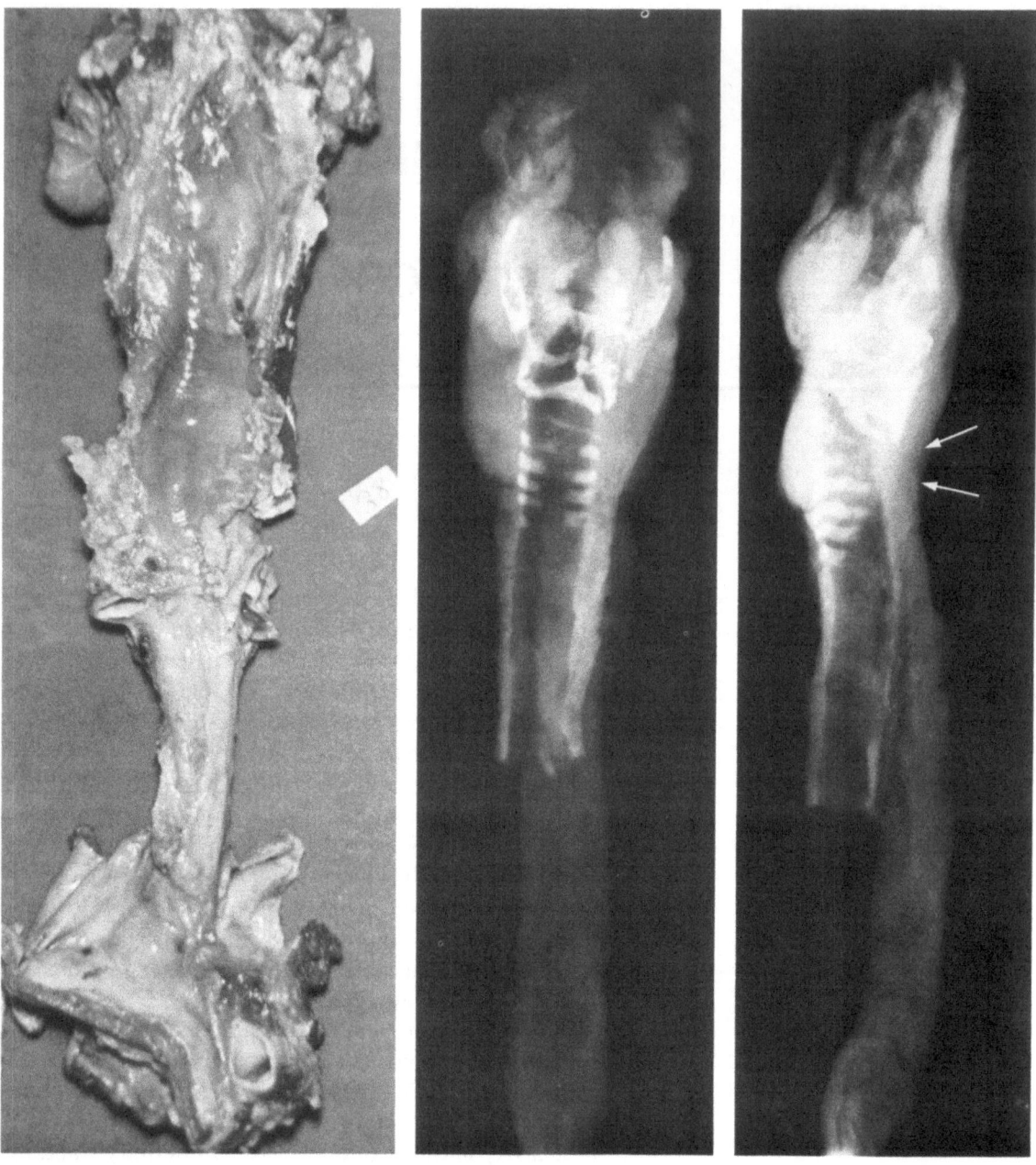

FIG. 15   FIG. 16A   FIG. 16B

FIGURE 15
Normal gross specimen showing posterior wall of hypopharynx and
esophagus.

FIGURE 16
Normal roentgenograms of a gross specimen. (A) AP view, (B)
lateral view. Note relationship of normal thyroid gland (soft tissue
mass) to sphincter zone (between arrows in B).

from the floor of the mouth. It consists of a tip, the body with a median sulcus, and a base or root which extends posteriorly to the anterior surface of the epiglottis. A median glossoepiglottic fold divides the retroglossoepiglottic recess into two symmetrical lateral pockets named valleculae. The muscles of the floor of the mouth are attached to the mandible, tongue, and hyoid bone. As a result, when the tongue is propelled posteriorly, as in swallowing, the hyoid bone is pulled anteriorly and upward.

The soft palate and uvula form the posterior wall of the oral cavity and separate it from the nasopharynx. The epiglottis is a thin leaflike symmetrical cartilage attached at its base to the superior angle of the thyroid cartilage of the larynx by the thyroepiglottic ligament. Anteriorly, the epiglottis is fixed by the hyoid epiglottic ligament at the hyoid bone. Laterally, the epiglottis is attached to the tongue and palate by the glossopalatopharyngeal folds. During swallowing, therefore, the base of the epiglottis moves with the larynx and hyoid bone anteriorly and upward, allowing the tip and body to fold over the opening of the larynx as the pressure of an advancing solid bolus reaches it. The epiglottis acts as a partial lid to the larynx during deglutition and represents a critical pivotal structure during swallowing. It directs the flow of fluids into the lateral channels and provides a chute for solid food, which slides over the anterior surface of the epiglottis while it folds over the larynx.

The nasopharynx is the recess that lies posterior and superior to the soft palate and uvula with a cephalic extension to the base of the skull and into the nasal cavities. It becomes part of the normal airway when the mouth is closed. The nasopharynx is occluded from the oropharynx during swallowing by the upward and posterior displacement of the soft palate and uvula. It is also occluded from the oropharynx by the anterior bulging of the posterior upper nasopharyngeal wall secondary to contraction of the superior constrictor, the palatine aponeurosis, and the palatopharyngeus muscles, as they form the "ridge of Passavant."

The oropharynx is a recess extending from the most inferior portion of the soft palate and uvula to the level of the hyoid bone. Its anterior wall is formed by the posterior border of the tongue and part of the epiglottis. Laterally and posteriorly the walls of the oropharynx consist chiefly of the constrictor muscles.

The hypopharynx is the recess immediately inferior to the oropharynx just lateral and posterior to the larynx and extending inferiorly to the pharyngoesophageal junction at the level of the inferior pole of the lamina of the cricoid cartilage. The anterior wall of the hypopharynx is formed by the laryngeal introitus superiorly and the inferior portion of the epiglottis, as well as the posterior wall of the cricoid lamina. Laterally and posteriorly the lower constrictor muscles complete the enclosed space.

The cervical esophagus extends from the pharyngo-esophageal junction to the thoracic inlet. It includes the pharyngoesophageal sphincter, a specialized transitional anatomic segment approximately 2 cm long which is actually a portion of the esophagus. Although this sphincter logically could be called the cervical sphincter or the upper sphincter, the term "pharyngoesophageal sphincter" is in use because some fibers of the cricopharyngeal muscle occasionally overlap the sphincter superiorly and become an integral part of it.

The thoracic esophagus extends from the thoracic inlet to the esophageal hiatus. It is divided into a number of segments which are described later.

The lower esophageal sphincter lies partly within the esophageal hiatus and corresponds to the abdominal segment of the esophagus. It is surrounded by and fixed to the esophageal hiatus by the phrenoesophageal membrane. This membrane permits considerable mobility of this segment of the esophagus above and below the level of the diaphragm, depending on the respiratory and swallowing phases.

The gastroesophageal junction can usually be detected on gross examination by a definite change in color corresponding to the confluence of the squamous epithelium of the esophagus and the columnar epithelium of the stomach (epithelial line). Occasionally, however, this mucosal junction may be located more proximally than the actual muscular sphincter.

The cardia of the stomach is that part of the stomach directly distal to the gastroesophageal junction. It forms the cardiac incisure laterally as it meets the fundus of the stomach. Medially the cardia is continuous with the lesser curvature of the stomach. Occasionally, an appearance simulating "shelving" may be noted, as an unusually high cardia extends around the abdominal segment of the esophagus.

The musculature of the pharynx, esophagus, and cardia

The pharynx and upper esophagus are formed of striated muscle. Although the level of transition from striated to smooth muscle varies, the transitional site usually begins gradually near the level of the aortic arch. A major physiologic difference between striated and smooth muscle is the rapid contraction of striated muscle compared to the slower contraction of smooth muscles which, in part, explains the rapidity of the initial swallowing contractions in the oropharynx. The posterior wall of the pharynx consists of an outer and inner layer of muscles. The outer and most complete layer is formed by three muscles, the superior, middle, and inferior constrictors. These muscle layers overlap one another. The inner layer is incomplete and formed superiorly and medially by the salpingopharyngeus muscle and inferiorly by the palatopharyngeus and stylopharyngeus muscles (185).

The superior constrictors arise bilaterally from the base of the skull and fuse posteriorly in a midline raphe. They are overlapped posteriorly by the middle constrictors, which arise from the hyoid bone, and the stylopharyngeus ligaments anteriorly, which also fuse with the central pharyngeal raphe (174).

The inferior constrictor muscles are divided into the thyropharyngeus and cricopharyngeus muscles. The thyropharyngeus overlaps the middle constrictors and arises from the thyroid cartilage. It also fuses posteriorly into the central raphe. The cricopharyngeus muscle is distinct from the more superiorly located thyropharyngeus. It is smaller and lighter in color and appears to emerge from beneath the fibers of the latter muscle. It has no central raphe. The cricopharyngeus originates laterally from the cricoid lamina and spreads out in a fan-shaped manner. Transverse bundles of fibers corresponding to the pars fundiformis (126) are not a constant feature (271). Some of these lower fibers blend or overlap with the outer musculature of the esophagus.

The inner muscular layer of the pharynx is formed by two longitudinal muscle bundles located bilaterally. The salpingopharyngeus muscle arises from the inferior part of the eustachian tube and blends inferiorly with the palatopharyngeus muscle. The palatopharyngeus muscle in turn arises from the pharyngeal aponeurosis and upper border of the base of the styloid process and spreads out caudad to join with some of the fibers of the salpingopharyngeus, also inserting into the pharyngeal aponeurosis (pharyngobasilar fascia). This aponeurosis corresponds to the submucosal layer of the esophagus. The fibers of both the stylopharyngeus and palatopharyngeus muscles occasionally extend inferiorly into the superior sphincter zone of the esophagus and reinforce the circular muscule layer.

Most of the muscles listed in the foregoing, in coordination with others attached to the hyoid bone, base of the tongue, and larynx, are instrumental in coordinating the upward and lateral shift of the larynx during deglutition, removing the larynx from the path of the oncoming bolus. The constrictor muscles also form the walls and recesses of the oronasohypopharynx.

The esophagus is a separate structure attached to the hypopharynx and larynx and does not represent a direct continuation of these various muscles. A uniform and continuous mucosal lining exists, however. The most proximal esophageal segment is the pharyngoesophageal sphincter, which forms an anatomic transitional area. The musculature between the hypopharynx and esophagus has been described variously. Anatomic studies have demonstrated a ring of circular fibers originating from the suspensory ligament of the cricoid cartilage which we believe to be the sphincter (Diagram 1). These fibers fuse posteriorly with, or may be partly overlapped by, the lower cricopharyngeal muscle. This description has been con-

ANTERIOR WALL OF HYPOPHARYNX
AND SPHINCTER ZONE

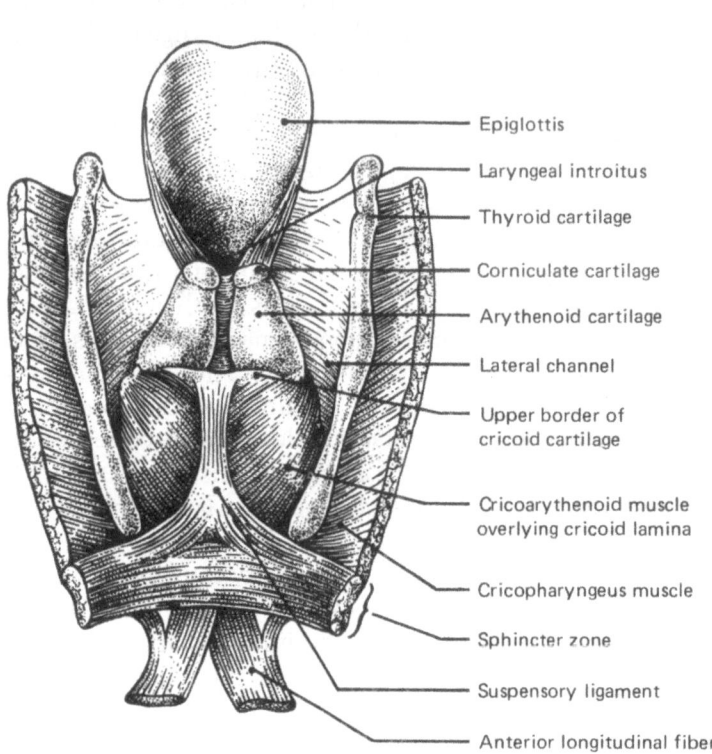

Epiglottis

Laryngeal introitus

Thyroid cartilage

Corniculate cartilage

Arythenoid cartilage

Lateral channel

Upper border of
cricoid cartilage

Cricoarythenoid muscle
overlying cricoid lamina

Cricopharyngeus muscle

Sphincter zone

Suspensory ligament

Anterior longitudinal fibers

DIAGRAM 1
Gross anatomy-origin of the pharyngoesophageal sphincter. From Zaino, C., et al. *The Pharyngoesophageal Sphincter, 1970.* Courtesy Charles C Thomas, Publisher, Springfield, Illinois.

firmed recently in the anatomic studies by Rodrigues (199). In addition, anteriorly longitudinal fibers originate from the cricoid lamina and surround the upper esophageal segment. A small, denuded posterior portion, known as Laimer's triangle, lacks longitudinal fibers. The rest of the esophagus is formed by an outer, irregular, longitudinal muscular layer and an inner circular or elliptical coat. Anteriorly, the esophageal wall is thinner and loosely attached to the trachea by fibrous tissue and slips of muscle fibers.

The lower esophageal sphincter has also shared in various descriptions. Anatomic studies have shown it to be a transitional zone 2 to 3 cm long, corresponding to Lerche's vestibule (140). The circular fibers of the distal end of the esophagus, at the site of the lower sphincter, are slightly thicker as they are reinforced by a number of extra muscle bundles (Laimer's bracket fibers). This segment is separated by the upper and lower attachment of the phrenoesophageal membrane (Diagram 2). A greater number of ganglion cells have been counted in this zone. The longitudinal muscle of the lower esophagus divides at the cardia into two main strips. One forms part of the lesser curvature and the other fuses with the greater curvature of the stomach. The circular fibers of the sphincter zone continue as the middle circular layer of the stomach. The cardia and fundus are surrounded by an additional oblique minor muscular layer, which has been designated as the collaris Helveti, Swiss tie, or constrictor cardia.

The mucus membrane and muscularis mucosa

The oral cavity, pharynx, and esophagus are carpeted by a continuous layer of mucus membrane composed of squamous eipthelium up to the gastroesophageal junction. In the hypopharyngeal area, the pharyngeal aponeurosis forms the submucosal layer, which becomes continuous with the muscularis mucosa of the sphincter zone and esophagus. Thus, the muscularis mucosa, composed of smooth muscle fibers, first appears in the sphincter zone with its own intrinsic innervation, including ganglion cells. This innervation continues inferiorly throughout the esophagus into the rest of the autonomically innervated digestive tract. A greater concentration of neurons has been found in the sphincter zone, accounting for the specialized function and reciprocal innervation of the pharyngoesophageal sphincter. Similarly, a greater number of ganglion cells, as compared to the rest of the esophagus, is present in the lower esophageal sphincter.

Membranous attachment of the orohypopharynx and esophagus

The fascial coverings of the pharynx consist of three layers superior to the level of the pharyngoesophageal junction and two layers inferior to this junction. The prevertebral layer covers the vertebral muscles and extends from the base of the skull to the mediastinum, above the level of the diaphragm.

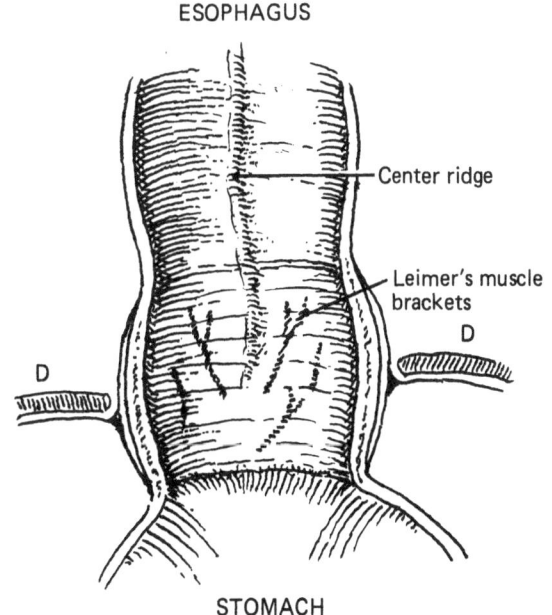

ESOPHAGUS

Center ridge

Leimer's muscle brackets

D

D

STOMACH

DIAGRAM 2
Gross anatomy—lower esophageal vestibular complex (between arrows). *From the Lower Esophageal Vestibular Complex, 1963. Courtesy Charles C Thomas, Publisher, Springfield, Illinois.*

The alar fascia also extends from the base of the skull to the lower mediastinum and covers the posterior hypopharynx and esophagus. A third layer, the buccinator fascia, extends from the middle constrictor muscles to the pharyngoesophageal junction and is strongly adherent to the hypopharyngeal musculature. The buccinator fascia fuses with the alar fascia, forming a very small retropharyngeal space lying anterior to the paravertebral space. This retropharyngeal space forms an accessory pocket posterior to the hypopharynx, permitting greater mobility during swallowing. Additional fibrotic bands immediately below the pharyngoesophageal junction and sphincter zone exist, bridging over the lobes of the thyroid gland and stabilizing the cervical esophagus.

The lower esophagus is fixed to the esophageal hiatus by the phrenoesophageal membrane. This membrane also separates the thoracic from the abdominal cavity. The upper and lower attachments of this membrane delineate the esophageal vestibular segment, which is the lower sphincter (Diagram 10A).

MEDIASTINUM AND DIAPHRAGM

The mediastinum is a long space within the central portion of the thoracic cavity, extending from the thoracic inlet to the diaphragm. It is arbitrarily divided into superior, inferior, anterior, middle, and posterior compartments. The superior compartment is separated from the inferior compartment by a plane drawn from the junction of the manubrium and body of the sternum (angle of Lewis) to the inferior margin of the fourth thoracic vertebral body. The inferior compartment is further subdivided into the anterior, middle, and posterior mediastinum. This volume chiefly concerns itself with the superior and inferior posterior mediastinal areas through which the esophagus courses. The esophagus is the most anterior structure within the posterior mediastinum, bordering upon the pericardial sac. Laterally, this posterior compartment is confined by the parietal pleura of both lungs and posteriorly by the bodies of the thoracic vertebrae. In addition to the esophagus, the posterior compartment contains the aorta, thoracic duct, azygous veins, sympathetic chain, vagus nerve, and posterior mediastinal lymph nodes.

The diaphragm limits the inferior extent of the mediastinal compartments. Of chief interest here is the right crus of the diaphragm, as it gives origin to the esophageal hiatus and tunnel. This crus is anchored posteriorly along the levels of the upper three lumbar vertebrae, arching over the aorta and dividing into a right and left sling, which forms the esophageal hiatus. Although a marked variation exists in the character of the interlocking muscular fibers, the esophageal opening is a distinct ring, unattached to the esophageal wall encircled at its distal end by the interlocking muscle fibers. The length of the tunnel depends on the thickness of the right sling or anterior lip of the esophageal opening. This right sling is wider anteriorly and becomes oblong and narrow posteriorly. The level of the esophageal hiatus, which varies, is 1.5 to 2.5 cm in diameter and is between the tenth and eleventh thoracic vertebrae, being located about 2 cm anterior and 1 cm to the left of the midline and below the dome of the diaphragm.

The Topographic anatomy of the orohypopharynx and esophagus

The topographic anatomy of these structures must be reviewed before the radiologic anatomy is considered (112). The length of the upper alimentary tract varies with the habitus of the patient. The average measurement from the incisor teeth to the gastroesophageal junction is 40 cm. The oral cavity and hypopharynx are approximately 16 cm long; the average length of the esophagus is 24 cm.

The hypopharynx and esophagus are flattened anteroposteriorly against the cervical and thoracic spine. Posteriorly, the hypopharynx is cushioned from the cervical spine and the adjacent muscles by the retropharyngeal fat and paravertebral spaces. Laterally, the carotid sheaths lie adjacent to its walls, whereas anteriorly the hypopharynx lies on the suspensory ligament and cricoarytenoid muscle of the cricoid lamina.

The sphincter zone of the cervical esophagus is partly surrounded by the thyroid gland, which may also extend posteriorly, separating this sphincter zone from the carotid sheaths. The rest of the cervical esophagus is loosely attached to the posterior wall of the trachea anteriorly and is partly surrounded laterally in its superior portion by the thyroid gland. The recurrent laryngeal nerves are located laterally between the trachea and esophageal wall. Inferior to the tracheal bifurcation, the esophageal lymph glands and vagal nerves are closely adherent to the esophagus.

The thoracic esophagus lies posterior to the trachea and extends to the tracheal bifurcation at approximately the level of the fifth thoracic vertebra. Here the left main bronchus crosses over the esophagus anteriorly. The thoracic esophagus enters from the thoracic inlet slightly to the left of the thoracic spine and swings slightly to the right at about the seventh thoracic vertebra to pass through the esophageal hiatus at the level of the first lumbar vertebra. At the fourth thoracic vertebra the arch of the aorta passes posteriorly and inferiorly alongside the esophagus, producing a left-sided indentation. The descending aorta courses along the left side of the esophagus and then swings to the right just posterior to the esophagus at the level of T-8.

Inferior to the level of the left main bronchus, the esophagus is in contact with the pericardial sac covering the left atrium of the heart. Superior to T-4 the esophagus is adjacent to the subclavian veins and parietal pleura. On the right side, the right parietal pleura lies lateral to the esophagus except where the azygous vein intervenes (near T-4). Inferior to the eighth dorsal vertebra, the esophagus turns laterally and is again in contact with the left parietal pleura until the esophagus passes through the esophageal hiatus of the disphragm on the left side. The esophagus is flattened anteroposteriorly in the thoracic cavity, with its resting width approximating 2 cm. The abdominal segment of the esophagus produces a groove on the under surface of the left lobe of the liver, which overlies it anteriorly.

RADIOLOGIC ANATOMY

The oral cavity is infrequently examined radiologically because of the relative ease of direct inspection. However, it is part of the upper gastrointestinal tract and is the proper place to begin fluoroscopic observations. At rest, with the mouth closed, the tongue lies in direct contact with the hard palate. As the mouth is opened to receive a thick barium bolus, the forepart of the tongue lowers to create room for the bolus, which is collected in a V-shaped groove at the center of the tongue. To begin the swallowing action, the mandibular teeth are braced against the maxillary teeth as the jaw and mouth are closed and the tongue propels the bolus against the hard palate. This stripping action propels the bolus into the hypopharynx (219).

If the thick barium bolus is large, part of it is retained in the lateral buccal space and swallowed by repetitive action of the tongue, after proper preparation by salibation and positioning of the bolus in the central groove of the tongue. As the barium is drunk from a straw or glass, the fluid collects in the front part of the mouth, with the tongue being lowered a considerable distance. Propulsion continues periodically without any bracing action of the teeth or jaw.

The radiologic examination of the oral cavity, orohypopharynx, and cervical esophagus, as observed on lateral and AP films of this region before, during and after a barium swallow, is considered next. In this connection, the lateral routine film of the neck, including the oral cavity, can be divided into a number of zones for detailed analysis (Fig. 17):

The oral cavity extends from the lips of the soft palate or uvula.
The nasopharynx lies behind the soft palate and extends from the base of the skull to the lowermost tip of the uvula.
The oropharynx extends from below the soft palate and uvula to the level of the hyoid bone.
The hypopharynx extends from the level of the hyoid bone to the pharyngoesophageal junction.
The sphincter zone extends 1 to 2 cm below the level of the pharyngoesophageal junction.
The cervical esophagus extends from the sphincter zone to the thoracic inlet.

FIGURE 17

Zones of the neck region. (A) Oral cavity and nasopharynx; (B) oropharynx; (C) hypopharynx; (D) upper sphincter, cervical esophagus, and thoracic inlet.

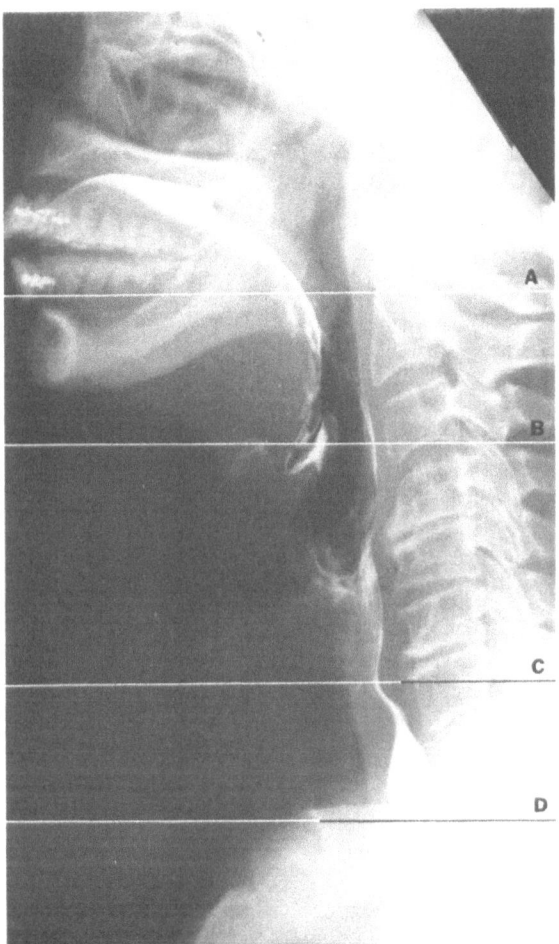

The oral cavity

On the plain lateral film of the neck the following are considered: the shape and contour of the oral cavity, including the mandible and maxillae; the presence or absence of teeth, dental plates, or fixed dentures; the presence or absence of malocclusion; the size and position of the tongue; the amount of air in the oral cavity; and the size and thickness of the soft palate and uvula.

After the ingestion of opaque material, but before a barium bolus is swallowed with the mouth closed, the bolus is lodged anteriorly, delineating part of the roof of the palate. The tongue is depressed and the floor is obscured by the barium, giving a "ragged" appearance inferiorly (Fig. 18A). At the beginning of the barium swallow, the bolus fills the entire oral cavity and begins to spill into the valleculae (Fig. 18B). The entire roof of the palate is sharply delineated. The bolus now lies chiefly in the central groove of the tongue, which is depressed, except for its anterior segment, as it begins its stripping action. Immedi-

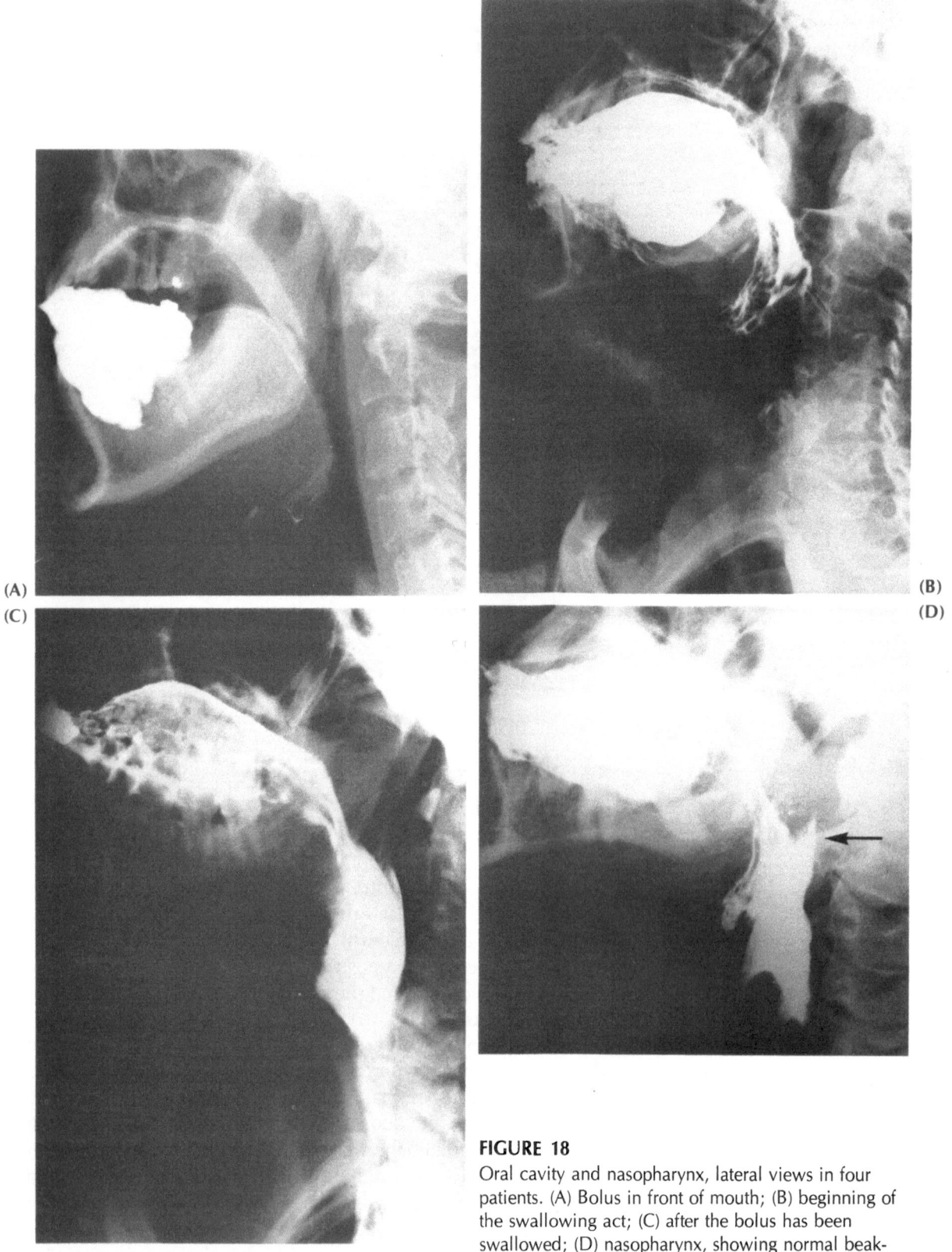

(A)

(B)

(C)

(D)

FIGURE 18

Oral cavity and nasopharynx, lateral views in four patients. (A) Bolus in front of mouth; (B) beginning of the swallowing act; (C) after the bolus has been swallowed; (D) nasopharynx, showing normal beak-like shadow (at arrow); also noted in C.

ately after the bolus has been swallowed, with the mouth closed, a coat of barium adheres to the roof of the mouth and the dorsal surface of the tongue. This barium coating is particularly well seen at the base of the tongue, where it is sharply accentuated down to the vallecula (Fig. 18C).

In the anteroposterior (AP) film of the neck, prior to ingestion of barium and with the mouth closed, the film is usually not informative because teeth, fixed bridges and/or dental fillings, and the cervical spine are superimposed. During the Valsalva maneuver, the vestibules are filled with air and occasionally abnormal soft tissue densities may be detected. With the mouth open, the tongue with its central groove and the inner portion of the oral cavity can be well delineated (Fig. 19). However, this AP view is seldom used except to confirm the presence of a particular lesion, previously identified. Another use of this projection lies in the detection of salivary calculi.

In the anteroposterior projection a barium bolus is observed to rest between the roof of the palate and dorsal surface of the tongue. Barium also fills the lateral gutters of the inner oral cavity (Fig. 20A). During a swallow, some of the barium may also be present in the lateral ventricles and in the oropharynx (Fig. 20B). After a swallow, a residual coating of barium outlines the dorsum of the tongue, the lateral ventricles, and the posterior molar recesses (Fig. 20C). Later, a thin coat of residual barium accentuates the dorsal surface of the tongue and oropharynx (Fig. 20D) Occasionally, the bolus is demonstrated as a

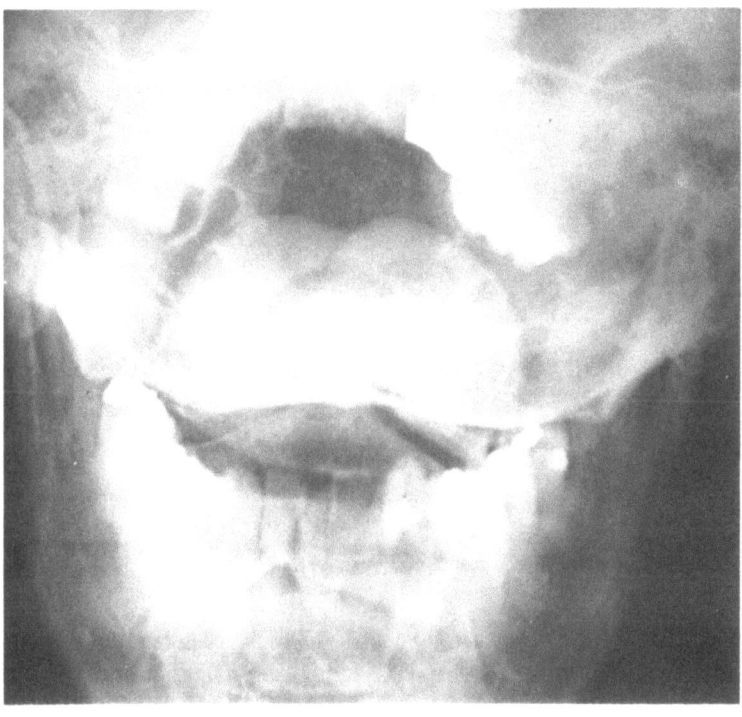

FIGURE 19
Oral cavity; plain frontal film with mouth open. Note central *groove of tongue.*

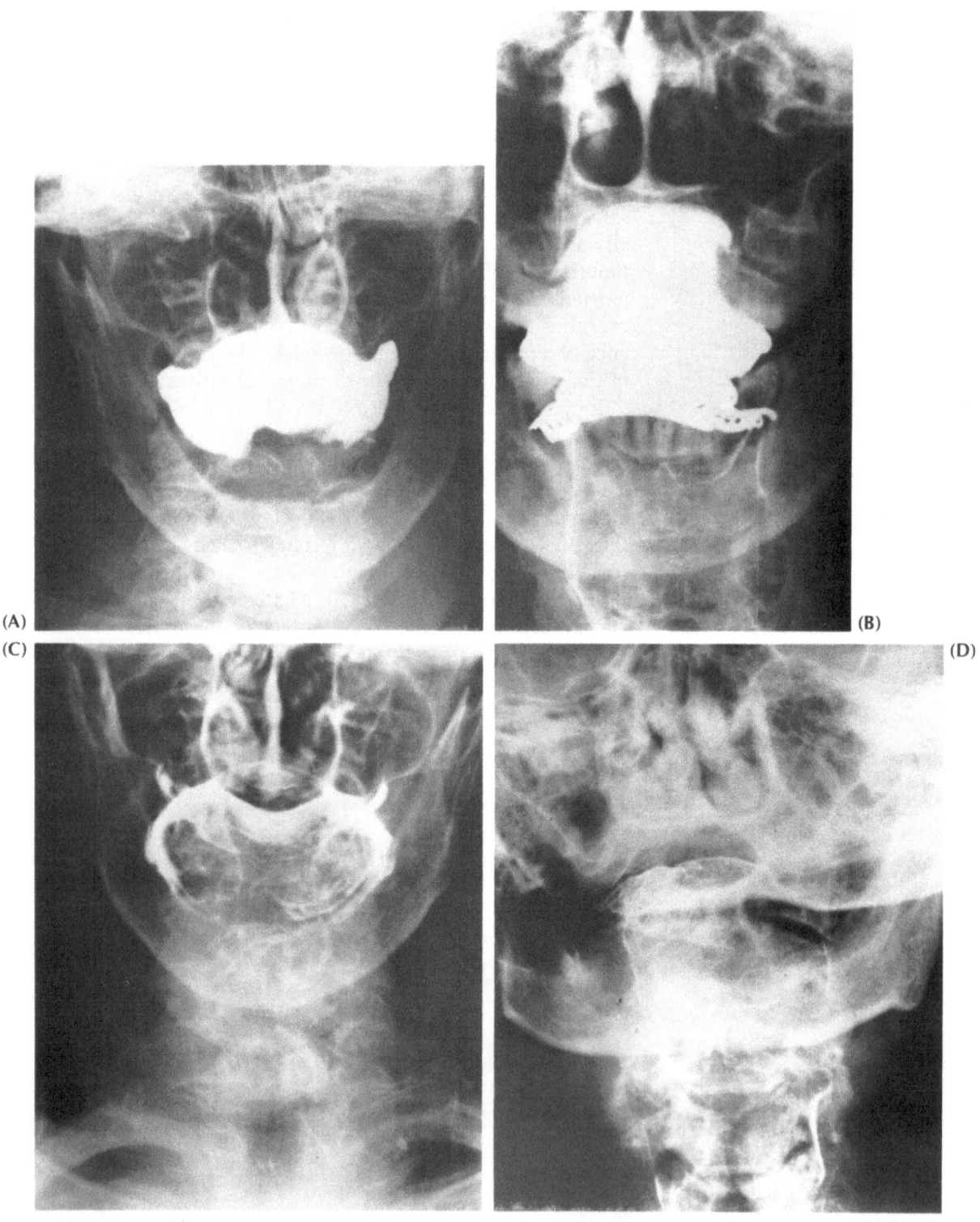

FIGURE 20
Oral cavity; frontal (AP) views in four patients. (A) With barium bolus in mouth; (B) beginning of swallowing action; (C) after swallowing of bolus; (D) residual thin coat of barium, mouth closed.

straight column as it descends into the oropharynx (Fig. 10A). Oblique films of the oropharyngeal area during and after a barium swallow are also very useful in detecting abnormalities. The normal appearance of this region in the RAO position is well illustrated throughout the text. (See Figs. 18C, 22AB, etc.)

The nasopharynx

The nasopharynx is usually outlined by air on a plain lateral film of the neck, with the mouth closed. The nasopharynx is a recess extending from the base of the skull behind the soft palate and uvula, continuing down into the oropharynx and hypopharynx. It may occasionally be bisected by a calcified stylohyoid ligament. Following ingestion of barium and especially at the height of the swallowing motion the nasopharynx is normally not opacified, except for a small segment directly posterior to the uvula at the point of contact between the soft palate and the posterior pharyngeal wall. This functional point may produce a beaklike shadow or a pseudodiverticulum (Figs. 18C and 18D). Regurgitation of barium into the nasopharynx implies impaired muscular coordination and is an abnormal finding. In the anteroposterior view of the mouth, the oropharynx, and nasopharynx are not well visualized because of superimposed shadows of the nasal cavity and cervical spine.

The oropharynx

The oropharynx is best defined on a plain lateral film of the neck. Films should be taken at rest and at the height of dry swallow. The tip of the epiglottis, the valleculae, the base of the tongue, and the posterior pharyngeal wall are usually well outlined by the air column in this area. At the height of the swallowing motion the degree of mobility may be assessed. Abnormal soft tissue masses can also be identified (Fig. 21). A film obtained during the Valsalva maneuver, which overdistends the oropharynx with air, is quite useful in delineating the surrounding soft tissues.

After the ingestion of barium, lateral films exposed at the height of a swallow also may demonstrate abnormal masses (Figs. 10B and 22A). At this time, the valleculae are opacified and the inverted epiglottis, which is folded over the introitus of the glottis, can be outlined within the barium column (Fig. 22B). After the bolus has been swallowed, residual barium will sharply delineate the posterior surface of the tongue, the valleculae, and the posterior pharyngeal wall (Fig. 17).

In anteroposterior plain films, the oropharynx is mostly obscured by the superimposed shadow of the mandible. During a

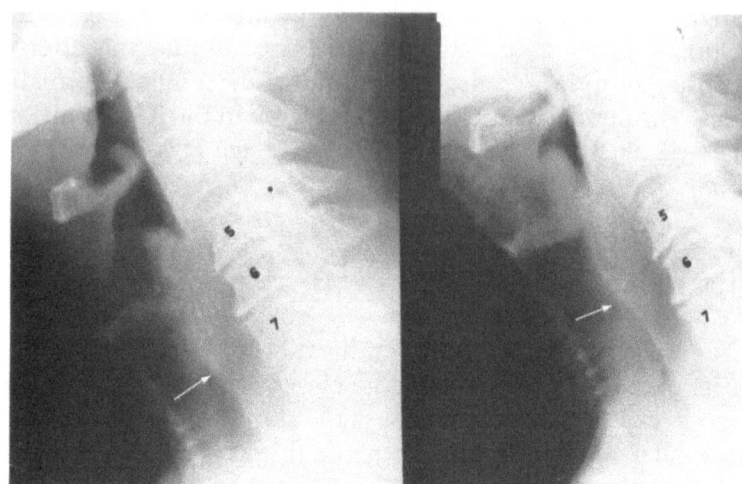

FIGURE 21

Oropharynx, plain film of neck. (A) At rest, (B) at height of dry swallow. Arrow at distal end of the cricoid lamina. From Zaino, C., et al. *The Pharyngoesophageal Sphincter,* 1970. Courtesy Charles C Thomas, Publisher, Springfield, Illinois.

FIGURE 22

Oropharynx during a barium swallow. (A) At height of barium swallow; (B) inverted epiglottis at arrow. From Zaino, C., et al. *The Pharyngoesophageal Sphincter,* 1970. Courtesy Charles C Thomas, Publisher, Springfield, Illinois.

(A)   (B)

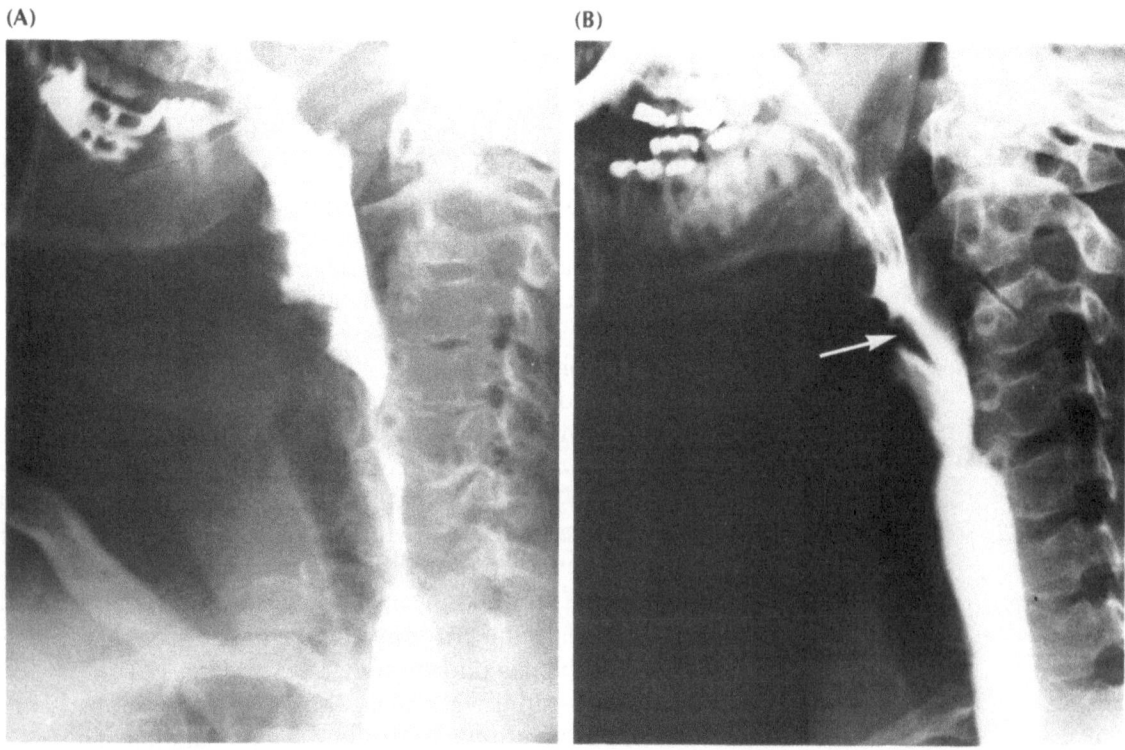

barium swallow, the oropharynx is represented by a solid, flattened column of barium as it descends to meet the posterior wall of the hypopharynx (Figs. 10A and 10C). After the passage of the bolus, residual barium coats this area, but the visibility of the oropharyngeal structures varies with the angle of projection, the thickness and length of the patient's neck, the amount of residual barium retained in the valleculae, and the degree of tonicity of the thyrohyoid ligaments.

The hypopharynx

The hypopharynx on the lateral plain neck film is divided into upper and lower sections. The upper section is filled with air, is continuous with the oropharynx, and extends into the open larynx and trachea. The valleculae, epiglottis, and laryngeal introitus are usually well delineated anteriorly. Posteriorly, the pharyngeal wall is continuous with that of the oropharynx.

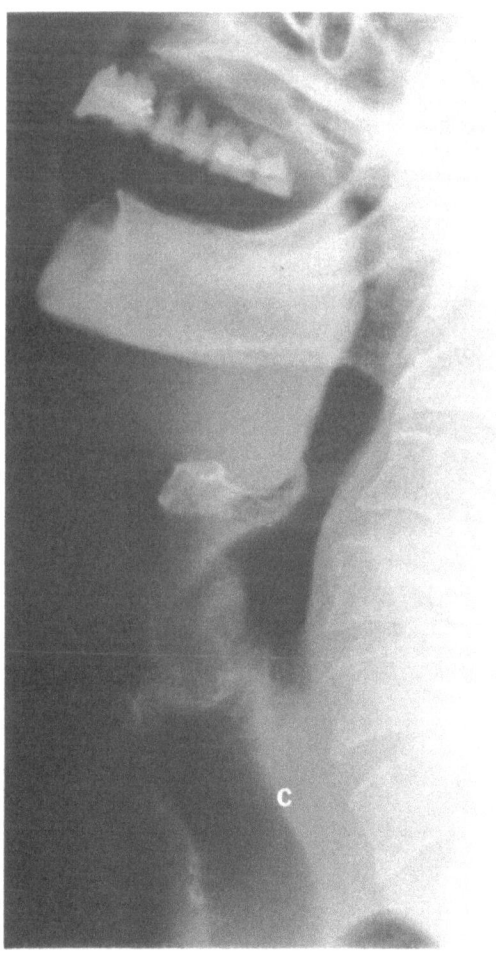

FIGURE 23
Hypopharynx, plain film of neck. C shows cricoid lamina.

The inferior portion of the hypopharynx is airless because it is compressed against the cervical spine by the larynx. It is usually visualized as a thickened postcricoid soft tissue density. The lower pole of the cricoid cartilage protrudes into the subglottic region posteriorly, producing a soft tissue impression within the air column even with absence of calcification of the cricoid cartilage (Fig. 23). In an anteroposterior plain film, the hyoid bone, laryngeal cartilages, and cervical spine are generally superimposed to such an extent that the hypopharynx is not delineated.

During the ingestion of a bolus, in the lateral position, the hypopharynx becomes distended at the height of swallowing, resembling an irregular funnel; this dilates superiorly and narrows inferiorly where it enters the gaping sphincter. The posterior wall of the hypopharynx presents a smooth, straight appearance except for the lowermost cricopharyngeal impression (Fig. 24B), which must be differentiated from an advancing peristaltic primary wave usually observed at a higher level (Fig. 24A). The upper segment of the anterior wall of the hypopharynx is irregular because of the closed laryngeal introitus. The lower portion of the anterior wall is also irregular because of the impression of the cricoid lamina and the superimposed shadows of the pyriform fossae or lateral channels. The impres-

FIGURE 24
Hypopharynx, during a barium swallow. (A) Advancing peristaltic wave (at arrow); (B) The cricopharyngeal impression (at arrow).

(A)

(B)

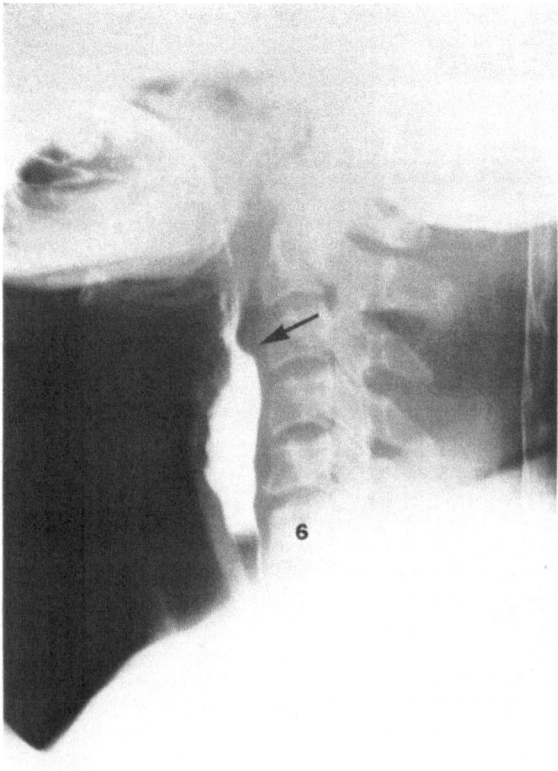

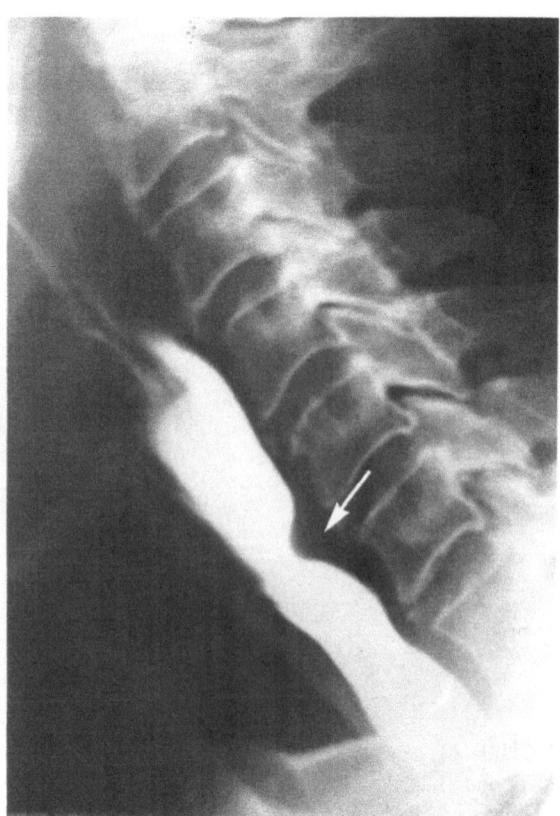

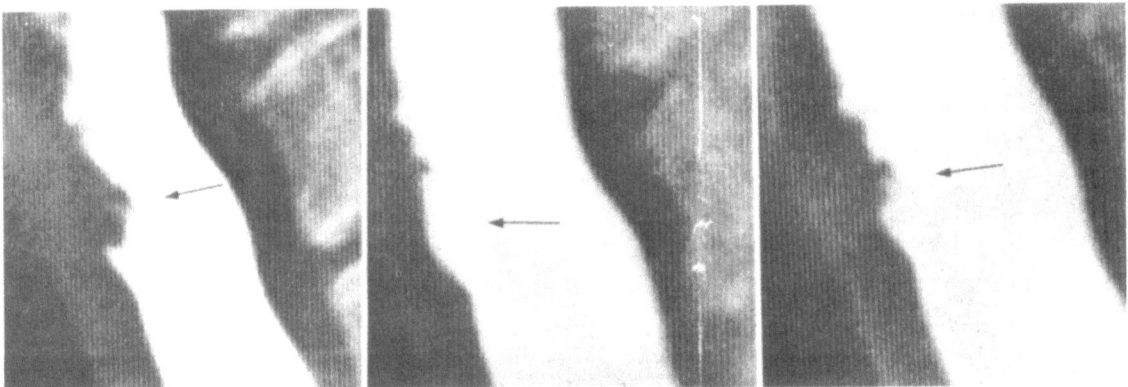

FIGURE 25
Hypopharynx, cricopharyngeal impressions (at arrow). From Pitman, R. G., and Fraser, G. M. The postcricoid impression on the esophagus. Clin. Radio., *16;* 37, 1965. E & S Livingstone Longman House, Essex, England.

sion of the cricoid lamina (188) may present as an irregular anterior mucosal defect and even simulate a neoplasm because of the thickened, redundant mucosa and the engorged venous channels which are often present normally in this area (Fig. 25) (89). At the level of the lower pole of the cricoid lamina, a small inconstant incisura or notch may be noted at the pharyngoesophageal junction (Fig. 26A). The cricopharyngeal

FIGURE 26
Pharyngoesophageal junction (A) showing normal notching (at arrow); (B) oblique view showing presence of pseudo-diverticula (at arrow). Note normal mucosal pattern at post cricoid region.

(B)

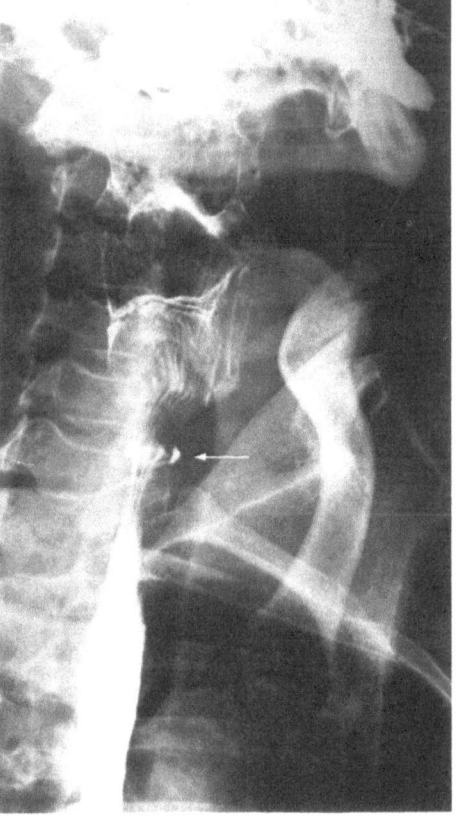

(A)

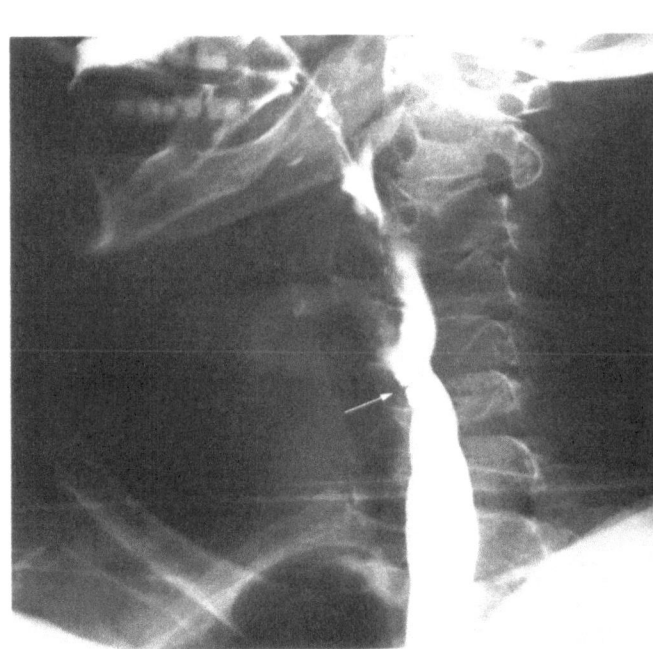

impression posteriorly can vary from a slight anterior bend in the posterior column to a pronounced semilunar indentation.

In the lateral view obtained shortly after the ingestion of the barium bolus with the mouth closed, the lower or postcricoid portion of the hypopharynx is visualized as a linear channel coated by the retained barium in the compressed mucosal folds. A small amount of retained barium at the lower end of this channel above the normally contracted pharyngoesophageal sphincter may resemble a pseudodiverticulum at the pharyngoesophageal junction (Fig. 26B).

In anteroposterior views barium in the area of the hypopharynx opacifies the valleculae, which appear as two opaque pockets. Below this site opacification is incomplete because of the "folded over" epiglottis. Laterally, in the frontal plane views, normal hypopharyngeal bulges, occasionally referred to as "ears" (Fig. 27A), may be identified. These "ears" are caused by stretching of the thyrohyoid ligaments leading into the pyriform fossae, which in turn lead into the terminal portion of the funnel-shaped segment of the hypopharynx and the area of the postcricoid lamina. Occasionally, lateral notchings which are normal may be noted in the area of the pyriform sinuses (Fig. 28A). These notches may be mistaken for webs if observed only on one side because of rotation and the possible asym-

FIGURE 27

Orohypopharynx, AP views in two patients. (A) Fully distended by barium showing bulging lateral "ears" (at upper arrow) and pyriform sinuses (at lower arrow); (B) during the Valsalva maneuver. Arrow at pharyngoesophageal junction. Note bulging ears with deviated and contracted upper sphincter immediately above arrow.

(A)

(B)

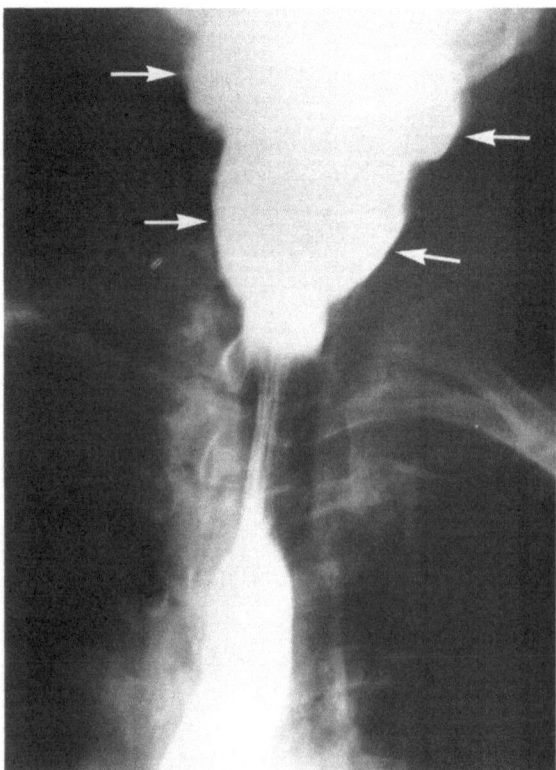
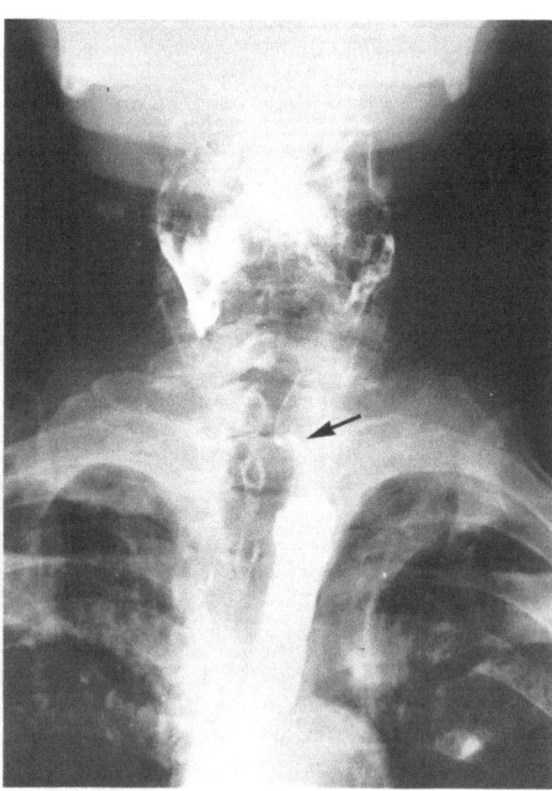

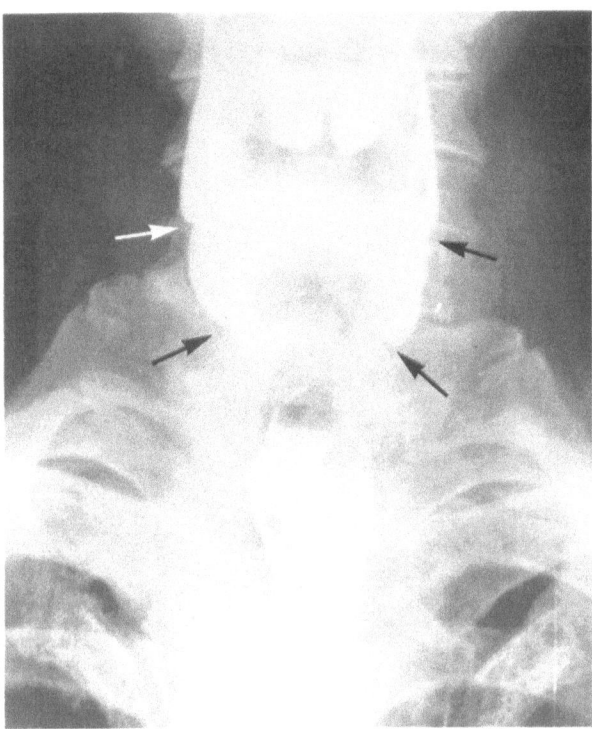

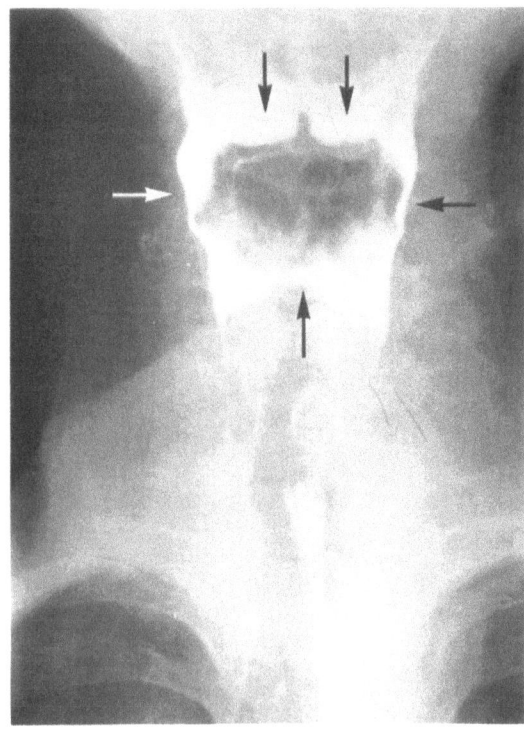

(A)

(B)

FIGURE 28
Orophypopharynx during barium swallow. (A) Normal bilateral notchings (at arrows). (B) The valleculae (upper arrows), lateral channels (middle arrows), and the cricoid line (lower arrow). From Zaino, C., et al. *The Pharyngoesophageal Sphincter,* 1970. Courtesy Charles C Thomas, Publisher, Springfield, Illinois.

metry associated with uneven retention of barium. The valleculae are usually clearly defined as two symmetrical pockets at the base of the tongue (Fig. 28B). At the height of a swallow the inverted epiglottis may appear stellar shaped (Fig. 29A). At rest, the normal epiglottis may be outlined occasionally if coated by residual barium (Fig. 29B). Films exposed during the Valsalva maneuver produce lateral air-filled bulges in the upper lateral channel, accentuating the lateral "ears" referred to earlier (Fig. 27B). These radiologic appearances of the normal hypopharynx in lateral and anteroposterior projections are demonstrated in Figs. 30 A–D, in films obtained at rest, after a barium swallow.

The pharyngoesophageal junction

The pharyngoesophageal junction is not normally visualized without ingestion of an opaque medium. In the lateral views, during the height of a barium swallow, a posterior indentation, representing the cricopharyngeal impression and corresponding in part to the cricopharyngeal muscle, may be noted. Recent anatomic studies (271) suggest that the cricopharyngeal muscle represents the uppermost level of the pharyngoesophageal sphincter, which extends 1 to 2 cm below the cricopharyngeus muscle. This posterior indentation may, in fact, be part of the posterior upper wall of this sphincter (see Diagram

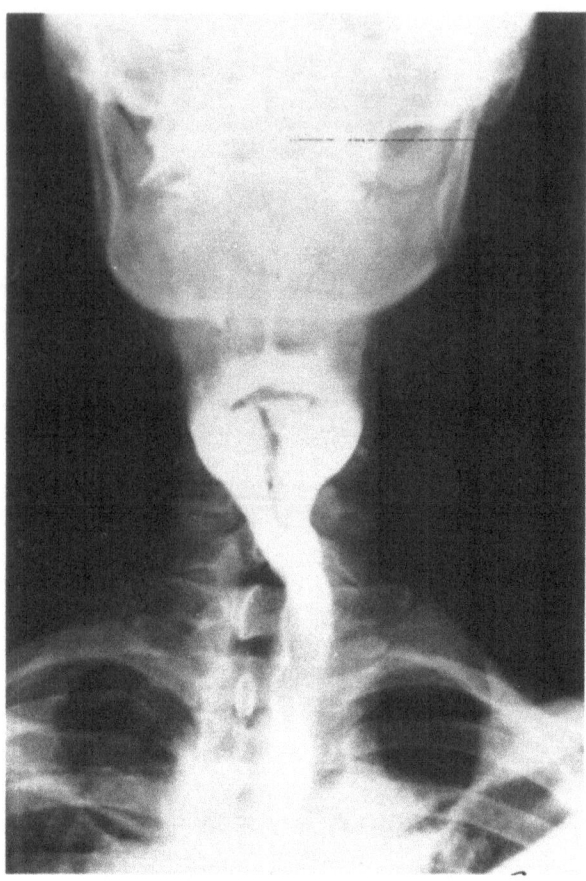

(A)

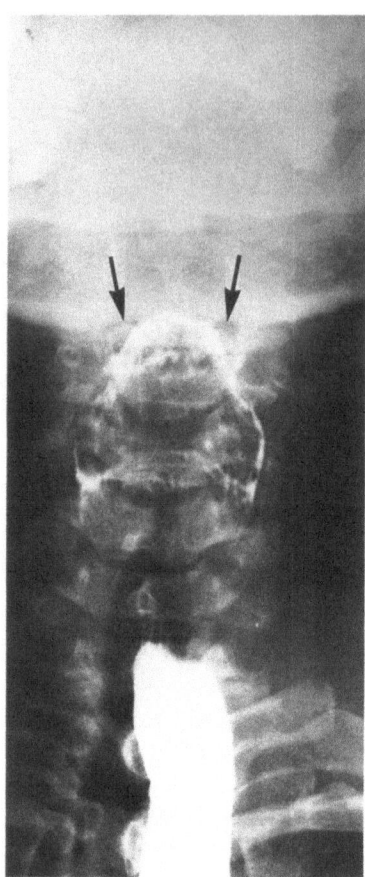

(B)

FIGURE 29
Hypopharynx, appearance of the epiglottis. (A) Inverted (star shadow); (B) at rest, upright. Epiglottis coated by barium (at arrows).

FIGURE 30
Orohypopharyngeal area and sphincter zone. (A) Lateral view after a barium swallow. (B) Tracing of A: 1, Valleculae; 2, Pyriform sinuses; 3, Compressed hypopharynx; 4, pharyngoesophageal sphincter (between arrows); 5, cricoid cartilage. (C) AP view after a barium swallow. Modified from Zaino, C., et al. *The Pharyngoesophageal Sphincter*, 1970. Courtesy Charles C Thomas, Publisher, Springfield, Illinois. (D) Tracing of C: 1, valleculae; 2, pyriform sinuses; 3, cricoid line; 4, hypopharyngeal area. Small arrows at site of normal notchings. Lowest black arrow indicates the pharyngoesophageal sphincter.

3). At rest, following the passage of the barium bolus, the pharyngoesophageal junction is identified by a small amount of retained barium above the level of the contracted sphincter (Fig. 31).

The pharyngoesophageal sphincter

The pharyngoesophageal sphincter, approximately 2 cm in length, is the most proximal segment of the cervical esophagus. In the lateral plain film of the neck, at rest, the sphincter zone corresponds to the thickened area of soft tissue which is present just below the level of the lower pole of the cricoid

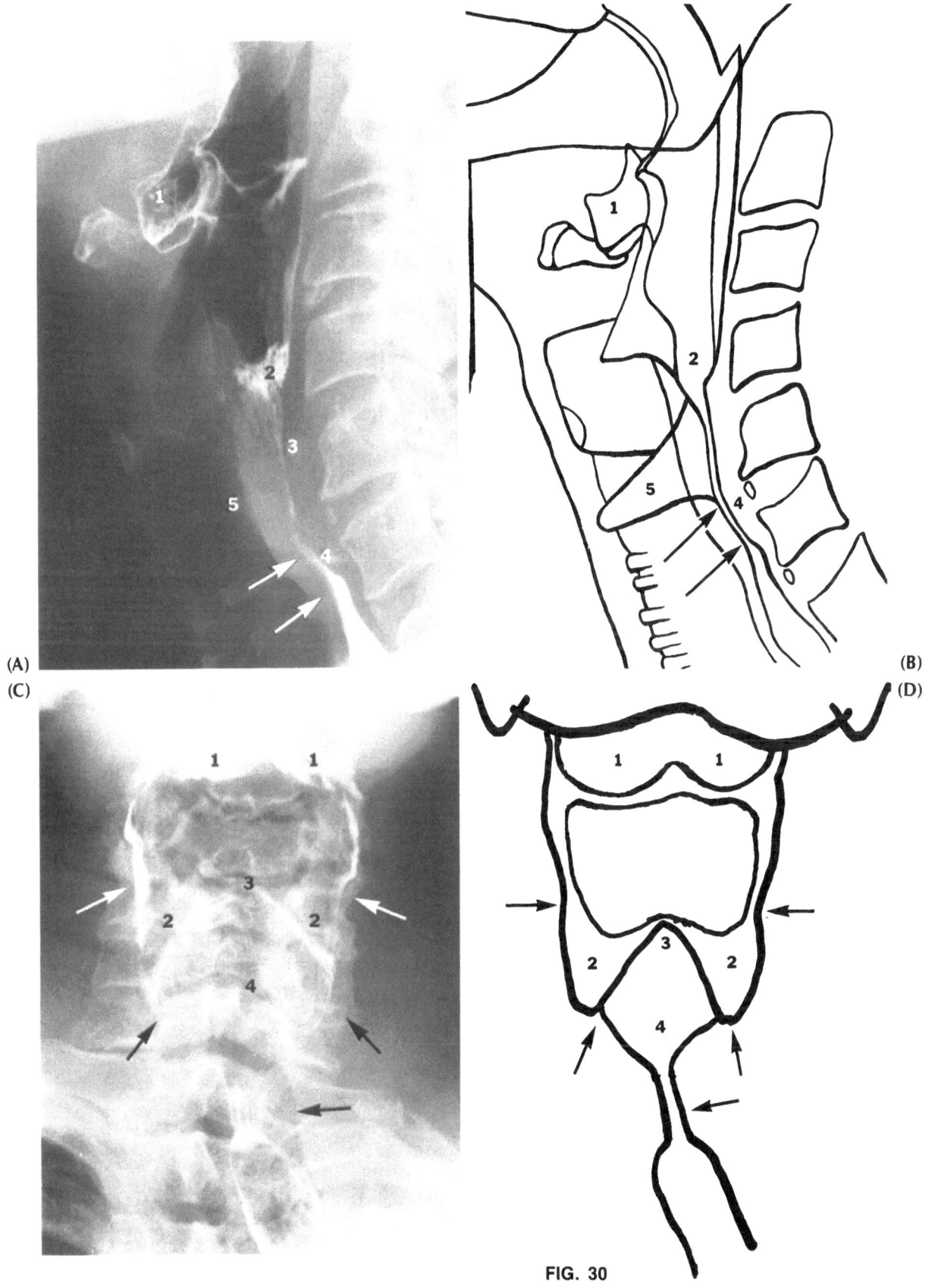

(A)

(B)

(C)

(D)

FIG. 30

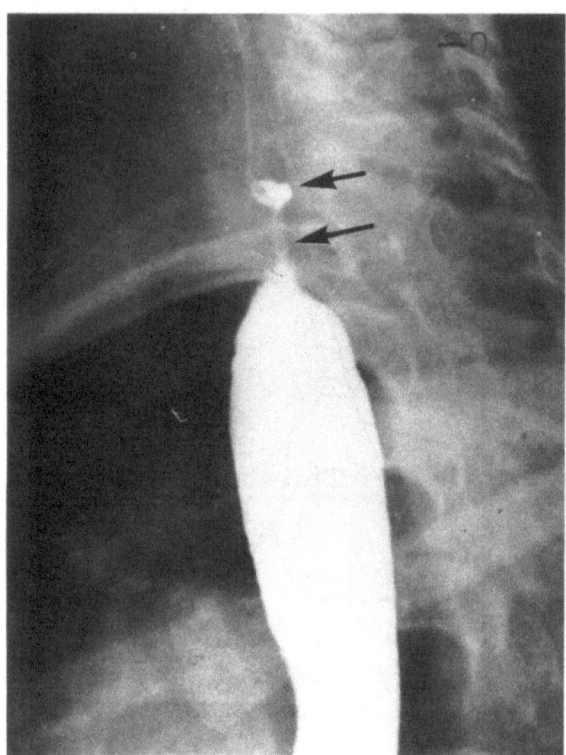

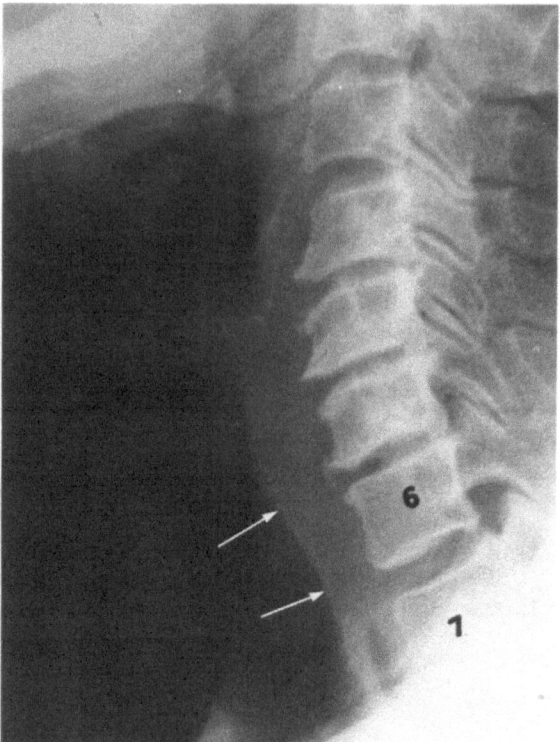

FIG. 31   **FIG. 32**

FIGURE 31
Normal contracted pharyngoesophageal sphincter (lower arrow).
Upper arrow at pharyngoesophageal junction.

FIGURE 32
Sphincter zone. Air trapped in the cervical esophagus below the location of the contracted upper sphincter (upper arrow at lower pole of cricoid lamina; lower arrow at distal end of normally contracted upper sphincter). From Zaino, C., et al. *The Pharyngoesophageal Sphincter,* 1970. Courtesy Charles C Thomas, Publisher, Springfield, Illinois.

cartilage and is continuous with the empty lower hypopharynx. Occasionally, the lower level of the normally contracted pharyngoesophageal sphincter, located several centimeters distal to the lower pole of the cricoid cartilage, is filled by air trapped in the cervical esophagus (Fig. 32).

Lateral films obtained after ingestion of a barium bolus usually visualize this contracted segment, corresponding to the sphincter zone (Fig. 31). The site of the distal end of the contracted sphincter may be recognized by the sudden distension with barium of the cervical esophagus directly below the contracted sphincter segment. When the sphincter segment is dilated it may be identified occasionally as a distinct bulge produced by the barium bolus as it passes through the sphincter at the height of the swallow (Fig. 33B). A crinkled mucosal pattern delineated by barium in the partly relaxed sphincter zone may be noted occasionally. This unusual irregularity disappears as the sphincter closes (Fig. 34). During the Valsalva maneuver, the visualized contracted sphincter occasionally forms a concave indentation at and below the level of the lower pole of the cricoid lamina. The upper portion of this con-

FIGURE 33

Upper and lower sphincters of the esophagus. (A) Upper sphincter contracted, (B) upper sphincter dilated, (C) lower sphincter contracted, (D) lower sphincter dilated. From Zaino, C., et al. *The Pharyngoesophageal Sphincter,* 1970. Courtesy Charles C Thomas, Publisher, Springfield, Illinois.

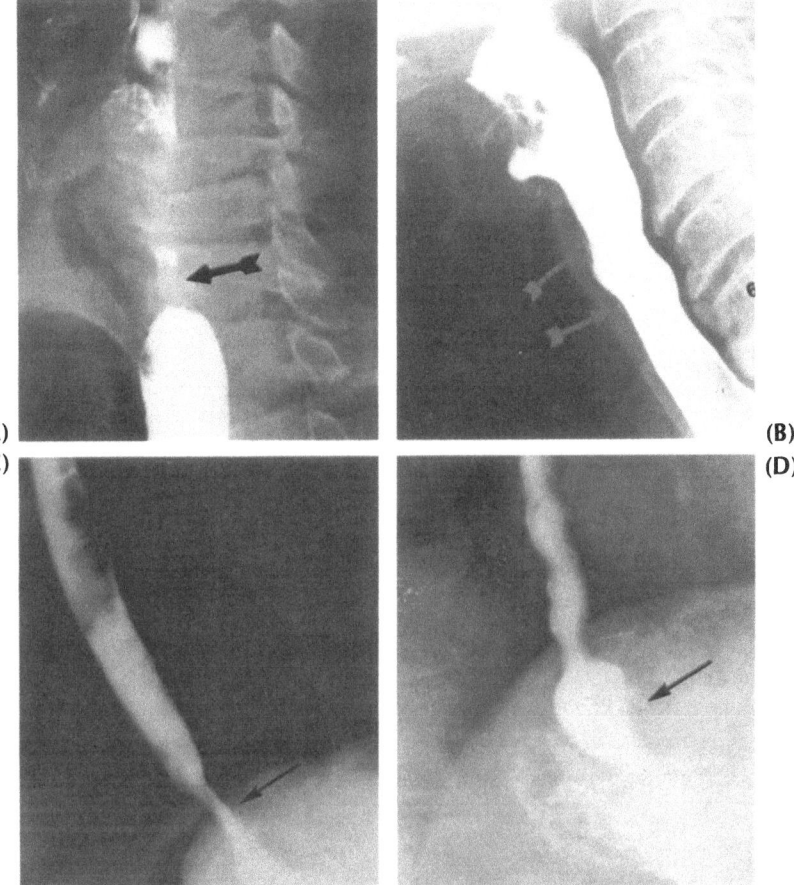

(A) (B)
(C) (D)

FIGURE 34

Mucosal pattern of the sphincter zone. (A, B) Crinkled mucosal pattern at height of a barium swallow. (C, D) At rest; normal smooth mucosal pattern in D. From Zaino, C., et al. *The Pharyngoesophageal Sphincter,* 1970. Courtesy Charles C Thomas, Publisher, Springfield, Illinois.

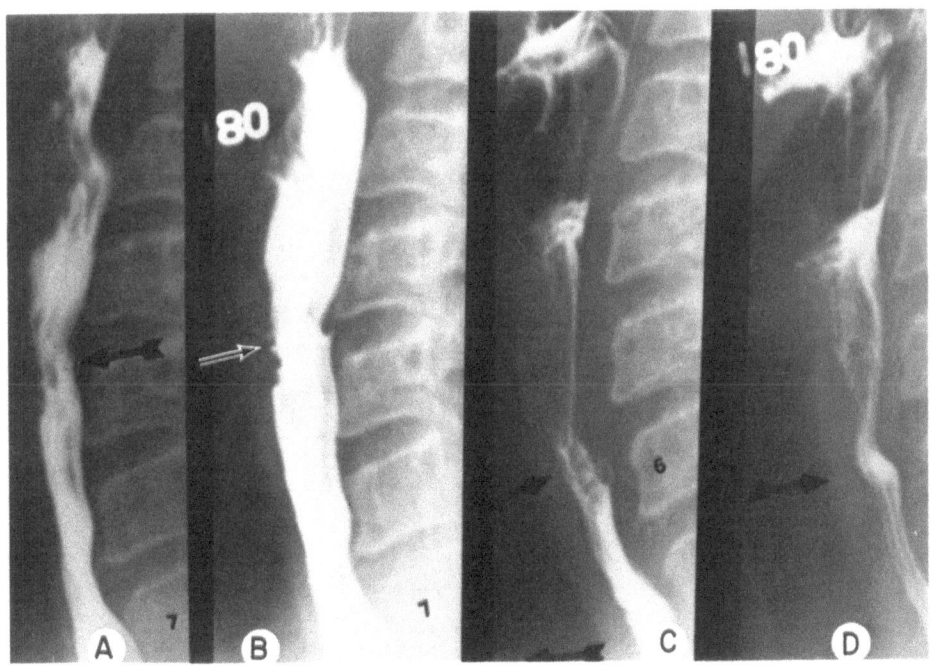

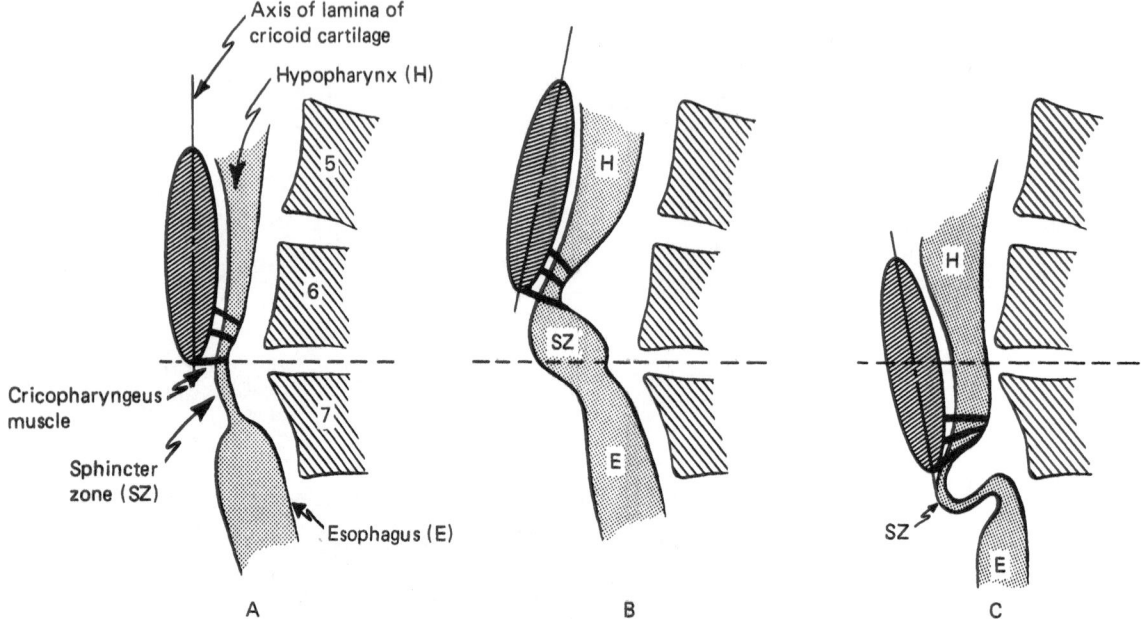

DIAGRAM 3
Gross anatomy-changes affecting the pharyngoesophageal sphincter (SZ) during swallowing and the Valsalva maneuver. (A) at rest, (B) at height of swallow, (C) during the Valsalva maneuver. From Zaino, C. et al. *The Pharyngoesophageal Sphincter*, 1970. Courtesy Charles C Thomas, Publisher, Springfield, Illinois.

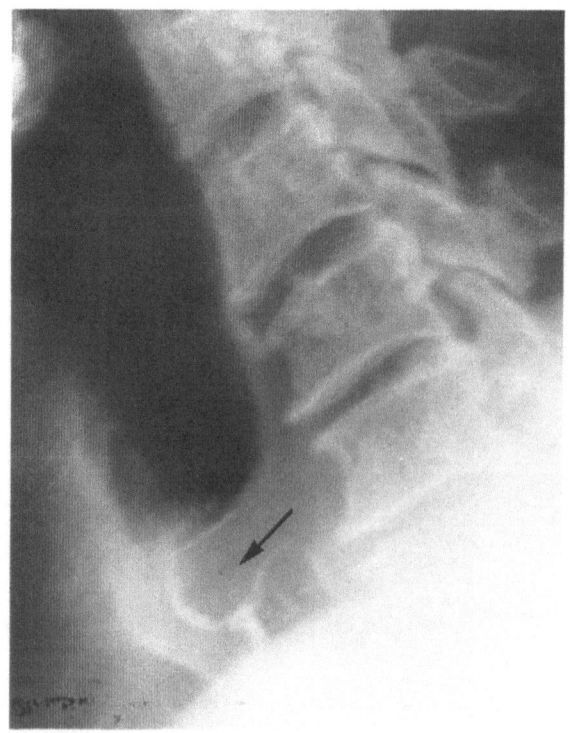

FIGURE 35
Sphincter zone. Lateral view during the Valsalva maneuver (at arrow).

cavity is created by the transverse fibers of the cricopharyngeus muscle, whereas the lower and longer segment is created by an acute flexion of the contracted sphincter segment as it is displaced downward by the larynx against the fixed cervical esophagus (Diagram 3 and Fig. 35).

In anteroposterior views, the nonopacified sphincter zone is not visualized. Following ingestion of barium, the sphincter is identified as a contracted, somewhat flattened segment at the level of the sixth and seventh cervical vertebrae. Stasis of barium at the upper level of the sphincter zone and distension of the lower cervical esophagus with barium immediately below the sphincter are commonly observed (Fig. 36). At the height of a swallow, the dilated sphincter zone, stretched by the bolus, simulates the nozzle of a funnel and rarely appears as a localized bulge. During the Valsalva maneuver, bilateral distension of the lateral channels and pyriform sinuses is noted. The flattened, contracted sphincter zone is identified at a slightly higher level during swallowing than at rest.

The cervical esophagus

The cervical esophageal region below the sphincter zone in plain lateral film of the neck can be completely obscured by the clavicle (in short-necked individuals). In the average pa-

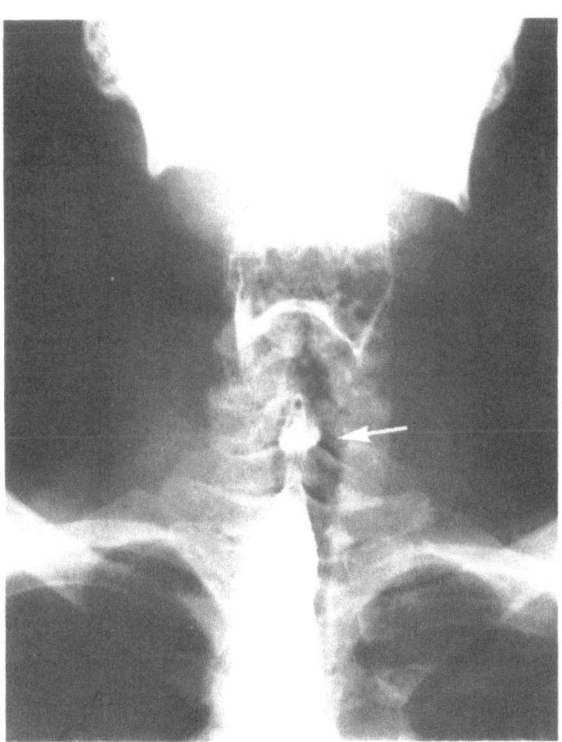

FIGURE 36
Sphincter zone, AP view. Arrow at pharyngoesophageal junction; contracted sphincter below arrow.

tient, a column of thickened soft tissue continuous with the sphincter zone and lying posterior to the trachea is noted. This feature may be obscured by the attachment of the outer long muscles of the neck. At the height of a dry swallow, the cervical esophagus is retracted superiorly so that it may be visualized if it contains air. The air-filled lung apices, incidentally, similarly may protrude above the thoracic inlet.

During the ingestion of barium, the cervical esophagus distal to the sphincter zone is distended by the bolus and appears as a solid opaque column continuous with the thoracic esophagus. Occasionally the dilated upper sphincter may be identified (Fig. 37). Rarely, oblique ridges have been noted above the inlet, possibly produced by the underlying musculature. After passage of the bolus, parallel mucosal folds outlined by barium and continuous with those of the thoracic esophagus are noted.

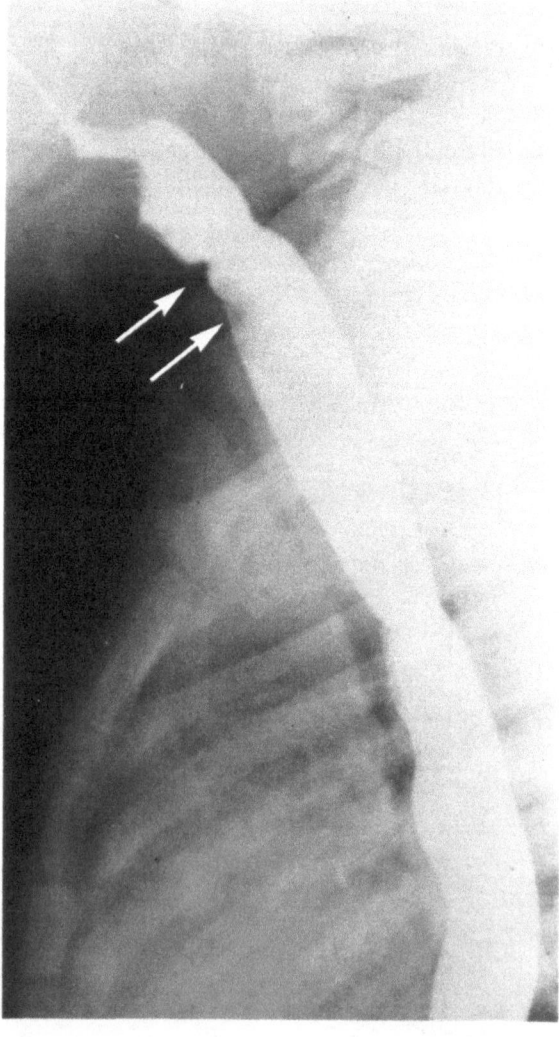

FIGURE 37

Cervical and thoracic esophagus. Note dilated sphincter zone between arrows and notch at the pharyngoesophageal junction (upper arrow).

FIGURE 38

Thoracic esophagus, AP, showing. D, thoracic inlet; E, supraaortic segment; F, aortic arch segment; G, bronchial triangle; H, retrocardiac segment; I, epiphrenic segment; J, lower sphincter zone.

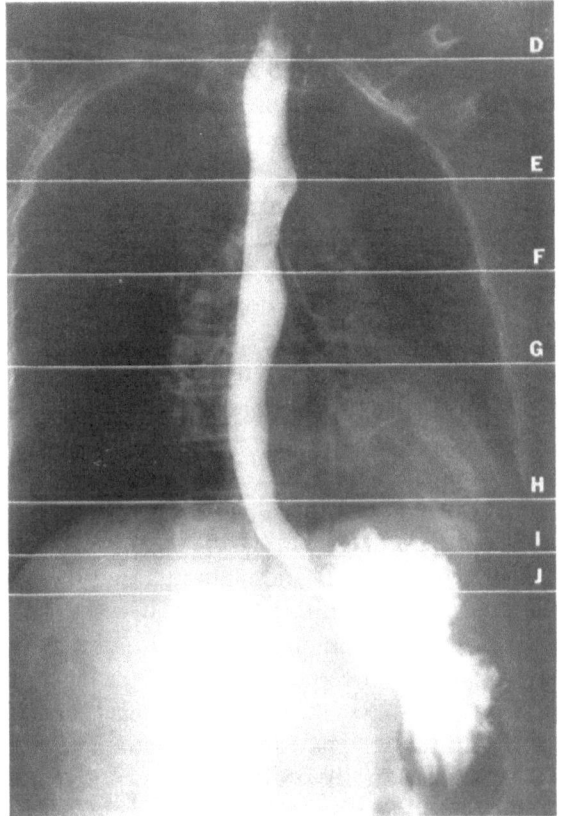

In anteroposterior views, the cervical esophagus is not visualized without opaque media. Following a barium swallow, the esophagus below the sphincter zone is seen as a dilated opaque column continuous with the thoracic esophagus, lying slightly to the left of the midline.

The thoracic esophagus

The thoracic esophagus is arbitrarily divided into the following segments (Fig. 38):

Supraaortic: extending from the thoracic inlet to the upper border of the aortic arch.

Aortic: extending from the upper border of the aortic arch to the upper border of the tracheal bifurcation.

Bronchial: extending from the upper border of the tracheal bifurcation to the lower border of the left main bronchus.

Retrocardiac: extending from the superior border of the left main bronchus to the level of the left lateral deviation of the lower esophagus.

Epiphrenic: extending from the left lateral deviation of the esophagus to the upper diaphragmatic level of the esophageal hiatus.

The lower sphincter zone (abdominal segment): lying partly within the diaphragmatic tunnel and the abdomen.

The contour and direction of the thoracic esophagus are determined by its surrounding structures. Several of these structures are responsible for normal indentations and compressions of the esophagus; these are reviewed as an aid in the subsequent localization and description of abnormal findings. In order to detect these normal indentations and compressions, a small amount of barium should be given to avoid their obliteration by overfilling of the esophagus.

THE SUPRAAORTIC SEGMENT The supraaortic segment of the thoracic esophagus, extending from the thoracic inlet to the aortic arch, rests on the prevertebral fascia posteriorly and the carotid sheaths and their vessels and pleura laterally. This segment is adherent to the trachea anteriorly and lies slightly to its left as it courses through the mediastinum. On radiologic examination, compression by the trachea of this segment of the esophagus occasionally produces an oblique, linear lucency on its right border. This finding is particularly apparent in the right anterior oblique position in individuals with narrow thoracic inlets (124) (Fig. 39).

THE AORTIC SEGMENT The aortic segment of the thoracic esophagus is characterized by the aortic arch impression at the level of the third and fourth thoracic vertebrae. On radiologic examination this aortic impression is reflected in a semilunar indentation on the left side of the esophagus. The degree of indentation varies with the age of the subject and the size of the arch. In infants and children, in whom the aorta is poorly developed, the indentation is small and inconspicuous. In the elderly individual and particularly in the presence of atheromatous changes, notching may be noted at the site of compression caused by wrinkling of the mucosal pattern (Fig. 40). In studying this area to exclude a vascular ring or anomalous vessels, standard PA frontal, right oblique, left oblique, and lateral views should be obtained (Diagram 7-A to follow—Chapter 3).

THE BRONCHIAL SEGMENT The bronchial segment of the thoracic esophagus can be subdivided into the aortic–bronchial triangle, the bronchial impression, and the interbronchial segment (29).

The aortic-bronchial triangle is the area of the esophagus partly partitioned by the lower border of the aortic arch and upper border of the left main bronchus as it crosses the esophagus from right to left. This segment becomes increasingly conspicuous in elderly patients, particularly in the presence of

FIGURE 39
Thoracic esophagus. Thoracic impression (upper arrow), aortic impression (middle arrow), and bronchial impression (lower arrow).

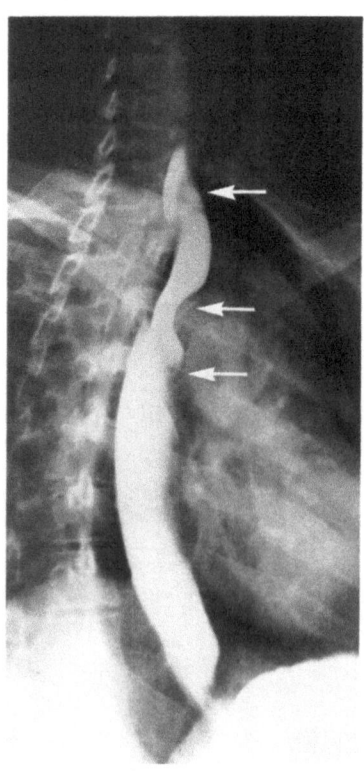

FIGURE 40

Normal aortic impression with irregular mucosal pattern. (A) At a higher level of projection, (B) at a lower level (upper arrow at tracheal impression.

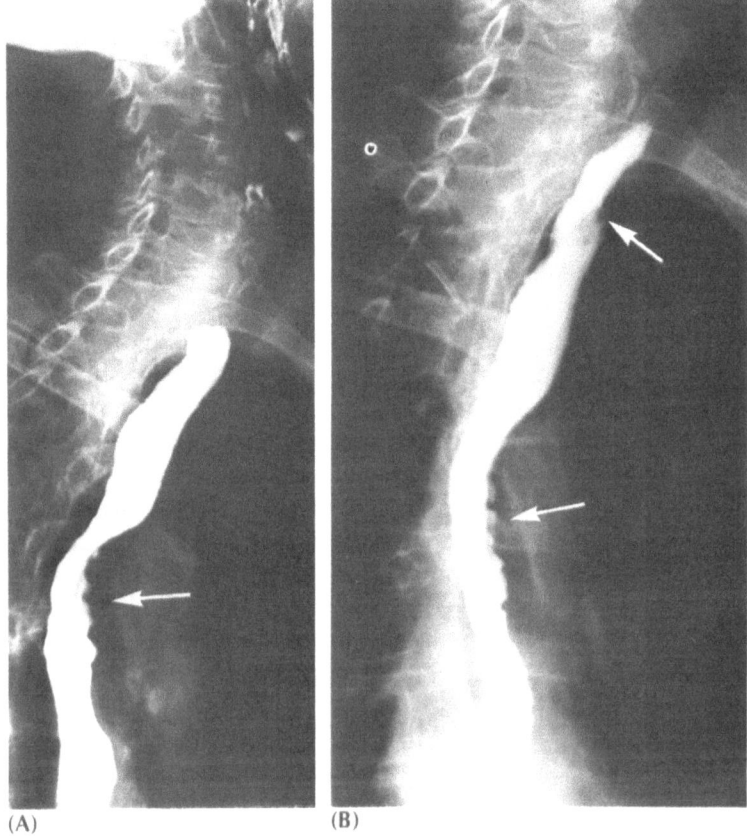

(A)   (B)

FIGURE 41

Normal bronchial segment. Arrow at bronchial triangle.

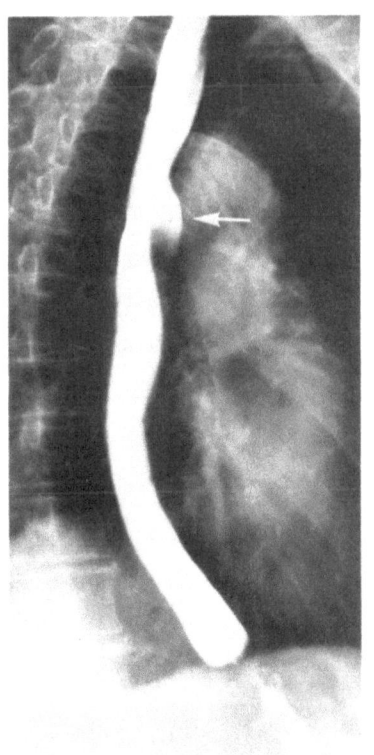

pulmonary emphysema when the bronchial impression is exaggerated. The indentations produced in this triangle result in a pseudo-diverticulum observed on a barium swallow, especially noticeable in the right anterior oblique position (Fig. 41).

The bronchial impression is produced by the left main bronchus as it descends obliquely to the left and posteriorly from the tracheobronchial bifurcation anterior to the esophagus (Fig. 39). This indentation is best observed at the level of the sixth to the eighth thoracic vertebrae. The left main bronchus, best visualized in frontal and right anterior oblique positions, produces a translucent tubular zone which is accompanied by an area of incomplete filling of the esophagus on barium swallow proportional to the degree and extent of the impression created by the bronchus. The more acute the angle at the tracheobronchial bifurcation, the greater will be the impression upon the esophagus.

The interbronchial segment extends from the level of the bifurcation of the trachea to the superior border of the left main bronchus. Chains of lymph nodes generally surround this area.

THE RETROCARDIAC SEGMENT The retrocardiac segment of the thoracic esophagus is close to that portion of the pericardial sac covering the posterior surface of the left atrium and left ventricle. Here, the esophagus traverses anterior to the thoracic aorta from left to right. Normally, esophageal compression is not produced in this region.

THE EPIPHRENIC SEGMENT The epiphrenic segment of the thoracic esophagus is the most inferior portion of the esophagus as it curves again to the left to enter the esophageal hiatus of the diaphragm. This segment is accompanied by the vagal nerves and is in contact with the pleura.

A characteristic dilatation, referred to as the "phrenic ampulla," is noted on barium swallow at the height of sustained full inspiration. The phrenic ampulla represents a physiologic dilatation of the lower end of the thoracic esophagus, observed best in the barium-filled esophagus, during sustained inspiration (242) (Fig. 42). The mucosa of the base of the phrenic ampulla, which is located at the level of the superior attachment of the phrenoesophageal membrane, usually appears puckered. This dilated segment is produced by (a) stasis of barium at this level caused by the occluding action of the inferior pull of the membrane that is fixed to the diaphragm; and (b) by the contraction of the lower esophageal sphincter within the esophagus hiatus. The base of the ampulla represents the upper portion of the sphincter zone. The shape and size of the ampulla vary with the degree of distension by the barium within it. The level of the apex of the ampulla depends also on the amount of barium in the distal esophagus.

The phrenic ampulla is best visualized in the prone right an-

FIGURE 42
Normal phrenic ampulla. (A) In full inspiration; (B) ampulla beginning to collapse.

(A) (B)

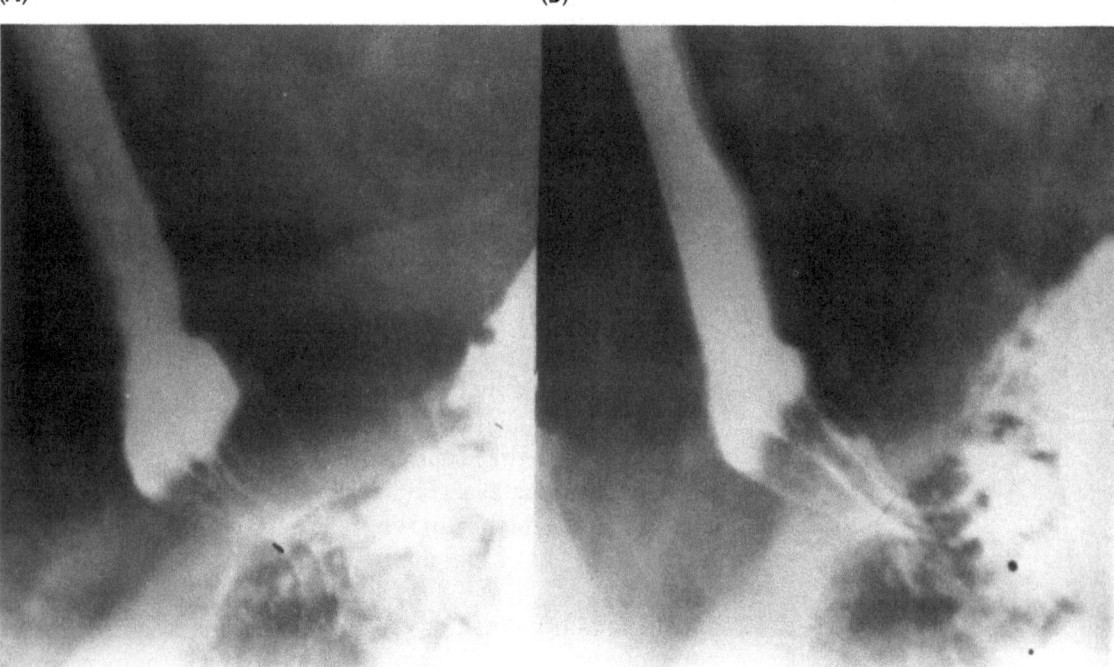

terior oblique position and may not even be demonstrated in erect individuals because of the effects of gravity. The ampulla is better demonstrated with thick rather than with thin barium and is more commonly observed in older people. Because the ampulla is produced by normal physiologic and anatomic factors, its demonstrated presence is of no clinical significance.

The lower sphincter zone

The lower esophageal vestibular complex or the lower sphincter of the esophagus corresponds to Lerche's vestibule, being located partly within the esophageal hiatus and partly within the abdomen (Diagram 10A; see Chapter 4). This lower esophageal sphincter corresponds to the abdominal segment of the esophagus. The sphincter zone extends from the superior attachment of the phrenoesophageal membrane to the inferior attachment of this membrane, which is at the site of the gastroesophageal junction. The sphincter is normally 2 to 3 cm long but may be longer, as demonstrated in pneumoperitoneum studies. However, it may appear shorter in the presence of an hiatal hernia. This sphincter is normally contracted, relaxing and opening completely as a bolus approaches it. This opening is caused partly by reflex action and also by the mechanical relaxation of the surrounding phrenoesophageal membrane. The lower sphincter in its dilated phase presents as an ovoid area directly above the gastroesophageal junction (Fig. 33D). The mucosal pattern of the sphincter zone is indistinguishable from the rest of the thoracic esophagus in its relaxed state, consisting of smooth, parallel folds (Fig. 1). The radiologic appearance of this segment may vary slightly with position or angulation and is observed best in the prone right anterior oblique position. In anteroposterior views, it can be partially or completely obscured if the gastric fundus is overfilled with barium (see Schonander studies, Fig. 11). In the right anterior oblique position this sphincter zone can be identified through the air-filled fundus of the stomach. In posterioanterior views the sphincter zone is generally obscured by the barium-filled cardia. The size of this sphincter is also affected by respiratory action because this segment is held in position by the phrenoesophageal membrane within the esophageal hiatus. To some extent, therefore, the position varies with the respiratory phase of the diaphragm. It can also be seen in various stages of contraction or dilatation (Fig. 43).

The esophageal hiatus

The esophageal hiatus is a fixed ring encircled by the phrenoesophageal membrane. It may be visualized, although rarely, during radiologic examination as an ovoid translucency, partic-

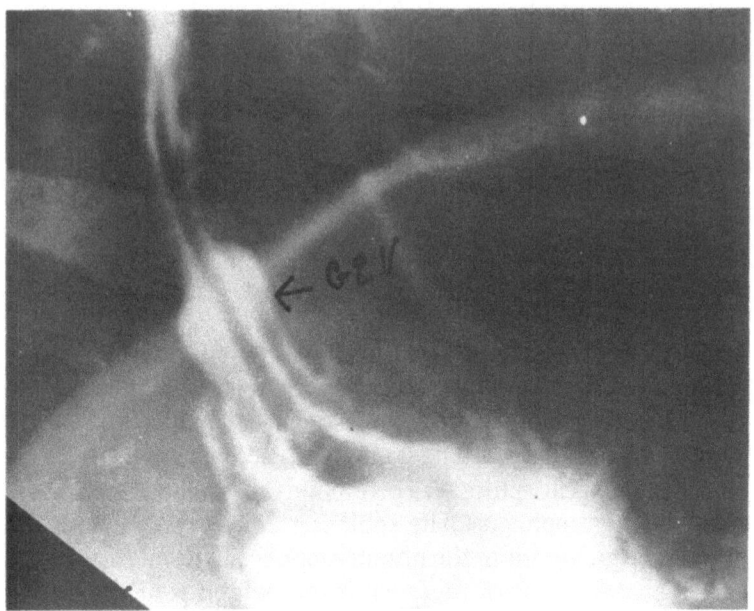

FIGURE 43

lower sphincter. G.E.V. at arrow (gastroesophageal vestibule) emptying into stomach.

ularly with tomography or in the presence of pneumoperitoneum (Fig. 44). The location of the esophageal hiatus varies with the respiratory phase and position of the patient. Thus the hiatus is not always located at the point where the esophagus crosses the dome of the diaphragm. Actually, in most instances, the hiatus is inferior to this site. The thickened lip of the esophageal hiatus may produce a tumorlike indentation of the fundal side of the cardiac incisura (Fig. 45).

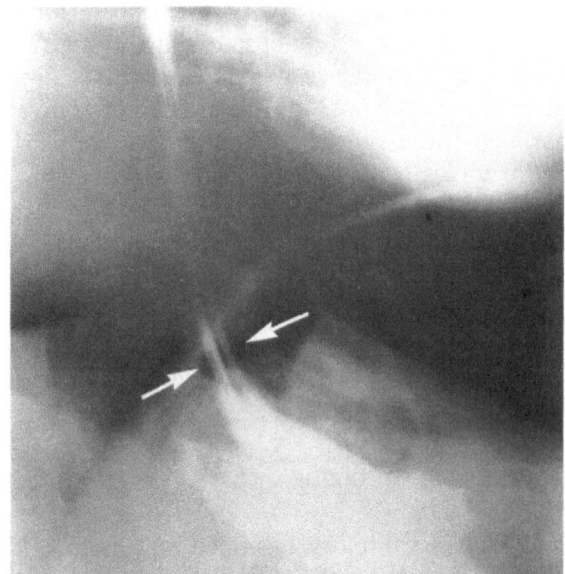

FIGURE 44

Esophageal hiatus (at arrow), prone, RAO, in presence of pneumoperitoneum.

FIGURE 45
Diaphragmatic impression at level of cardiac incisura (at arrow).

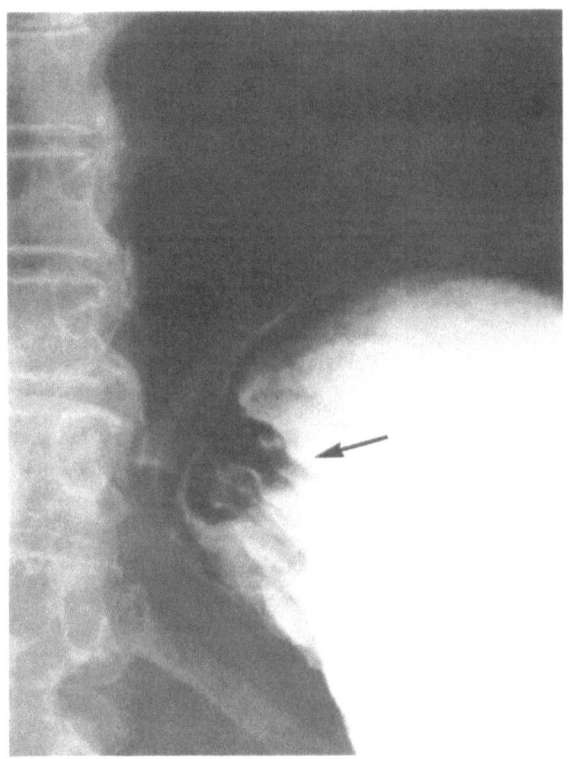

The gastroesophageal junction

The gastroesophageal junction corresponds to the site of the lower attachments of the phrenoesophageal membrane and to Lerche's constrictor cardia. This point is also referred to as the "epithelial line." It may be observed radiologically as a ring, star, or spherical area through the air-filled cardia of the stomach especially in the prone right anterior oblique position (Fig. 46). Various stages of contraction often are noted (269). The radiologic junction is accompanied by the "sign of the burnous" a cloaklike mucosal pattern caused by contraction of the underlying oblique fibers of the stomach (Fig. 47).

The gastric cardia and incisura

The cardia is that part of the stomach directly inferior to the gastroesophageal junction. The fundus corresponds to the lateral and apical region of the stomach, usually separated by the cardiac incisura. A cardiac shelf that pools barium may be present. This shelf may be mistaken for part of the esophagus, especially when the stomach is unfolded. A high cardia also can produce a medial pouch that has been mistaken for a hiatal hernia.

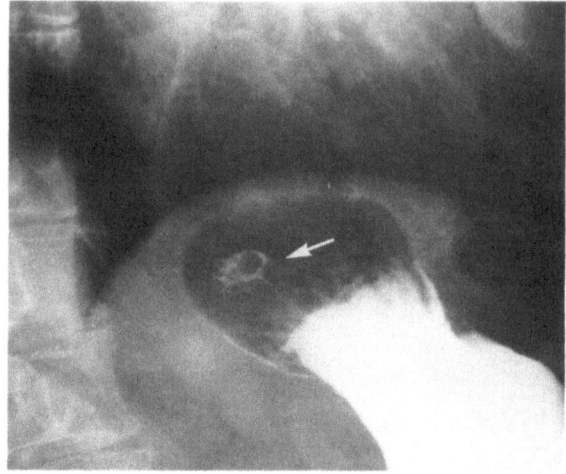

(A)

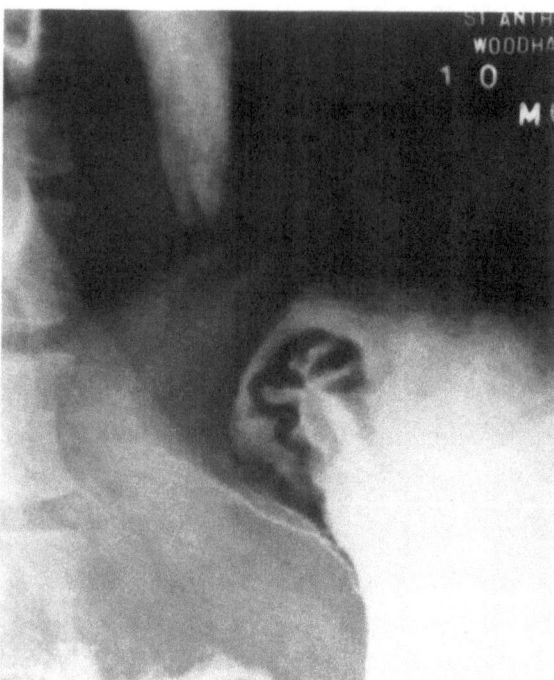

FIGURE 46
Gastroesophageal junction. (A) Ring-like shadow
(at arrow); (B) star-like shadow.   **(B)**

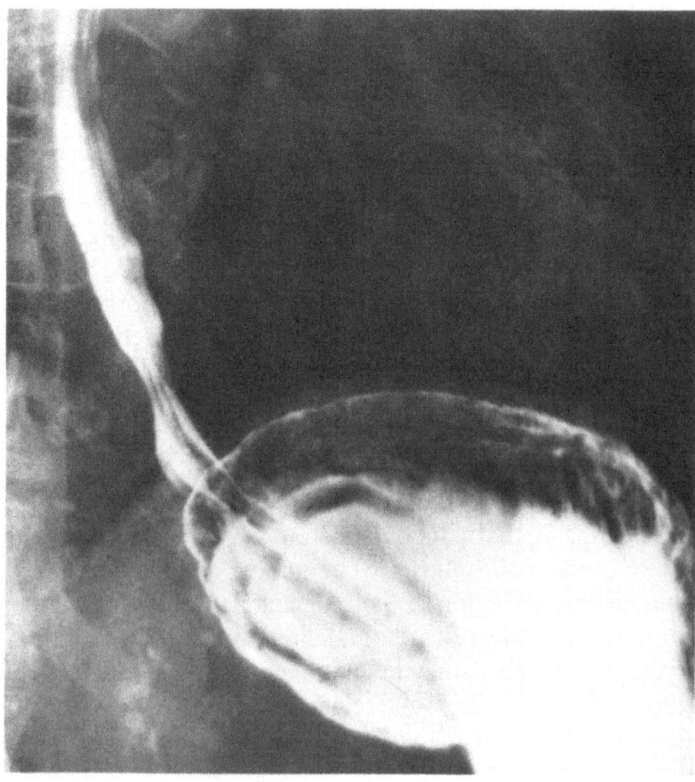

FIGURE 47
Sign of the burnous. Cloak like
folds surrounding the
gastroesophageal junction. From
Zaino, C., et al. *The Lower
Esophageal Vestibular Complex,*
1963. Courtesy Charles C
Thomas, Publisher, Springfield,
Illinois.

FIGURE 48

Cardiac incisura (at arrow). From Zaino, C., et al. *The Lower Esophageal Vestibular Complex,* 1963. Courtesy Charles C Thomas, Publisher, Springfield, Illinois.

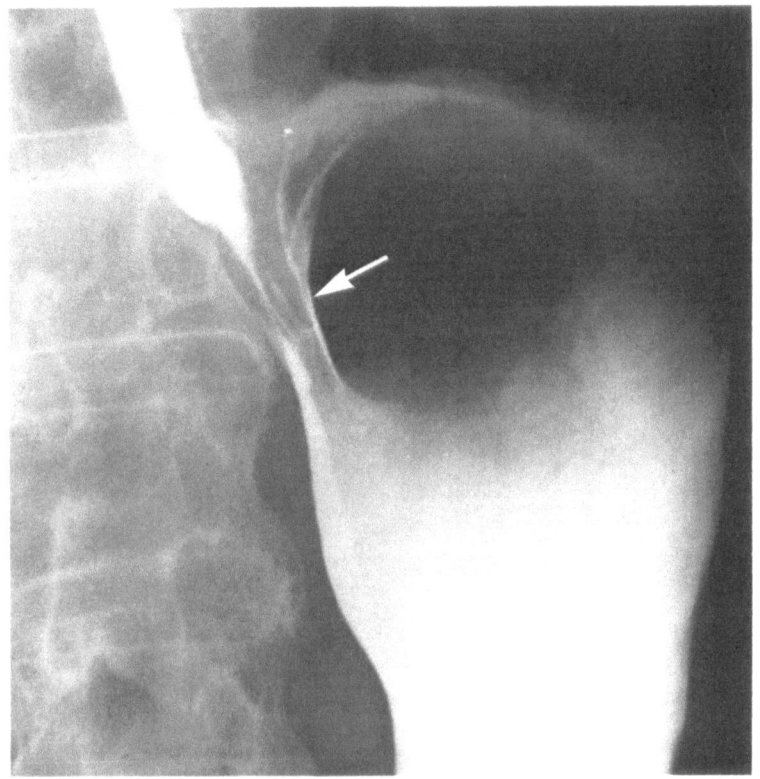

The cardiac incisura is the angle produced by the fundus of the stomach and abdominal esophagus. It differs with the habitus of a patient from an almost vertical to a horizontal position. In the oblique views the cardiac incisura may present as a notch or groove separating the barium-filled cardia and fundus (Fig. 48).

Cervical and esophageal stripes

The cervical prevertebral fat stripe represents adipose tissue in the retropharyngeal and retroesophageal spaces (258). On radiologic examination of a plain lateral film of the cervical region, this stripe is observed as a longitudinal translucent line anterior to the cervical vertebrae (Fig. 49). Its importance rests in its altered position secondary to spondylosis deformans, tumors of the cervical vertebrae, hemorrhage, or edema. Inflammatory changes of the prevertebral space may result in the blurring and forward displacement of the stripe. Calcifications posterior to the stripe should not be mistaken for foreign bodies of the orohypopharynx.

Certain important mediastinal lines and stripes which can occasionally be identified on a PA view of the chest are related to the esophagus.

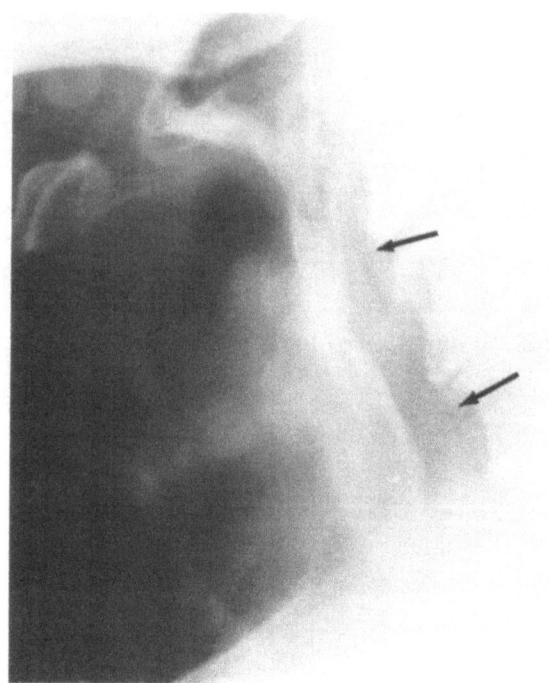

FIGURE 49
Cervical stripe (at arrows).

The posterior mediastinal line is observed in the superior aortic triangle and is formed by the apposition of the pleural surfaces to the esophagus on the right side as projected through the air-filled trachea. The posterior mediastinal line is also referred to as the posterior superior esophageal pleural stripe (87).

The anterior mediastinal line, formed by the combined densities of the visceral and parietal pleura of the right upper lobe, must be differentiated from the posterior mediastinal line. Although this anterior mediastinal line is also projected through the air-filled trachea, it lies more medial and nearer to the midline than the posterior mediastinal line.

The posterior inferior stripe is projected in the retrocardiac space and is produced by the intimate contact of the esophagus with the pleura on the right side. These stripes are observed optimally on tomographic examination rather than on plain chest films. Displacement of some of these stripes may occur in the presence of esophageal disorders.

The orohypopharynx and esophagus as a functional unit

In connection with these anatomicoradiologic observations, the orohypopharynx and esophagus may be described as a physiologic unit (260) as observed during fluoroscopy or during review of motion studies (i.e., tape or film). With the patient in the prone right anterior oblique position the following observations during fluoroscopy upon ingestion of a barium bolus warrant a detailed description.

As the thick barium bolus is held in the oral cavity, it is

noted to lie anteriorly in the central groove of the tongue with the mouth and lips closed. As the patient swallows the barium, it is propelled posteriorly by the sweeping action of the tongue, first initiated by a forward and upward motion of this structure against the hard palate. The soft palate or uvula moves posteriorly to abut against a fold of the posterior wall of the pharynx (the ridge of Passavant), occluding the nasopharynx.

The posterior border of the bolus may appear somewhat irregular in contour as barium fills a small recess posterior to the uvula in the nasopharynx. Opacification of this recess results in a beaklike or pseudo-diverticular appearance—a normal finding. As the bolus glides on the posterior wall or root of the tongue, it flattens this structure and pools in back of the epiglottis filling the valleculae. As the swallowing act progresses the larynx moves upward and anteriorly under the floor of the tongue, away from the path of the approaching bolus. This permits the epiglottis to be folded over posteriorly by the bolus, forming a partial lid to the laryngeal introitus. The bolus slows momentarily at this site because of the narrowed anterioposterior lumen produced by the folded epiglottis.

As the bolus is propelled downward by the contractions of the superior constrictors and passes beyond the level of the epiglottis, this structure returns to its normal position. The bolus then enters the hypopharynx and open sphincter zone. The posterior advancing edge of the bolus passes across a broad indentation of variable length and depth, corresponding to the degree of prominence and contraction of the terminal fibers of the cricopharyngeus muscle (cricopharyngeal impression), just above the sphincter zone. A posterior wall impression in this region may also be produced by spondylosis of the cervical spine.

The anterior edge of the bolus is observed posterior to the cricoid lamina. A number of normal irregularities that may produce a variable irregular anterior border can be identified as postcricoid impressions. Occasionally, at the lower pole of the cricoid lamina, a small inconsistant notch or incisura is noted.

The bolus is then funneled into the open sphincter zone, with the posterior wall of the hypopharynx acting as a chute. The sphincter occasionally opens with a configuration resembling two open arms. This pattern is more often detected during repetitive swallows, when the mucosal lining has been coated with barium. The filled sphincter zone occasionally appears as a dilated ovoid shadow below the pharyngoesophageal junction. This junction is estimated to be at the level of a small anterior notch, directly below the level of the cricopharyngeal impression or at the lower pole of the cricoid lamina.

As soon as the bolus has passed the sphincter zone, the sphincter contracts, producing a narrowed segment several centimeters long and below the level of the lower pole of the cricoid lamina. Above the level of the contracted sphincter, retained barium may simulate the appearance of a diverticulum at the pharyngoesophageal junction. Below the level of this contracted segment, the esophagus remains distended as the transit of the bolus is slowed at the thoracic inlet.

As the bolus enters the supraaortic segment of the thoracic esophagus an oblique ridge occasionally is noted below the thoracic inlet. This ridge is produced by compression by the trachea as the esophagus veers to the left. This is followed by the aortic impression. The bolus hesitates momentarily at the aortic impression, especially if prominent tortuosity of the aorta exists. As the bolus progresses down the esophagus, the typical concave density of the aortic arch is observed, with its attendant aortic pulsations. Directly below the aortic impression a pseudodiverticular pocket occasionally may be noted, especially in the elderly, because of retained barium in the esophageal aortic–bronchial triangle. The next impression is that of the left main bronchus as it crosses obliquely against the esophagus, producing a translucent tubular ridge.

The bolus then reaches the retrocardiac segment of the esophagus, which is characterized by the presence of cardiac pulsations. Here the barium bolus hesitates again, but momentarily, at the lower end of the thoracic esophagus, above the level of the diaphragm. If the patient then inspires deeply, the bolus usually does not enter the stomach but collects in the lower esophagus above the level of the diaphragm, producing a pear-shaped opacity with its apex at the top—the phrenic ampulla. This ampulla collapses suddenly when normal respiration is resumed. An additional dilated pocket occasionally is noted directly below the phrenic ampulla, corresponding to the dilated vestibule or lower sphincter zone. This secondary pocket is normally within the esophageal hiatus or below the diaphragmatic dome and represents the abdominal esophageal segment. After this segment contracts, the bolus has entered the stomach. The contracted lower sphincter is now observed as a narrowed segment several centimeters long, similar in appearance to the contracted upper sphincter. The gastroesophageal junction can then be identified as the most distal end of the contracted segment, resembling a small star or a ring density through the air and barium-coated mucosal pattern of the stomach. This anatomic finding is most apparent after the bolus has descended well beyond the cardia of the stomach.

The oblique fibers surrounding the cardia of the stomach occasionally produce characteristic mucosal folds (sign of the burnoose). The cardiac incisura occasionally is noted through the air- and barium-filled stomach as a small vertical notch. Occasionally, a tumorlike indentation is noted on the fundal side of the cardiac incisura, because of a prominent lip of the anterior border of the right crus of the esophageal hiatus of the diaphragm.

All these observations generally are not apparent during one primary peristaltic wave, following the synchronous contractions of the constrictors of the pharynx. Additional swallows and changes in position may be necessary. As the thick bolus is propelled along, secondary waves appear, permitting complete expulsion of the barium after the bolus has emptied into the stomach. The presence of these secondary waves, producing total expulsion of the barium into the stomach, may be helpful in evaluating the normal functional response of the esophagus and in visualizing the normal mucosal pattern.

CHECKLIST OF OBSERVATIONS DURING AND FOLLOWING A BARIUM SWALLOW

Age, sex, habitus of patient, and relevant history (including previous surgery) should be obtained before the examination is begun.

1. *Oral cavity*
   Shape and contour
   Presence of malocclusion
   Presence of teeth, fixed bridges, or dentures
   Amount of air present
   Size of tongue and presence of central groove
   Size of bolus
   Posterior displacement and elevation of soft palate on swallowing
   Size and thickness of soft palate and uvula
   Forcefulness of swallowing action
   Presence of repetitive swallowing motions
   Rate of swallowing
2. *Oropharynx*
   Approximation of posterior pharyngeal wall (fold of Passavant) and soft palate
   Presence of nasopharyngeal beak of pseudo-diverticulum
   Absence of regurgitation of media into nasal cavity
   Presence of bulges or pockets on posterior wall of tongue or lateral walls of pharynx
   Nature and presence of peristaltic action in posterior wall of the pharynx
   Presence of thickening of retropharyngeal soft tissues
   Demonstration of bilateral filling of valleculae (normal)
   Demonstration of folding over of the epiglottis
   Absence of spillage of barium into larynx or trachea
3. *Hypopharynx*
   Mobility of larynx on swallowing
   Presence of ballooning or widening of hypopharyngeal walls
   Emptying rate of lateral food channels (pyriform fossa)
   Presence of postcricoid impressions, notches, webs, and incisura
   Presence of cricopharyngeal muscle impression
   Presence of abnormal stasis, bulges, or pockets
   Presence of abnormal calcifications

4. *Upper sphincter and cervical esophagus*

Demonstration of elevation and opening of sphincter to receive advancing bolus

Presence of delayed opening and closing of sphincter

Length of sphincter

Presence of abnormal angulation of sphincter zone segment

Presence of pseudo-diverticula at pharyngoesophageal junction

Demonstration of abnormal deviations, angulations, or compressions of the cervical esophagus

Appearance of the cervical spine

5. *Thoracic esophagus*

Presence of thoracic inlet compression or displacement of the esophagus

Demonstration of tracheal esophageal impression

Demonstration of aortic and bronchial impressions

Presence of abnormal deviations, compressions, displacement, torsion, or angulation of esophagus

Appearance of the thoracic spine

Demonstration of calcification of the thoracic aorta and relationship to the esophagus

Nature of peristaltic waves

Presence of abnormal peristaltic waves, contraction, or segmentation

Demonstration of redundancy or foreshortening of esophagus

Degree of distensibility of esophagus

Determination of thickness of the esophageal wall

Presence or absence of a phrenic ampulla

Appearance of mucosal pattern of emptied esophagus

6. *Lower esophageal sphincter*

Appearance of dilated and contracted sphincter

Relationship of sphincter to diaphragm and esophageal hiatus

Effects of full inspiration and expiration

Rate of emptying of sphincter

Appearance and effect of cardiac pulsations

Presence of eventration of diaphragm

Degree of mobility of diaphragm

Presence of periesophageal basal pleural adhesions, effusion, or compression by an enlarged liver or spleen

Presence of funneling, herniations, or invaginations

7. *Cardia*

Demonstration of esophageal hiatal impression

Appearance of gastroesophageal junction

Appearance of cardiac incisura

Appearance of fundal impression secondary to the anterior lip of the esophageal hiatus

Demonstration of the sign of the burnoose

Demonstration of shelving

Presence of abnormal pockets

CHAPTER

3

CONGENITAL ANOMALIES AND DEVELOPMENTAL ABNORMALITIES

NORMAL EMBRYOLOGY The primitive foregut, which is a straight blind tube of entoderm, is in contact at its cephalic end with ectoderm separated from the foregut by the pharyngeal membrane at the floor of the oral fossa or stomodeum. At the beginning of the fifth week of development the pharyngeal membrane ruptures and the foregut becomes continuous with the oral cavity. The oral fossa develops into the oral cavity and becomes lined with ectoderm. The cephalic portion of the foregut develops into the pharynx and esophagus, being of entodermal origin. As development progresses, the branchial grooves and arches appear and eventually form part of the face and neck (7). These arches are barlike prominences, separated by grooves corresponding to the gills slits of fish; they are part of a vestigial transition. The germ layers of the branchial arches develop into the various structures of the oral and hypopharyngeal portion of the upper gastrointestinal tract (3).

The mouth, tongue, and muscles of mastication are formed from elements of the first and second branchial arches. The foramen caecum at the base of the tongue represents the proximal opening of the thyroglossal duct. The distal end of the foramen caecum gives rise to the thyroid gland, lying at the level of the base of the tongue where the primitive stomodeal–pharyngeal musculature was located initially. The pharyngeal structures also arise from the four main and one rudimentary branchial arches (Diagram 4). From the third arch, the mesoderm gives origin to the superior constrictors and the entoderm to the epithelial lining of the roof of the tongue, pharynx, and part of the epiglottis and pyriform sinuses. The inferior con-

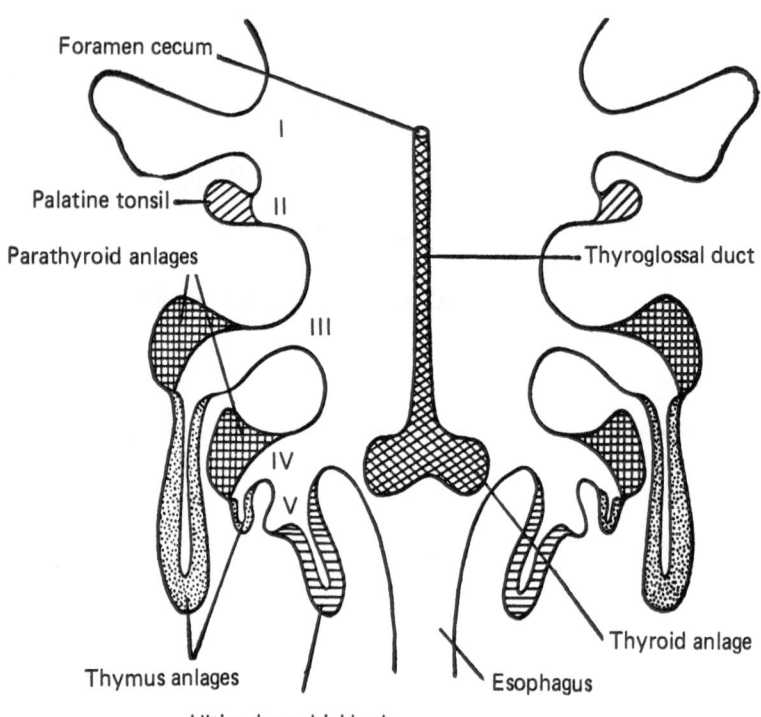

Foramen cecum

I

Palatine tonsil II

Parathyroid anlages

Thyroglossal duct

III

IV

V

Thyroid anlage

Thymus anlages

Esophagus

Ultimobranchial body

DIAGRAM 4.
Embryology–the pharyngeal pouches and their derivatives. From L. B. Arey's *Developmental Anatomy*. Philadelphia, W. B. Saunders Co., 1926.

strictors and aortic arch are formed from the mesoderm of the fourth arch. The entoderm at this level produces the remaining epithelial lining of the hypopharynx. Six vascular arches surround the five branchial pouches. These arches and pouches develop at different times. The carotid artery arises from the third aortic arch. The normal left aortic arch and right subclavian artery develop from the fourth arch, whereas the pulmonary arteries and ductus arteriosus develop from the sixth arch.

The heart originates from a single endothelial tube lying in the folds of the splanchnic mesoderm. This tube subsequently folds on itself, fuses, and rotates to form the normal four-chambered heart, connected by the four valves of the developed heart.

In early fetal life, the trachea and esophagus comprise one structure. The anterior part of the foregut, the laryngotracheal ridge, develops into the larynx, trachea, and lungs. The posterior part of this portion of the foregut develops into the esophagus. Both parts are separated by a complete septum distally. The esophagus anlage becomes filled with proliferating cells, which subsequently fenestrate and produce a central lumen. The original cells are small, ciliated, and columnar in type; they become vacuolated and later are replaced by squamous cells. This process starts in the middle of the esophagus and spreads to both ends. Some of the original cells persist at both ends of the esophagus and develop into superficial (cardiac) glands which secrete serous fluid in the adult. The deep glands of the esophagus develop somewhat later and are located in the submucosa; they are found particularly in the vestibular or lower segment of the esophagus, where they secrete mucus.

Mesodermal tissue condenses around the esophagus, ultimately becoming its smooth muscular coat. This coat fuses with the striated muscle bundles of the branchial mesoderm of the pharynx. A definitive esophagus is observed in the 4 to 5 mm long embryo (Diagram 5), being attached initially to a dorsal mesentery which rapidly thins out as the esophagus elongates and migrates downward (Diagram 6). At an early stage, the distal end of the esophagus enters the stomach in an almost vertical position. With formation of the fundus of the stomach, the esophagogastric junction takes shape. The vertical entrance of the terminal esophagus changes to a gentle curve directed caudad and finally resumes a more acute bend below the esophageal hiatus of the diaphragm.

The diaphragm originates partly from the septum trans-

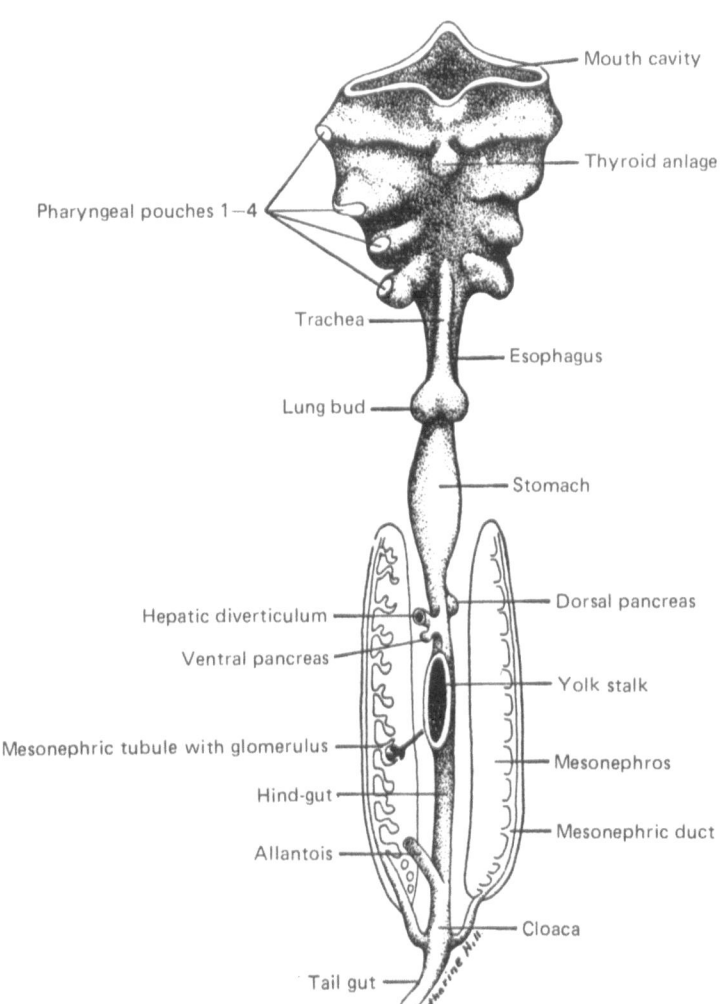

DIAGRAM 5.
Embryology—4 to 5 mm embryo showing esophagus. From L. B. Arey's *Developmental Anatomy*. Philadelphia, W. B. Saunders Co., 1926.

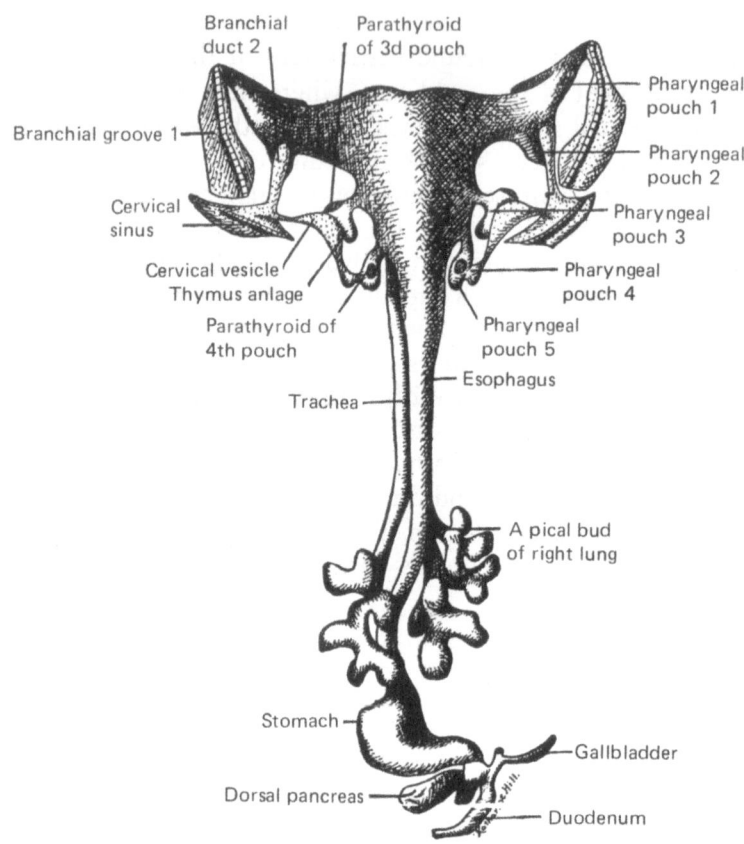

DIAGRAM 6.
Embryology–12 mm embryo showing development of the esophagus. From L. B. Arey's Developmental Anatomy. Philadelphia, W. B. Saunders, Co., 1926.

versum, which precedes the descent of the esophagus and stomach. Eventually the diaphragm encompasses the lower end of the esophagus. Prior to the complete formation of the diaphragm, a cranial extension of the omental bursa is observed, becoming separated by the full development of the diaphragm and then ultimately being obliterated. Occasionally, this bursa, located to the right of the end of the esophagus just above the diaphragm, remains patent, persisting as the pneumoenteric recess or infracardiac bursa. A congenital paraesophageal hernia may be present at birth at this site or a similar hernia may develop in later years.

The phrenoesophageal membrane appears after the normal rotation of the stomach and angulation of the terminal esophagus have occurred. This membrane anchors the terminal or sphincter segment of the esophagus within the esophageal hiatus and seals off the esophageal hiatus.

Analysis of pressure patterns in infants transmitted from the stomach and esophagus indicate that the tone of the lower esophageal sphincter is poor during the first week of life, improving progressively throughout the first year of life. The lower sphincter also appears to be located at a higher level at birth in contrast with later years.

CONGENITAL ANOMALIES OR MALFORMATIONS
Branchial anomalies

Branchial anomalies (3) are congenital aberrations originating from the grooves, ridges, or pouches of the branchial area, resulting in residual cystic tumors and fistulous tracts in the neck. They are characterized microscopically by the presence of Hassall's corpuscules (7).

Cysts

Branchogenic cysts, with or without the presence of fistulous tracts, may communicate with the pharynx, the skin, or both. These cysts are located in the midline or in the lateral aspect of the neck (Fig. 50).

The thyroglossal cyst, with or without a fistulous tract, is usually found in the midline immediately below the hyoid bone. Such cysts communicate with the pharynx when there has been incomplete obliteration of the thyroglossal duct. Injection of the fistulous tract from the skin opening with a water-soluble opaque medium will opacify the extent of the tract and its opening into the pharynx near the foramen caecum. A thyroglossal cyst may be recognized on a plain lateral film of the neck as a midline soft tissue mass at the base of the tongue, compressing the valleculae and displacing the epiglottis posteriorly. Visualization of such a mass may be enhanced by ingestion of barium. A thyroglossal cyst must be differentiated from an ectopic or aberrant thyroid gland, which

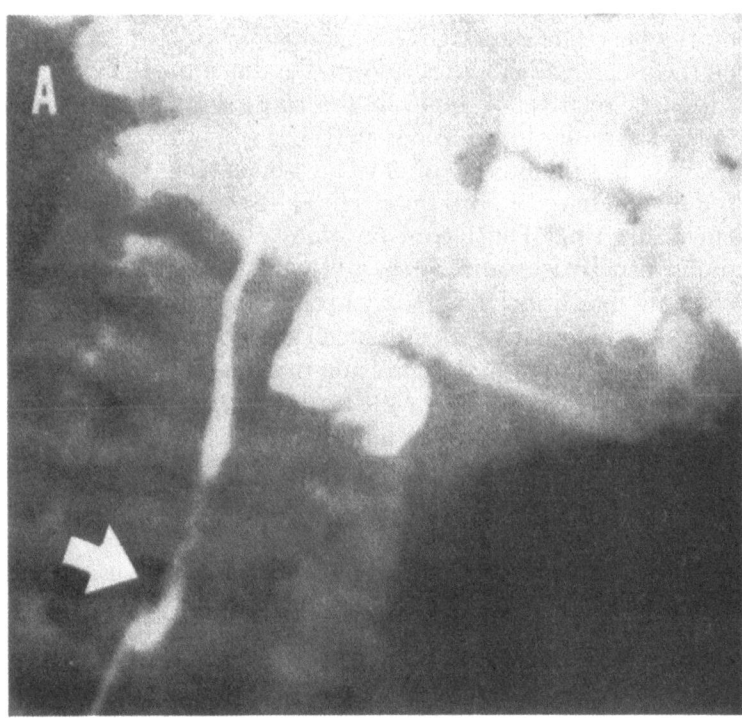

FIGURE 50.
Branchogenic fistula. Opening in side of neck (at arrow). Reprinted from *JAMA, 183;*112, 1963. Copyright 1963, American Medical Association. Albers, G. D., Bronchial Anomalies.

may present a similar radiologic appearance. A radioactive iodine scan will help in establishing the diagnosis. An enlarged lingual tonsil or an aryepiglottic cyst may also be located in this area. Aryepiglottic cysts do not extend into the epiglottis.

Branchial cysts found in the lateral aspect of the neck may also have fistulous openings into the pharynx, which occasionally may be identified following the injection of water-soluble media.

Congenital pharyngeal diverticula

Congenital pharyngeal diverticula are remnants of the third and fourth branchial clefts (Fig. 51). Their roentgenologic appearance may be similar to Zenker's diverticula. The congenital pharyngeal diverticula must also be differentiated from a high esophageal atresia, especially in the newborn. Diverticula of the pyriform fossa usually are the result of a small invagination of the ectoderm of the third arch. Congenital posterior hypopharyngeal diverticula are caused by abnormal ectodermal invagination of the fourth branchial arch. Congenital diverticula of the pharygoesophageal junction are rare, being observed following a barium swallow in the first few months of life (38). The radiologic diagnosis of a pharyngeal diverticulum is relatively simple and is described in the section on acquired diverticula (see Chapter 7).

CARDIOVASCULAR ANOMALIES
Vascular rings

In order to diagnose correctly abnormal vascular compressions on the opacified esophagus, the normal vascular indentations on the esophagus should be known (see Chapter 2). Their delineation is relatively simple in the adult, but in infants the normal vascular indentations are small and often obscured by the enlarged thymus gland. A true vascular ring is detected by the compression of both the trachea and the esophagus by the encircling ring. The lateral position, using a high-kV technique, usually is required to best visualize the trachea. A bronchogram may even be necessary to confirm the presence of tracheal compression. In infants such compression is difficult to demonstrate. A normal impression may be present on the left side of the trachea caused by the aortic arch. On full expiration, this tracheal compression is longer because the trachea is narrowed; in full inspiration the compression is shorter because the trachea widens. Slight buckling of the trachea and esophagus also may occur normally.

In the presence of abnormal compression of the esophagus (and trachea) in infants, the symptoms are usually of respiratory obstruction because of the softness of the tracheal rings. In the adult, the symptoms of compression are chiefly of dys-

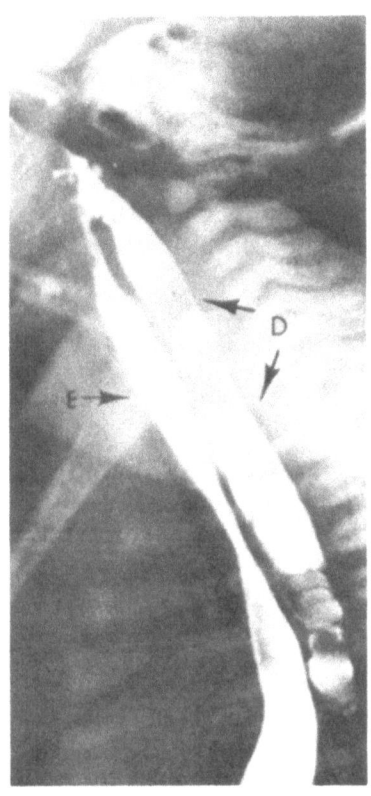

FIGURE 51.
Congenital pharyngeal diverticulum as indicated by arrows (D). From MacKellar, A., and Kennedy, J. C. Congenital diverticulum of the pharynx simulating esophageal atresia. J. Pediatr. Surg. 7:409, 1972. By permission Grune & Stratton, New York.

phagia. Various vascular rings and related malformations result from partial or complete regression of the vascular embryonal arches or associated segments. A large number of malformations exists but only the most important types which produce abnormal compression or displacement of the opacified esophagus are considered here. The radiologic diagnosis depends on evaluating the opacified esophagus at fluoroscopy as well as the films obtained in various projections (130).

Berdon and Baker (18) have described four patterns of vascular compression involving the trachea and esophagus which may be observed on a lateral projection of the opacified esophagus.

1. Compression of the posterior wall of the esophagus and anterior wall of the trachea produces a true ring and is caused chiefly by a double aortic arch.
2. Compression of the anterior wall of the trachea with no compression of the esophagus, caused by an aberrant innominate artery.
3. Posterior esophageal compression without tracheal compression, caused by an aberrant right subclavian artery.
4. Compression of the posterior wall of the trachea and anterior wall of the esophagus, caused by an aberrant left pulmonary artery.

A detailed evaluation is possible upon viewing the opacified esophagus in four main projections (see Diagram 7-A). The chart published in Klinkhamer's monograph *Esophagography in Anomalies of the Aortic Arch System* has been modified in order to summarize graphically the various vascular rings and aberrant vessels compressing the esophagus and/or trachea (Diagram 7).

Double aortic arch

The double aortic arch is the most common of the vascular rings (154). In considering its pathogenesis it must be kept in mind that the ascending aortic arch divides into two arches. The anterior and usually smaller arch passes anterior to the trachea, whereas the posterior arch loops behind the esophagus. These two arches then fuse to form a single descending aorta. A ring is formed consequently which encircles the trachea and esophagus. Although, in addition, a left- or right-sided descending aorta, a left-sided ductus, or an aberrant left subclavian artery may be present, the radiologic appearance usually only indicates the vascular ring as the prominent feature.

In infants, a plain chest film is usually not helpful except in detecting a right-sided descending aorta. Esophagograms yield

A. Normal

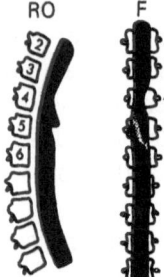 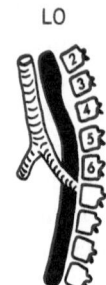 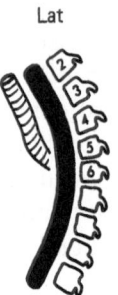

RO = Right oblique
F = Frontal position (AP)
LO = Left oblique
Lat = Lateral position

B. Vascular Rings
   1. Double aortic arch

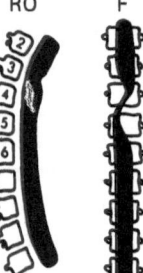 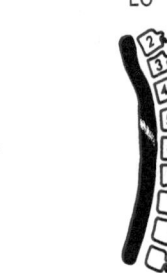 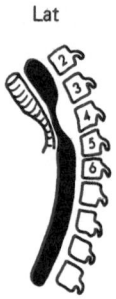

   2. Right sided aortic arch
      a) with right descending aorta and posterior ductus arteriosus

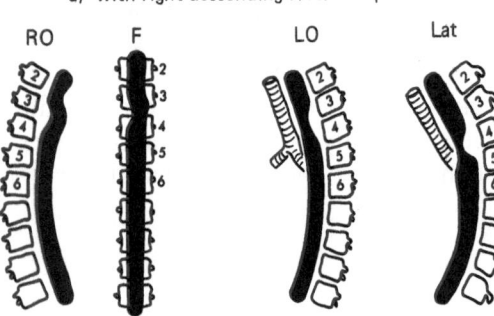

      b) with right descending aorta and left posterior subclavian

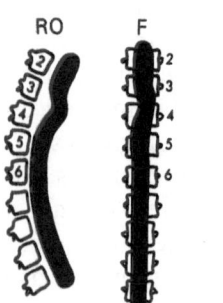 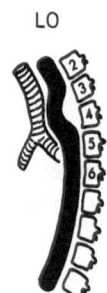 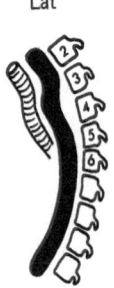

DIAGRAM 7.
Esophagograms in the diagnosis of vascular rings and other vascular abnormalities. From Klinkhamer, A. C. Chart of aberrant arteries in the superior mediastinium, 1969, Courtesy of Agfa-Gavaert, Mortsel, Belgium.

c) with a left descending aorta

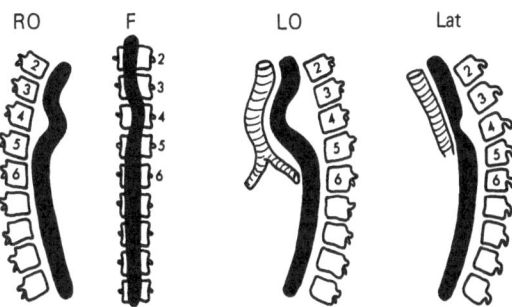

C. Other Vascular abnormalities
  1. Right sided aortic in the presence of a ductus arteriosus (no vascular ring)

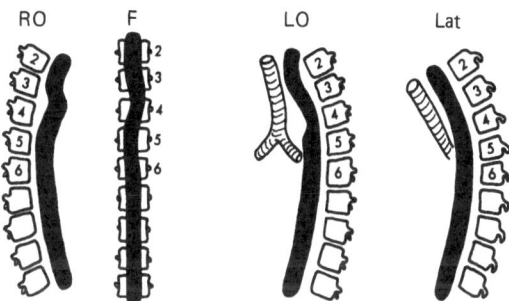

  2. Aberrant right subclavian (Arteria Lusoria)

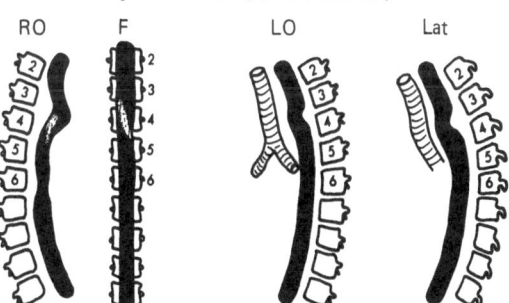

  3. Aberrant left pulmonary artery (Pulmonary Sling)

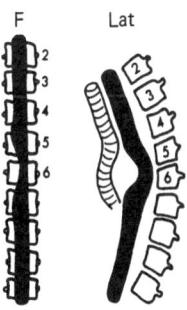

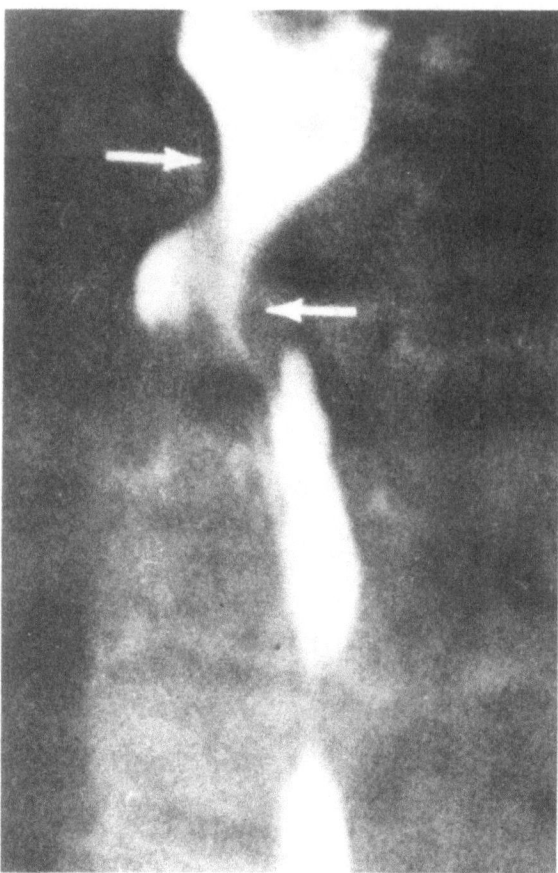

(A)

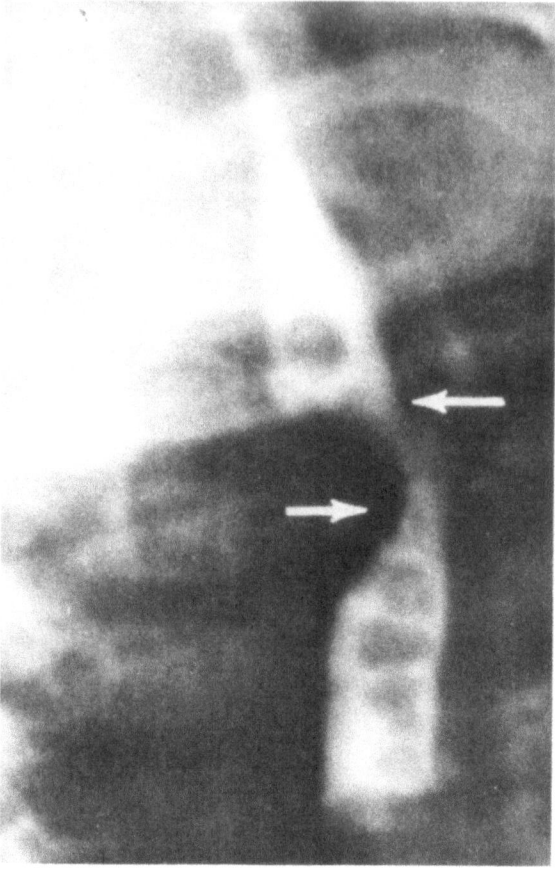

(B)

FIGURE 52.
Vascular rings, double aortic arch. (A) Frontal view, (B) lateral view. Arrows at site of vascular compression. From Stewart, et al. *Atlas of Vascular Rings,* 1964. Courtesy Charles C Thomas, Publisher, Springfield, Illinois.

variable findings, depending on the degree of compression of the trachea and esophagus. When two arches are present, kinking of the esophagus produces a sinuous, contracted esophageal segment. The classic radiologic findings in frontal plain films after ingestion of a barium bolus demonstrate a high esophageal indentation on the right and a somewhat lower left-sided impression (233) (Fig. 52). In addition, in the lateral view, a posterior esophageal compression is noted (Diagram 7-B1). The tracheal impression, when present, is located on the anterior wall at the level of the carina. When both arches are at the same level, a bilateral indentation of the opacified esophagus is produced, also observed in a right-sided aortic arch with an aberrant subclavian artery. In oblique views, a posterior compression of the esophagus is defined, usually poorly demonstrated in infants. Lateral views will best show these indentations of the esophagus and trachea. Difficulty may exist in differentiating a ring from a right subclavian artery. In the latter anomaly, the posterior compression on the esophagus is usually lower than with an aortic ring and no tracheal indentation is identified.

Right-sided aortic arch

A right-sided aortic arch may be associated with congenital heart disease. Other anomalous vessels may coexist that in various combinations can produce a true ring, with compression of the trachea and esophagus.

A right aortic arch and a right-sided descending aorta with an associated ductus originating from the main pulmonary artery, an aortic aneurysm, or directly from the aorta, will produce a true ring by passing behind the esophagus and trachea. On radiologic examination in the frontal view, a shallow right-sided indentation on the opacified esophagus secondary to the right-sided aorta and an additional impression on the left side, caused by the ductus, may be noted. In the right anterior oblique position a posterior esophageal indentation is observed, caused by the aortic arch. In the lateral position, a marked indentation on the posterior wall of the esophagus is noted, secondary both to the aortic arch and the ductus (Fig. 53). The trachea becomes flattened against the anterior wall of the esophagus by the pulmonary artery (Diagram 7-B2a).

A ring is also formed when an aberrant left subclavian artery crosses the esophagus posteriorly from right to left after origin from the aortic arch. The barium esophagogram will show indentations from the right-sided aorta and retroesophageal subclavian artery (Diagram 7-B2b; Fig. 54). These indentations may be sufficiently extensive to resemble a stricture. A right aortic arch with an isolated left subclavian has also been described (221).

Right-sided aortic arch and left-sided descending aorta exist in two forms producing essentially identical radiologic findings (175). In one type, the ductus extends from the left pulmonary artery to the left-sided descending aorta, with the left subclavian and left carotid arteries arising from a common stem. In the second type, the left subclavian artery arises from the aorta. Consequently, a ring is formed around the trachea and esophagus. An impression is produced on the right side of the trachea at the point of its bifurcation. Esophagograms, in the frontal view, demonstrate a right-sided aortic indentation with displacement of the esophagus medially (Diagram 7-B2c). Oblique views will show a marked posterior impression produced by the aortic arch, without deviation of the esophagus, particularly in the presence of compression. In the absence of compression by the ring, the trachea and esophagus may be angled anteriorly at the site of the impression by the aortic arch.

A left aortic arch and a right descending aorta in the presence of an aberrant right subclavian artery and right ductus (a rare anomaly) will also produce a complete vascular ring. Esophagograms demonstrate an almost horizontal vascular impression on the posterior wall of the esophagus at the level of the aortic arch in this anomaly.

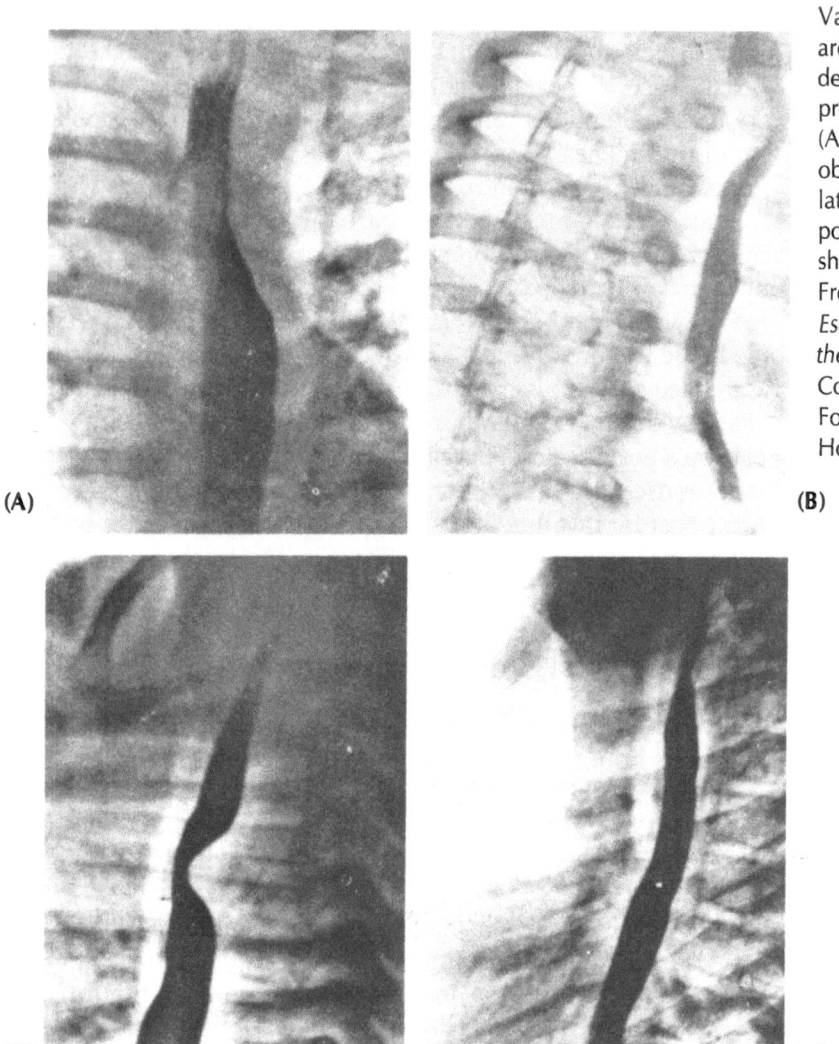

(A)

(B)

(C)

(D)

FIGURE 53.
Vascular ring. Right-sided aortic arch with a right-sided descending aorta in the presence of a posterior ductus. (A) Frontal esophagram, (B) oblique esophagogram, (C) lateral esophagogram, (D) postoperative film in lateral view showing normal esophagus. From Klinkhamer, A. C. *Esophagography in Anomalies of the Aortic Arch System,* 1969. Courtesy Excerpta Medica Foundation, Amsterdam, Holland.

OTHER MISCELLANEOUS VASCULAR ANOMALIES
Right-sided aortic arch

A right aortic arch crosses anteriorly or posteriorly to the esophagus. The anterior aortic arch is located anterior to the trachea and esophagus and is usually associated with congenital heart disease (particularly the tetrology of Fallot) (79). In addition, a situs inversus may be present. On radiologic examination, both the esophagus and the trachea are displaced posteriorly at the level of the arch and are best observed on oblique and lateral views.

The posterior aortic arch is identified generally as an isolated anomaly, although infrequently it may be associated with a patent ductus or coarctation. The arch may have an aortic diverticulum. On roentgenologic examination, a posterior esophageal indentation is observed at the level of the arch in the oblique and lateral views. There is no compression of the trachea unless a ring is also present.

Right-sided aortic arch with a ductus

The right-sided aortic arch in the presence of a ductus arteriosus can show abnormal esophageal compressions even without an actual ring being present. The ductus can arise from the right pulmonary artery crossing the right main bronchus to join the right-sided aorta or the ductus can arise from the left pulmonary artery to join the left subclavian artery. The left subclavian artery originates in both instances anteriorly from the right aortic arch. Esophagograms in the right oblique projection reveal a long, shallow, dorsal impression and the trachea and esophagus are bent slightly forward. However, on the lateral film, there is no posterior esophageal compression (Diagram 7-C1).

Coarctation and pseudo-coarctation of the aorta

Coarctation of the aorta is a congenital malformation characterized by stenosis of the aorta between the left subclavian and a point just distal to the insertion of the ductus or ligamentum arteriosum. There is great variability or narrowing at the site of the stenosis with resultant secondary changes. Anterior retraction of the aorta toward the midline at the site of the stenosis and a poststenotic dilatation of the descending aorta are present. On routine radiologic examination, the diagnosis of coarctation of the aorta is not easily made in infants. Rib notching which develops in late childhood and often not until adulthood is a clue to the diagnosis. If an aberrant right subcla-

(A)   (B)

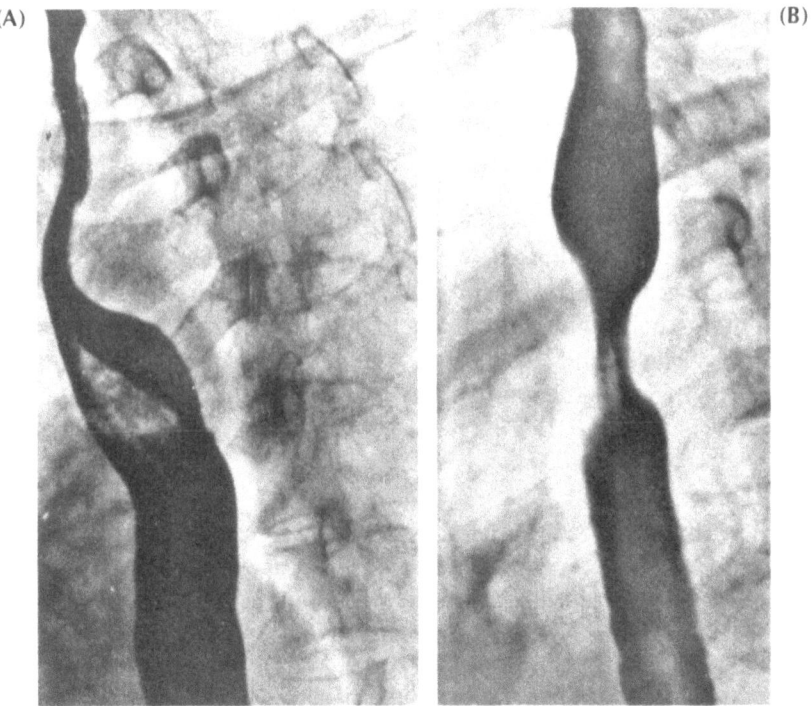

FIGURE 54.
Vascular ring. Right-sided aorta and aberrant left subclavian artery. From Klinkhamer, A. C. *Esophagography in Anomalies of the Aortic Arch System*, 1969. Courtesy Excerpta Medica Foundation, Amsterdam, Holland.

vian artery is also present, rib notching is more extensive and may be observed in younger individuals. On a plain film of the chest, an inverted 3 sign may be identified on the left border of the aortic arch caused by contraction of the aorta at the site of the stenosis and as a result of the poststenotic dilatation. Esophagograms reveal a slight or absent aortic arch indentation. Occasionally the dilated poststenotic aortic segment displaces the esophagus anteriorly and to the right. Marked esophageal indentation by the left main bronchus and multiple fixed indentations on the middle third of the esophagus can occur because of congested collateral vessels compressing the esophagus. Because hypertension is usually present, left ventricular enlargement generally is associated. Coarctation may be present with other cardiac and vascular congenital irregularities. Angiocardiograms will confirm the diagnosis.

Different types of coarctation exist. The most common form consists of a ligamentous coarcted segment and an obliterated ductus. Other varieties include a patent ductus or a hypoplastic descending aorta below the level of coaractation. Clinically, the discrepancy between the elevated blood pressure of the upper and the reduced blood pressure in the lower extremities is most useful diagnostically.

Pseudo-coarctation of the aorta (231) is associated often with congenital heart disease. The radiologic appearance in this disorder is secondary to kinking or buckling of the aortic arch at the level where true coarctation is expected. Notching of the ribs and aortic dilatation are absent. Esophagograms demonstrate the "reverse 3" sign reminiscent of a true coarctation, along the left border of the esophagus in the posterior–anterior and left anterior oblique views (Fig. 55). Slight enlargement of the left ventricle is often present.

Coronary sinus enlargement in infants is an anomaly secondary to a persistant left superior vena cava or anomalous pulmonary venous return. A dilated coronary sinus produces an esophageal impression on the anterior wall of the barium-filled esophagus at the level of T-7 and T-8, best observed in the lateral view as well as the right anterior oblique projection. The esophageal impression must be distinguished from left atrial enlargement, which produces a larger impression, more proximally placed and less discrete than an enlarged coronary sinus (78). Angiographic confirmation is essential.

ABERRANT VESSELS

The aberrant right subclavian artery is referred to as the "arteria lusoria," producing dysphagia lusoria. The aberrant right subclavian artery arises as the last major vessel of the aorta sweeping upward to the right just posterior to the esophagus and trachea (195). Atresia of the esophagus may be an associated anomaly (27). Esophagograms show a typical abnormal

FIGURE 55.
Pseudo-coarctation of the aorta.
(A) Arrow at site of
pseudo-coarctation of the aorta:
oblique view of chest. (B)
Esophagogram showing the
reverse "3" sign in some
patients.

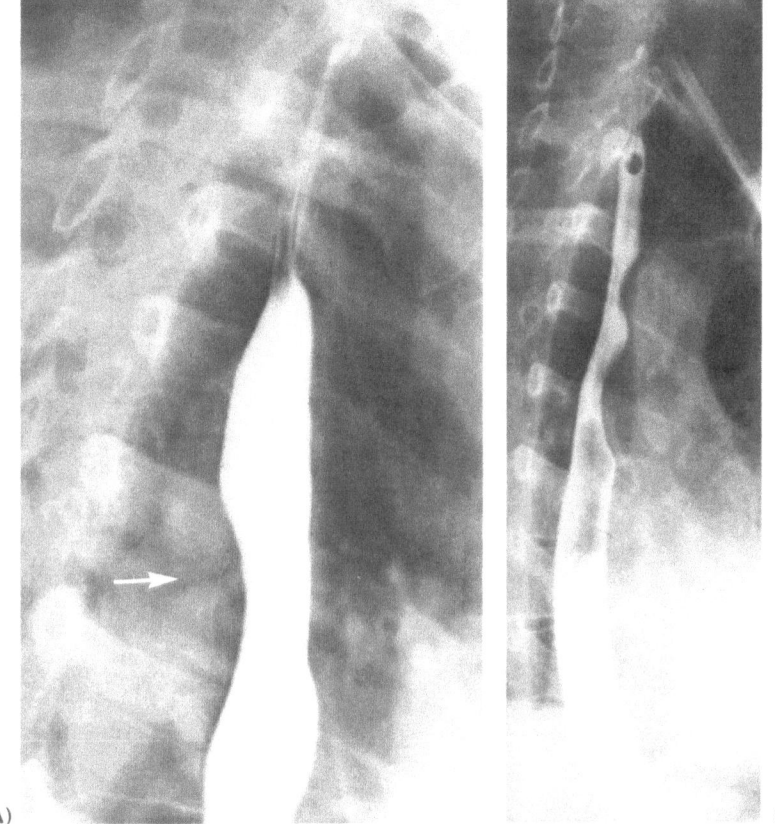

(A)   (B)

impression (Diagram 7-C2; Fig. 56). In the frontal esophagogram, the vascular indentation on the esophagus runs from its
left inferior border to its right upper border. In the right anterio-
oblique view a spiral impression of the esophagus is noted,
which must be differentiated from the left main bronchus. In
the left anterior oblique and lateral views, when the anomalous
vessel is located between the trachea and esophagus, the esophageal impression is located anteriorly. If a bicarotid type of
truncus is also present, anterior flattening of the trachea is observed. In the elderly, because of the wide aortic arch, it may be
difficult to make the diagnosis.

Congenital subclavian steal syndrome with a right aortic
arch (250) is a rare entity. The right aortic arch in this syndrome usually is associated with a decreased pulse pressure on
the left side. Three types of abnormal vascular arrangements
exist: (1) The left subclavian artery is isolated from the aortic
arch steming from the pulmonary artery by way of the ductus
arterious; (2) a mirror image of the first type exists, with the
left common and subclavian arteries being atretic; (3) an aberrant left subclavian artery originates from a retroesophageal
aortic diverticulum, producing a loose vascular ring.

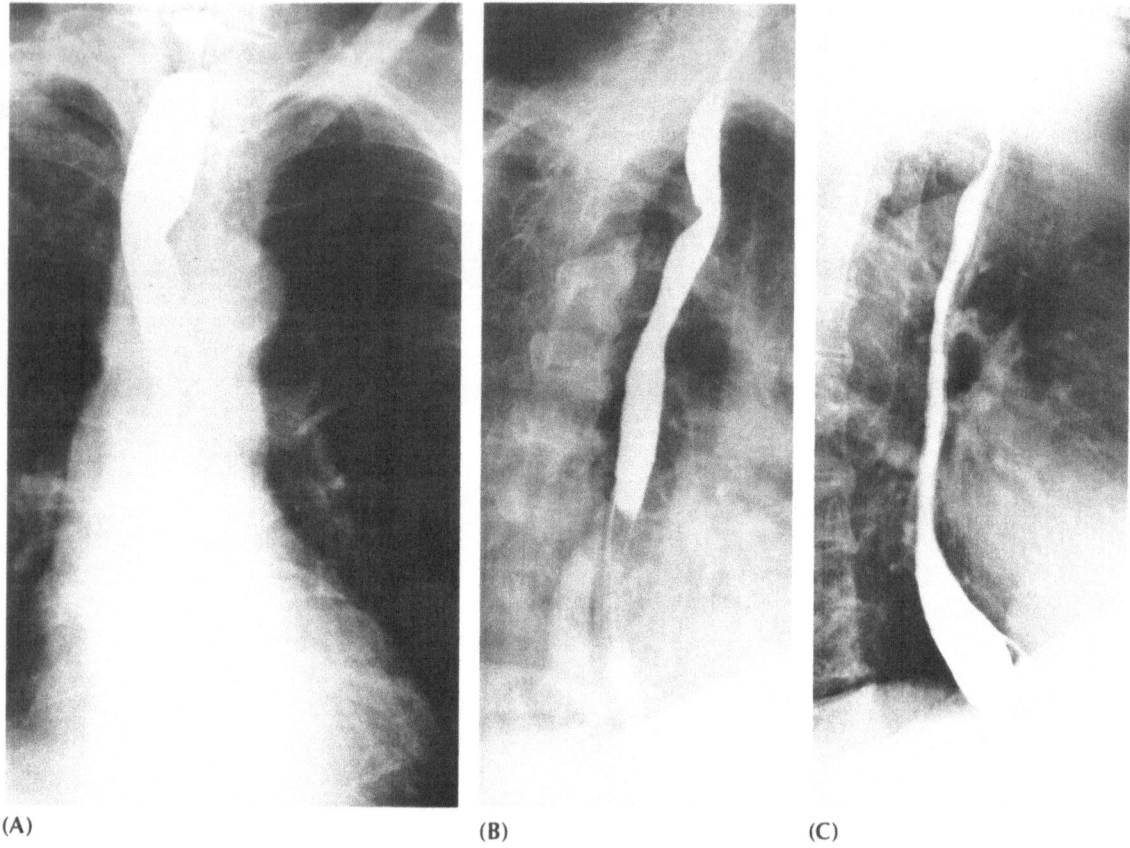

(A) (B) (C)

All three types show a right-sided aortic compression on the barium-filled esophagus. However, in the first two types, the lateral view shows no retroesophageal indentation or notch. In the third type the aortic diverticulum produces a wide concave impression on the posterior surface of the barium-filled esophagus, suggesting the presence of a ring. This feature, in addition to the diminished pulsations in the left arm caused by the stenosis of the left subclavian artery, is diagnostic. The presence of a right-sided aorta, absent retroesophageal compression of the esophagus, and diminished pulsation in the left arm and the carotid artery indicate a type 1 or type 3 defect. The diagnosis, however, is substantiated by selective aortography.

Aberrant left pulmonary artery (pulmonary sling) arises from the right pulmonary artery and passes between the trachea and esophagus from right to left. This anomaly may produce respiratory symptoms, depending on the degree of compression of the trachea. An anterior wall compression at the level of the tracheal bifurcation is visualized on the frontal and lateral views of the barium-filled esophagus. An impression in the posterior surface and right side of the trachea at the level of the carina is identified. In addition, an oval shaped density may be interposed between the trachea and esophagus at this level,

FIGURE 56.

Aberrant right subclavian artery (arteria lusoria). (A) Frontal esophagogram, (B) RAO esophagogram, (C) lateral esophagogram showing shallow vascular compression at upper end of the esophagus.

resembling a mediastinal bronchogenic cyst (Diagram 7-C3). The diagnosis is made definitively after an angiogram. This entity is referred to as a pulmonary sling because of the accompanying compression of the trachea and main bronchi. This developmental abnormality may also be associated with other congenital anomalies.

An aberrant innominate artery or a common trunk for the innominate and left carotid artery produces an anterior compression on the trachea above the level of the carina, with a normal esophagogram. This abnormality may be responsible for stridor and respiratory symptoms, especially in infants.

CONGENITAL HEART DISEASE

An enlarged and distorted cardiac silhouette on radiologic examination of the chest in infants and children usually indicates congenital heart disease, particularly when associated with cyanosis. The delineation of the type of abnormality is aided by a barium swallow. The esophagogram may demonstrate accompanying vascular abnormalities and/or enlargement of the cardiac chambers. The radiologic appearances of individual chamber enlargements as they compress the opacified esophagus are presented in Chapter 4. The size and shape of the heart itself is, of course, most helpful in establishing a diagnosis.

In the presence of a right aortic arch, a congenital cardiac disorder should be suspected even when the cardiac silhouette appears normal. Opacification of the esophagus will determine whether the aortic arch is anterior or posterior to the esophagus. If the arch is anterior to the esophagus, cyanotic heart disease, such as truncus arteriosus or tetralogy of Fallot, is usually present and often associated. With a posterior aortic arch, cyanotic heart disease generally is absent. Any associated anomalies involve chiefly the great vessels, such as patent ductus or coarctation of the aorta. Many relatively simple or multiple combinations of congenital abnormalities of the heart caused by abnormal embryologic development may exist with or without abnormalities of the great vessels. The limited scope of this book in this area does not permit a detailed diagnostic description of such cardiac lesions, even though compression of the opacified esophagus may be present. Angiographic studies are usually definitive in establishing the type of cardiac anomaly (64).

A simple classification of congenital heart disease is based on the presence or absence of cyanosis. In the absence of cyanosis, commonly encountered lesions include patent ductus arteriosus, patent interventricular or interauricular septum, subaortic and valvular stenosis, and isolated pulmonary artery stenosis. The more common abnormalities associated with cyanosis include tetrology of Fallot, truncus arteriosus, Eisenmenger complex, tricuspid stenosis and atresia, transposition of great vessels, and Ebstein's malformation of the tricuspid valve.

A few of more commonly encountered congenital cardiac abnormalities are reviewed briefly with special reference to their impact on the barium-filled esophagus.

The tetrology of Fallot is the most common congenital cyanotic heart abnormality. Although a number of subtypes exist, the syndrome is characterized by a primarily high, large ventricular septal defect, and varying degrees of stenosis of the pulmonary artery infundibulum and/or pulmonary valve. Each type combination of the various abnormalities usually produces a more or less identifiable radiologic pattern. The commoner subtypes include tetrology with a third ventricle secondary to stenosis of the mouth of the infundibulum, tetrology with infundibular and valvular stenosis, and tetrology with an overriding aorta with or without a right-sided aortic arch.

The classic form of Fallot's tetrad is characterized by a "wooden shoe" appearance of the cardiac silhouette on a plain film of the chest. This configuration is produced by the concave upper left border of the heart resulting from the absence of normal pulmonary vessels and an elevated and rounded cardiac apex secondary to right ventricular hypertrophy and infundi-

FIGURE 57.
Dextrocardia. (A) Chest film. (B) esophagogram, frontal view. Courtesy of S. Glasser and P. L. Clemetson of Sunnyvale, Calif.

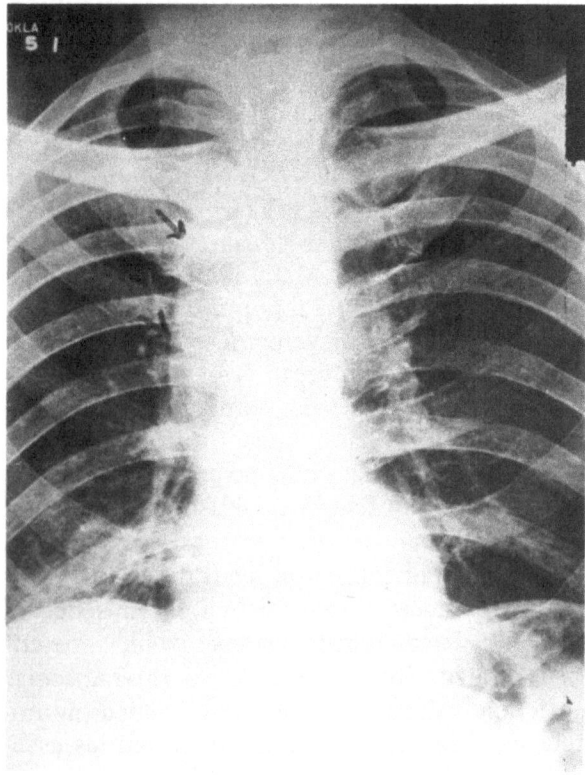

(A)

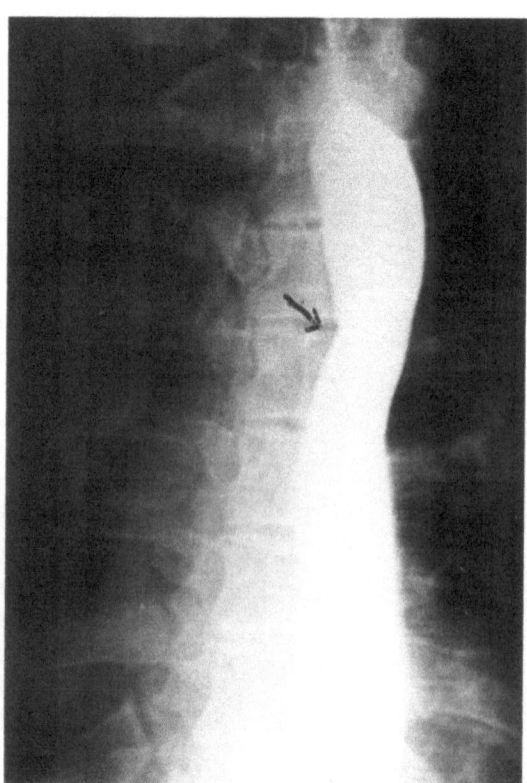

(B)

bular stenosis. The heart generally is not grossly enlarged. The pulmonary arterial vasculature is usually diminished in size.

Approximately 25% of cases are associated with a right-sided aortic arch. Right ventricular enlargement can be seen as the disease becomes more chronic. The esophagogram is of value in demonstrating the arch indentations as well as the location of specific heart chamber enlargement. The typical right ventricular enlargement and the diminished size of the pulmonary vasculature is diagnostic.

Truncus arteriosus is anatomically different but usually demonstrates the same radiologic findings as in tetrology of Fallot. Instead of pulmonary stenosis, as in Fallot's tetrad, atresia of the pulmonary valves is present. A right aortic arch may be present. The arterial circulation to the lungs occurs through the bronchial arteries, which dilate and may produce esophageal compression. In the frontal view, these vessels are noted to be distal to the tracheal bifurcation, thus eliminating the possibility of a posterior indentation secondary to an aberrant subclavian artery.

Patent ductus arteriosus often is an isolated congenital defect but may be associated with other cardiac acyanotic congenital disorders. On radiologic examination, the findings vary with age and the size of the shunt. Enlargement of the pulmonary arteries and pulmonary conus, arterial overcirculation, right ventricular, and eventually left ventricular enlargement are characteristic. The esophagogram is helpful in evaluating individual chamber enlargements (see Chapter 4).

ABNORMALITIES OF POSITION

In dextrocardia, the heart and great vessels are reversed in position as in a mirror image of the normal. This abnormality may be associated with visceral situs inversus or may be an isolated finding. The normal esophageal impressions are reversed on the esophagogram (Fig. 57).

Dextro position of the aortic arch may be present without any other abnormality. The esophagogram will show a right aortic and a left bronchial impression. The position of all other structures is unaltered (Fig. 58).

A cervical aortic arch is rare. In this condition, the arch is located at a higher level in the cervical region and usually is associated with a right-sided aorta. Esophagograms demonstrate the absence of the normal aortic impression in its usual location. Fluoroscopic examination shows a pulsating mass in the apices of the lungs and in the cervical region where a right-sided esophageal impression caused by the right aortic arch is to be noted. A high vascular ring may be present because of a patent ductus arteriosus. Angiocardiography is necessary to confirm the diagnosis and to differentiate a cervical aortic arch from an abnormally elongated aortic arch.

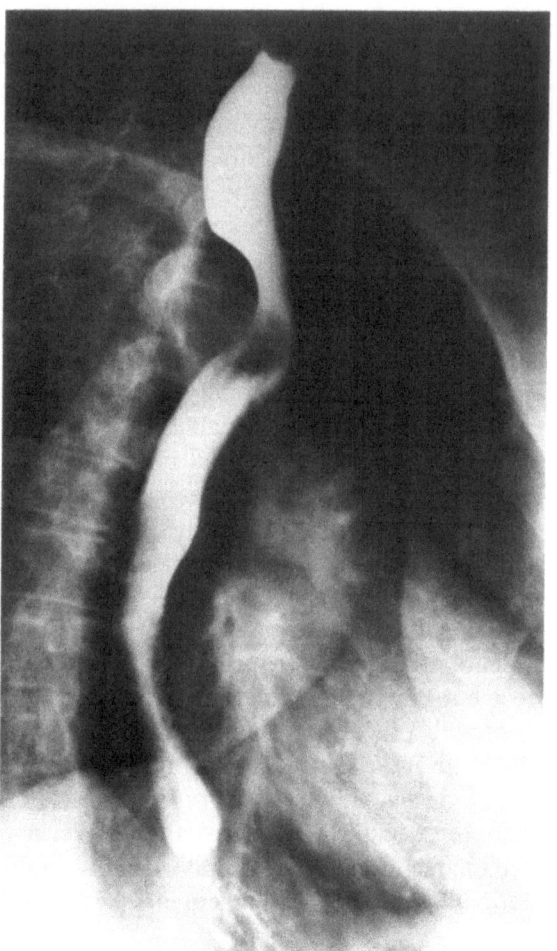

FIGURE 58.
Right-sided aortic arch. See posterior aortic esophageal compression.

ORAL AND PHARYNGEAL
DYSPHAGIA IN
INFANCY

Suckling is one of the most important reflexes of the infant. It facilitates swallowing which, in turn, inhibits respiration, momentarily permitting normal passage of food from the oral cavity to the esophagus, the mechanism for which is controlled cerebrally. Fluoroscopic observations of the suckling and swallowing mechanisms in infants is valuable in detecting abnormalities (149). Normally, the bolus being sucked from a bottle collects anteriorly between the tongue and hard palate, with the soft palate and dorsum of the tongue isolating the bolus until swallowing begins. Swallowing is carried out at regular, short intervals, with the sweeping action of the tongue pushing the bolus against the soft palate. The soft palate is elevated and moved backward, sealing off the nasopharynx. The larynx is simultaneously pulled anteriorly and upward away from the oncoming bolus, which then enters the esophagus. Respiration takes place between suckling while swallowing ceases temporarily. Abnormal suckling and swallowing patterns result in nasal regurgitation, tracheal spillage, and motor disturbances of the hypopharyngeal sphincter and upper end of the esophagus.

Abnormal suckling and swallowing disorders are serious problems and should be differentiated according to their oral, pharyngeal, or esophageal origins. These distinctions are made chiefly on clinical grounds. The dysphagia of suckling results from malformations or dysfunction of the tongue, palate, or pharynx, principally caused by disorders of the facial and oral skeletal muscles or cerebral lesions. Oral defects are usually recognized at birth. These include harelip, cleft palate, an excessively small or large tongue, neoplasms, or fistulae. Pharyngeal disorders can be demonstrated with a barium swallow. In sucking difficulties, barium may be instilled orally through a nasal catheter to determine the site and nature of specific abnormalities.

The Pierre–Robins syndrome is a rare oral malformation of unknown cause, characterized by congenital micrognathia, macroglossia, glossoptosis, and a palatine fissure. This disorder produces an acute oral dysphagia, dyspnea, and cyanosis which worsens when the patient is supine or when feeding is attempted. The cyanosis is secondary to the tongue blocking the airway as it prolapses through the fissured hard palate. The condition gradually improves with proper treatment. The child is kept prone with the tongue fixed to the lower lip while feeding is accomplished by a nasal catheter (67). Radiologic examination is helpful in excluding the presence of other anomalies.

Neurogenic and muscular abnormalities affecting the oro-hypopharynx and esophagus are discussed in Chapter 6. A number of other congenital syndromes affect this area. Because these disorders are rare and no radiologic observations related to these rare entities have been recorded, either in the literature or personally, they are not discussed here.

ATRESIA AND AGENESIS OF THE ESOPHAGUS

Incomplete canalization or defective unfolding of the walls of the foregut results in atresia of the esophagus. Incomplete separation of the tracheal bud from the esophagus produces fistulous tracts between the trachea and esophagus. Incomplete canalization or defective unfolding of the foregut and incomplete separation of the tracheal bud produce atresia and fistulous tracts. Rarely, complete absence of the middle of the esophagus or of the entire esophagus (agenesis) may be encountered.

Classification (see Diagram 8)

A. Complete absence of the mid-esophagus without any connective tissue between the two blind ends (agenesis) and no fistulae

A. Agenesis of mid esophagus

B. Atresia of mid esophagus

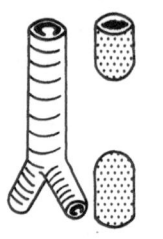
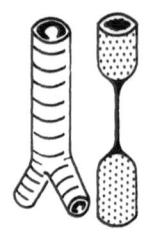

DIAGRAM 8.
Agenesis atresia and fistulae of the esophagus. Compiled from previous drawings by numerous authors.

C. Atresia of the esophagus in the presence of fistulae

Type 1 Type 2 Type 3

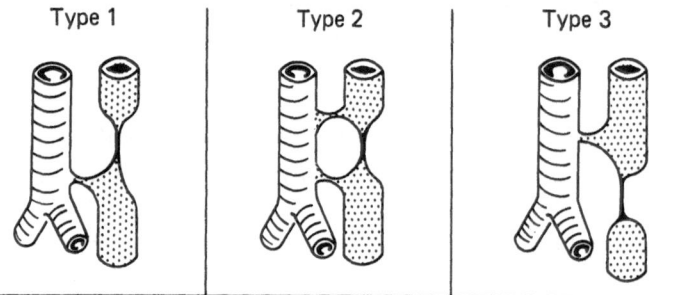

D. Fistula without atresia (H-type)

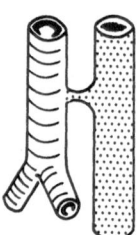

B. Absence of the mid-esophagus in the presence of a fibrous connection between the two blind ends (atresia) and no fistulae

C. Esophageal atresia in the presence of a fistulous tract (three types):
   1. Atresia of the mid-esophagus with lower end connected to the trachea or main bronchus (most frequent)
   2. Atresia of the mid-esophagus with both ends connected to the trachea
   3. Atresia of the mid-esophagus with upper end connected to the trachea

D. Fistulous connection between the esophagus and trachea without atresia (H-type tracheoesophageal fistula)

Agenesis

Congenital absence of the entire esophagus and absence of the mid-esophagus are rare. Associated atresia in the absence of fistulous tracts is also rare (248). These two types cannot be dif-

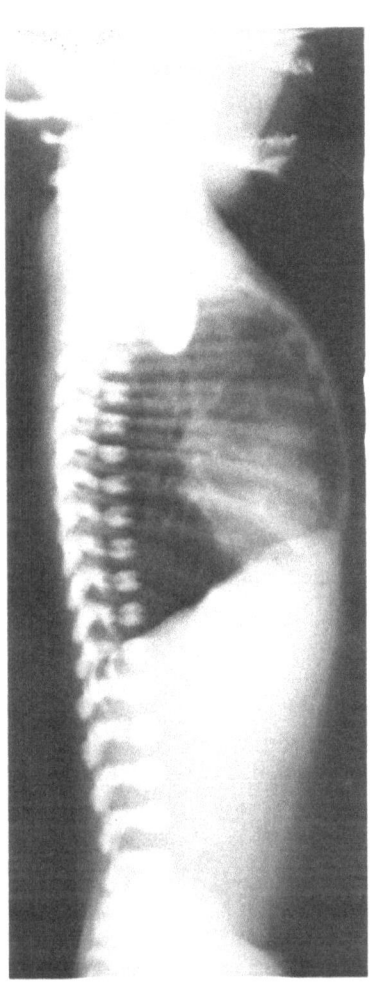

FIGURE 59.

Agenesis of mid-esophagus. Opaque media in blind esophageal pocket; no air in the digestive tract. Courtesy of G. S. Marchese and E. Grassi, Regina Margerita Hospital, Torino, Italy.

ferentiated radiologically. At birth, infants commonly aspirate during swallowing. A plain film of the abdomen generally reveals no air in the digestive tract in the newborn. When an 8–10 French catheter is passed through the nose with fluoroscopic guidance, the tip of the catheter coils in the closed end of the upper esophagus or hypopharynx. Injection of a small amount of contrast medium opacifies the cul-de-sac of the atretic esophagus, which may extend to the middle third of the mediastinum (Fig. 59). This examination is best performed with the infant prone in the right anterior oblique position, which best excludes an associated fistulous tract. The contrast medium should be injected in small quantities to avoid overdistension with overflow into the larynx and bronchial tree, which may be confused with a fistula. Many laterally situated inconstant furrows at the distal blind end of the upper portion of the esophagus are observed caused by peristaltic waves, which may cause overflow of the contrast medium into the trachea with spillage into the lung. The blind pouch must be differentiated from a congenital diverticulum of the orohypopharynx. The diagnosis of congenital diverticulum presents no problem because contrast eventually trickles into the esophagus outlining it in the entire length. A film of the abdomen will also show air in the stomach and intestines in an infant with a congenital diverticulum.

Atresia

Atresia of the esophagus is associated with tracheoesophageal fistula in approximately 90% of cases and is frequently accompanied by other anomalies, resulting in a high morbidity or mortality (139). At birth, affected infants are unable to swallow without choking. A plain film of the abdomen will usually show a gas-filled stomach.

The most common form of fistula and atresia is type C-1 (see Diagram 8) in which an upper blind esophageal pouch exists and the trachea or left main bronchus communicates through a fistulous tract with the distal patent esophageal segment. Free passage of air into the stomach and bowel is therefore possible. Following a barium swallow the upper esophageal pouch is visualized and a fistulous tract outlined by air is observed, leading to the lower esophagus. Air often outlines the stomach (Fig. 60). The upper blind esophageal stump is often dilated with air and fluid, resulting in a fluid level in the upright position. Anterior displacement and narrowing of the trachea caused by pressure from this dilated stump frequently are observed. As an 8–10 French catheter is passed through the nose into the esophagus, it stops or coils within the upper blind pouch. As contrast is injected in small amounts, the presence or absence of a fistulous tract between this pouch and the trachea should be ascertained.

In type C-2 defect (see Diagram 8), fistulous tracts are

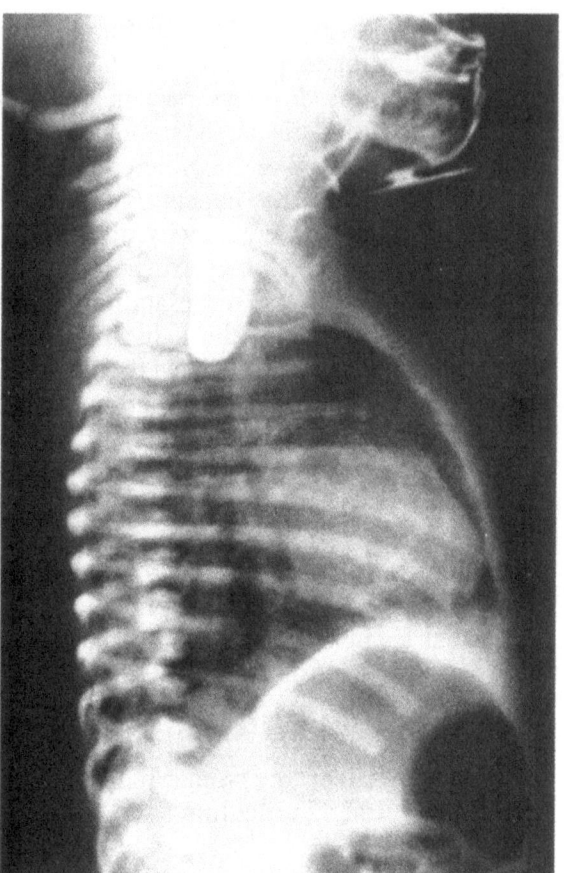

FIGURE 60.
Atresia of the esophagus in the presence of a fistula. Blind upper esophageal pocket with air-filled fistulous tract leading to stomach, which is dilated. Courtesy of John Caffey, M.D.

present above and below the area of atresia. The upper fistula is usually located in the midline of the posterior surface of the trachea, well above the level of the carina. When high in position, the fistula may be difficult to detect because of aspiration of the contrast medium into the trachea, secondary to regurgitation and peristaltic action of the stump. However, small amounts of the contrast may be observed passing into the stomach via the lower fistulous tract. Occasionally a catheter can be threaded through both fistulous openings and directed into the stomach.

In the rare, type C-3 fistula (see Diagram 8), only a tract at the base of the upper esophageal stump exists. Pulmonary damage generally is present at birth, in contrast to the other types in which the lungs usually are normal.

H-type tracheoesophageal fistula

An H-type tracheoesophageal fistula without atresia (159, 243) can also be suspected when unexplained pulmonary disease, including frequent attacks of pneumonia and atelectasis, occurs in infants who "choke" during feeding (Fig. 61). This type D (see Diagram 8) occasionally may be an isolated congenital abnormality.

Embryologically the H-type fistula is probably a result of faulty separation of the trachea and esophageal septum at its epithelial margin. Most of these communications are located in the region of the cervical esophagus and are single. They may, however, vary from pin size to several millimeters in diameter and usually extend from the anterior wall of the esophagus to the posterior wall of the trachea. This type of fistula can be difficult to demonstrate radiologically. Distension with air of the gastrointestinal tract (particularly the stomach) often

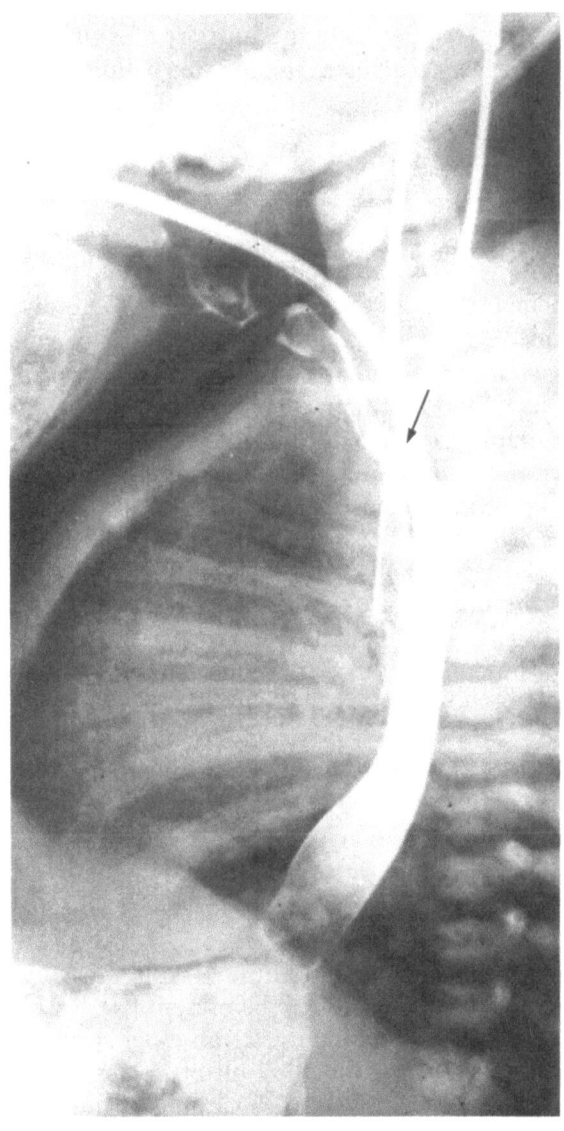

FIGURE 61.
H-type fistula (at arrow).

is present on a plain film of the abdomen. A chest film usually reveals some degree of pneumonia.

For optimal delineation using fluoroscopic examination and cineradiography, barium is injected through a nasal catheter into the esophagus at a level above the carina with the patient in the prone and right anterior oblique positions. If a tract is not demonstrated, then esophagoscopy and bronchography may be performed simultaneously. In addition, methylene blue is injected into the esophagus and can be identified in the trachea if an H-type fistula is present. Alternatively a tracheogram can be obtained with the patient supine and rotated to the side, following the injection of barium or a water-soluble medium. Interval films which follow the contrast into and through the fistulous tract are then obtained.

A new technique to demonstrate such fistulae has been described. With the patient in the Trendelenburg position the proximal portion of the esophagus is occluded by a Foley catheter in order to prevent aspiration of the contrast medium. Another small catheter is used distal to the inflated balloon to introduce the contrast agent (81b).

Congenital bronchogenic cyst

Congenital (cystic) tumors of the posterior mediastinum

Bronchogenic cysts result from an abnormality of budding of the tracheobronchial tree from the primitive foregut. This division forms a dorsal segment, which becomes the esophagus, and a ventral segment, giving origin to the larynx, trachea, and lungs. These cysts may be found in the posterior, middle, and anterior mediastinum. Because of the scope of this monograph, only cysts that may compress and even displace the esophagus are considered. Posterior mediastinal cysts are located in the retrocardiac area. The typical cyst is a round or oval, well-defined solitary mass, occasionally multilocular. It seldom communicates with the bronchial tree, even when attached by a stalk. The cyst usually is lined with respiratory epithelia and the wall contains mucus glands, cartilage, and smooth muscle fibers.

On radiologic examination a homogenous, round or oval mass in the region of the carina is observed to compress the esophagus. A cyst may be located between the esophagus and the trachea, resembling a pulmonary sling. It may also mimic displacement of compression of the esophagus by an enlarged left atrium. Cysts located in the lower esophageal region may resemble intramural lesions (76a).

In infants, the chief symptoms are those of respiratory distress, whereas in adults dysphagia may be present (106).

Enteric cyst of the esophagus represents an esophageal duplication that results from the pinching off of an embryonal diverticulum (63, 137). Enteric cysts of the esophagus are inti-

FIGURE 62.
Enterogenous cyst (at arrow).
From Reed, J. C., and Sobonya,
R. E. Morphologic analysis of
foregut cysts in the thorax. Am.
J. Roentgenol., *120*:858, 1974.

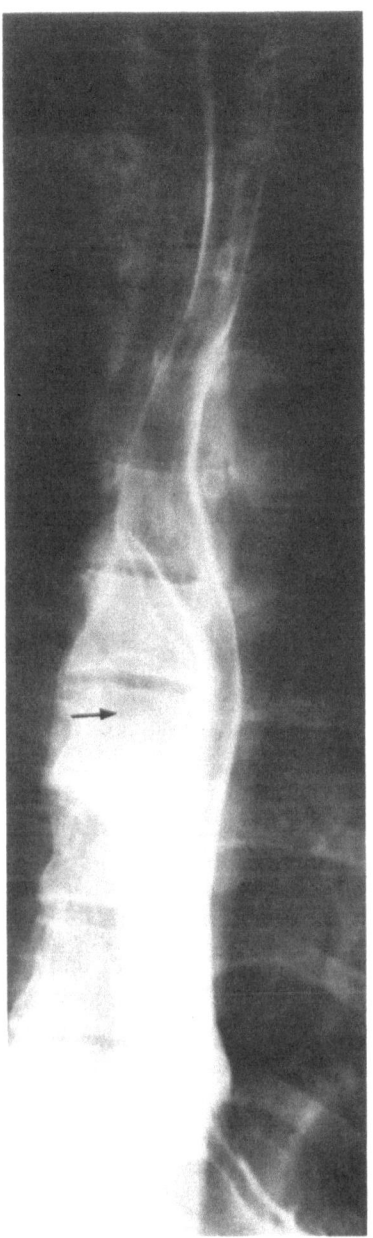

mately attached to the esophagus in a submucosal, intramural
position (196) (Fig. 62). They usually have no fistulous connection with the esophagus and produce a flattening of one side of
the esophagus. These cysts vary in size, being as large as 5 cm
in diameter (222). The lesion is grossly similar to a bronchogenic cyst but is lined with esophageal, intestinal, or a
mixed type of epithelium. The typical cyst has a two-layered
muscular wall resembling the esophagus, but the serosa is
missing, being replaced by part of the pleura. The cyst contains

a substance resembling gastric juice. This lesion is most frequently located in the posterior mediastinum but may also present in the middle or lower mediastinum, extending commonly into the right hemithorax. This cyst generally is larger and located further posteriorly than the bronchogenic cyst.

Radiologically, the typical features are those of a mediastinal mass which is spheroid or tubular in shape and homogenous in density. The lesion usually produces an intramural type of defect of the esophagus (see Chapter 7). Lobar or segmental pulmonary collapse with an ipsilateral mediastinal shift may be produced by pressure of the cyst on a bronchus.

Bronchography may show compression and displacement of a bronchus which does not occur in a bronchogenic cyst. The differential diagnosis from other mediastinal masses and other "wall" lesions of the esophagus may, on occasion, present difficulties.

Neurogenic cysts

These cysts are located in the posterior mediastinum, compressing or displacing the esophagus, related in degree to their size and location.

Neurenteric (archenteric) cyst (66) arises from incomplete separation of the endoderm of the notochord. The wall of the cyst contains both gastrointestinal and neural elements. The cyst is connected by a stalk to the meninges but rarely to the esophagus. On radiologic examination, a sharply defined, round or oval loculated, posterior mass of homogenous density is frequently associated with a defect of the thoracic spine. If sufficiently large, the lesion can compress and displace the esophagus, as well as other posterior mediastinal structures.

Meningocoele (meningomyelocoele) develops from herniation of the leptomeninges through an intervertebral foramen. Associated vertebral and rib abnormalities usually are present. Neurofibromatosis is associated commonly. Meningomyelocoele contains spinal fluid and nerve elements resembling solid neurogenic neoplasm. The lesion will displace and compress the posterior mediastinal structures, including the esophagus, depending on its size and location. On myelography, contrast often will opacify a meningomyelocoele.

Cystic lymphangioma (Hygroma)

The cystic variety, often present at birth, occurs in infants and extends into the neck (not true of the adult variety). This lesion is lobulated, is lined by endothelium, and contains lymph. On radiologic examination, a soft tissue mass is noted in the neck or anterior segment of the upper mediastinum.

Congenitally short esophagus (brachyesophagus)

A short esophagus may be the result of failure of growth of the subtracheal portion of the embryologic esophagus. This results in a portion of the stomach being located within the thorax, as the stomach fails to descend to its normal position below the diaphragm. Prior to the 12 to 18 mm embryologic stage, the caudal migration of the septum transversum exceeds the passive descent to the stomach to such an extent that the stomach is cephalad to the future diaphragm. At this stage, if the stomach does not descend, a congenitally short esophagus will result (187). Variations in growth of the length of the esophagus or in the descent of the stomach may ensue, so that all or part of the stomach remains in the thorax above the level of the esophageal hiatus, with the esophagus diminished in length. The portion of the stomach above the diaphragm does not represent a true hernia, because it has no serous sac, nor is the phrenoesophageal membrane normally attached to the lower esophageal sphincter. The esophageal hiatus is usually abnormally large because it is formed around a segment of the stomach that is much greater in caliber than the normal esophagus. If the stomach later descends, the enlarged esophageal hiatus persists, predisposing to the formation of a sliding hiatal hernia in young individuals (31).

Radiologic examination demonstrates a short esophagus and a thoracic stomach. The gastric fundus is not delineated and the esophagus opens like an inverted funnel into the cardia of the stomach at about the level of the fourth thoracic vertebra. If the esophagus is longer, the gastroesophageal junction may be at the seventh or eighth thoracic vertebral level. The esophagus descends almost vertically to enter the stomach in its uppermost part. This superior aspect of the stomach resembles a dilated portion of the esophagus. The esophageal sphincter can be recognized as a contracted area between the lower end of the esophagus and the stomach. The sphincter is not fully competent because the normal phrenoesophageal membrane attachments are not present. Reflux and free flow of barium may be noted between the thoracic stomach and esophagus.

Congenital hiatal hernia

A hiatal hernia in an infant or young child is principally associated with excessive width of the esophageal hiatus in combination with laxity of the attachments of the phrenoesophageal membrane. The hernia is a true one if a sac is present. A congenital paraesophageal hernia is also a true hernia, protruding through an unfused or persistant infracardiac bursa or pneumoenteric recess to the right of the esophagus. On radiologic examination, in a congenital hiatal hernia, the stomach remains, at least in part, constantly within the thorax, unlike an acquired hiatal hernia. (The exception occurs in adults where a large sliding hiatal hernia has become incarcerated above the diaphragm.) Both the short esophagus and congenital hiatal hernia must be differentiated from an acquired lesion. Gross anatomic and microscopic studies may be necessary for this distinction.

The incidence of hiatal hernia in infants and children is probably higher than statistics suggest (88), a result, in part, of difficulty of the diagnostic examinations, especially in infants. However, in the presence of symptoms of persistant vomiting, regurgitation, frequent respiratory infections, and failure to thrive, congenital esophageal hernia should be considered in the differential diagnosis. Most of the radiologic diagnostic criteria presented in Chapter 5 also pertain to infants and children. Certain differences in children are worth noting, however. In children, more rapid emptying of the esophagus occurs and all structures are smaller, including the herniated segment of the stomach. Additional findings to be anticipated in children are: absence of peristalsis in the terminal esophagus, indicating the presence of a collapsed or empty herniated gastric segment; an apparently long contracted sphincter zone partly caused by an empty or collapsed herniated gastric segment; an unusually high level of the sphincter zone; and the presence of gross reflux.

Darling (54) has recently added to the radiologic criteria in the diagnosis of hiatal hernia in infancy and childhood. He describes a "beak sign," which represents an early form of funneling of some of the barium into the herniated stomach through the esophageal hiatus, with the child being examined in the supine position. He also refers to a "hole" sign in the frontal view in the region of the esophageal hiatus, which is the result of an air-distended small segment of stomach within the hiatal tunnel.

If the hernia is not detected in an early stage, subsequent inflammatory changes may occur, resulting in esophagitis. A "congenital stricture" may be the end result of an unidentified esophagitis secondary to a small hiatal hernia.

Sandifer's syndrome

Hiatal hernia associated with torticollis and athetoid body movements in children has been reported (127). These abnormal motions appear to be directly related to the hernia, because they appear during eating and have been cured following surgical repair of the hernia.

On fluoroscopic examination, during a barium swallow, the body contortions are initiated when the bolus reaches the gastroesophageal junction and enters the herniated gastric segment. The athetoid motions appear to be related to the activity of the diaphragm. The children maintain these contorted positions in an effort to obtain relief from the spasm of the cervical muscles brought on by eating.

Webb and Sutcliffe (252) have suggested an explanation for this rare condition. They presume a neurogenic pathway between the diaphragm and the neck muscles. This permits reflex contractions of the neck muscles in these children, produced by abnormal stimuli secondary to the presence of the hiatal hernia.

Congenital presence of ectopic glands and mucosal epithelium in the esophagus

In the human embryo, columnar epithelium initially lines the esophageal lumen, being eventually replaced by squamous cell epithelium. However, a columnar-type epithelium may occasionally persist in the lower esophagus, referred to as congenital heterotopia. Aberrant cells may also be present in isolated portions of the esophagus (ectopia). In addition, ectopic gastric glands may also be present in the lamina propia of the esophagus. True esophageal glands normally are located in the submucosa and deep within the muscularis mucosa. Ectopic gastric glands are located above the level of the muscularis mucosa where the superficial cardiac glands are normally placed. Ectopic or heterotopic mucosal epithelium or glands cannot be demonstrated on radiologic examination directly but indirectly their presence may be suggested on the delineation of an acquired ulcer or stricture (see section on Barrett ulcers, Chapter 7).

Congenital stenosis

As a result of inadequate canalization of the esophagus, mild to marked narrowing of the esophageal lumen, involving short or relatively long segments, may be present at birth. In severe and extensive stenosis, the symptoms at birth include difficulty in swallowing and vomiting, which simulates esophageal atresia. Fluoroscopic examination usually reveals a long, narrowed segment located in any area of the esophagus. Spasm is absent, with some distension of the segment noted above the level of obstruction (Fig. 63). In milder cases, symptoms do not become manifest until solid food is added to the infant's diet (usually around the age of 8 months). Impaction of food may occur above the level of stenosis.

Congenital web and diaphragm

As a result of incomplete vacuolization of the epithelial lining of the esophagus, single or multiple thin, smooth membranes may occlude the lumen of the esophagus, caused by semilunate-shaped septa that produce thin, ringlike densities. Radiologically, during the active phase of swallowing, these septa (rings) appear as thin incisura-like defects. These rings must be differentiated from acquired webs, which occur chiefly in adults (156). Complete or partial rings of the esophagus must be differentiated from webs, congenital stenosis, and atresia of the esophagus. Rings are slightly thicker than webs but not as long as strictures and are ringlike in appearance (see Chapter 7).

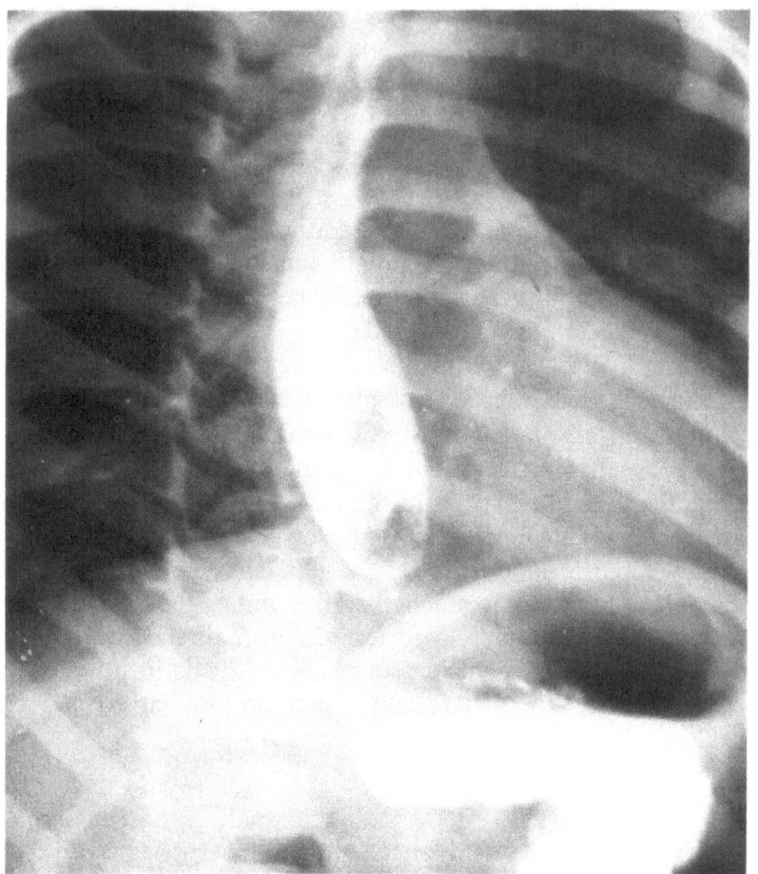

FIGURE 63.
Congenital stenosis at distal end of esophagus.

These diverticula are secondary to invaginations of residual buds into the esophageal wall during the embryonal process of separation of the laryngotracheal ridge into the esophagus and trachea (239). This is a true diverticulum because it involves the entire wall of a segment of the esophagus. False diverticula are acquired and consist only of mucosa and muscularis mucosa herniating through a defect or a weak area in the esophageal muscular wall. These two types of diverticula cannot be differentiated radiologically but when such diverticula are demonstrated in infants or children a congenital origin is suggested.

Congenital esophageal diverticulum

This condition, which has been reported in siblings (189), is rare in children under the age of 14 years. It may be caused by congenital absence of ganglion cells in the sphincter zone (similar to Hirschsprung's disease) and represents a neuromuscular disorder. A familial infantile achalasia inherited as an autosomal recessive disorder has been described, associated with short stature, vitiligo, and muscular wasting, in three siblings of an Apache indian kindred (263b). Congenital (amyenteric) (1)

Familial or congenital amyenteric achalasia of the lower esophagus

or acquired achalasia cannot be differentiated radiologically. The criteria for the diagnosis of this entity are discussed in Chapter 5.

Congenital varices

Varices of the esophagus have also been reported (117) in the early months of life unrelated to portal stasis. Esophageal varices should be suspected in instances of small, frequent hemetemesis (148). The criteria for their radiologic diagnosis are presented in Chapter 7.

Congenital esophageal cartilagenous rings

The presence of these rings has been reported by Anderson et al. (4). They produce a localized, funnel-shaped area of stenosis in infants and children, producing vomiting and dysphagia during the ingestion of solid food. These rings are the result of tracheobronchial remnants within the esophageal wall, secondary to a defective separation of the tracheal and esophageal components during embryonal life. The radiologic findings are those of an area of localized, fusiform narrowing in the distal end of the esophagus, with proximal dilatation. Small clefts or diverticula are present in the stenotic area (Fig. 64). The relationship of these congenital clefts to intramural diverticula (which are acquired) still must be determined (see Chapter 6).

Air esophagograms

Air esophagograms in the neonate may be normal findings but are also associated with severe respiratory distress, especially in infants with impaired respiratory excursion of the chest wall, e.g., hyalin membrane disease (123). On the lateral chest radiograph, the esophagus is partly or entirely filled by air and generally distended and noncollapsable. The gas-filled esophagus returns to normal when the underlying cause of the respiratory distress is ameliorated or disappears. In adults, re-

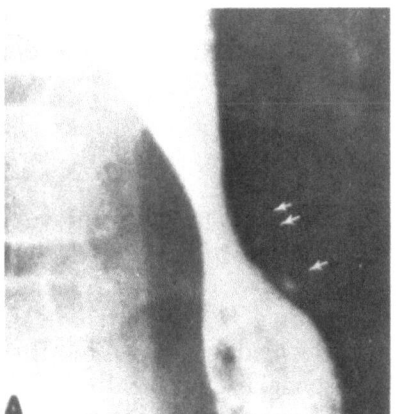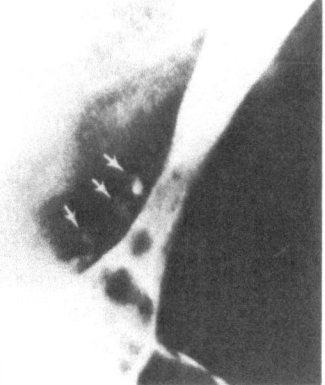

FIGURE 64.
Congenital cartilagenous rings (arrows) in lower esophagus. From Anderson, L. S., et al. Cartilagenous esophageal ring: A cause of esophageal stenosis in the infants and children. Radiology, *108*:665, 1973.

tained air in the esophagus is usually abnormal but may be present following surgical procedures on the chest, still without clinical significance.

Delayed development of the neuromuscular mechanism of the pharyngoesophageal sphincter produces swallowing and respiratory difficulties until the sphincter assumes its normal function (85). This abnormality can be suspected clinically in infants with frequent regurgitation, difficulty in swallowing, or passage of orally ingested liquids into the respiratory tract. Cineradiography is helpful in making the diagnosis. An opaque medium is seen to reflux into the nasal cavity during attempts at swallowing, or passage into the trachea and bronchi may occur, together with pooling of barium in the hypopharynx because the sphincter zone fails to open properly. In addition, esophageal incoordination can produce ineffective peristaltic activity, with reflux of the opaque medium into the hypopharynx. This incoordination is more frequent in premature infants and in infants with cerebral damage (222).

DEVELOPMENTAL DISORDERS
Pharyngeal incoordination in the newborn

In infants, disorders involving the lower sphincter are caused by delayed neuromuscular coordination. In relaxation of the lower sphincter (chalasia) with the absence of normal tone, excessive gastroesophageal reflux occurs. Effortless vomiting, at times projectile, is observed several days after birth, especially with the infant in supine or decubitus position (17). Vomiting does not occur with the infant held erect. This disorder is temporary and as the tone of the sphincter assumes a normal status, the symptoms disappear (Fig. 65).

On cineradiography, free regurgitation of opacified formula from the stomach to the esophagus is noted. The esophagus is dilated and peristaltic waves are few. Lower sphincteric action is absent. In mild forms, abdominal palpation with the gloved hand readily produces regurgitation, particularly in the Trendelenburg position. Persistent vomiting and regurgitation of gastric contents can produce inflammatory changes in the esophagus, with subsequent scarring and shortening of this structure.

Gastroesophageal incoordination (chalasia)

This familial disease is characterized by an autonomic nervous system dysfynction, with superimposed motor and sensory abnormalities involving the swallowing mechanism. A lack of endogenous catecholamines is reported (12). Delayed relaxation of the upper sphincter and disturbed esophageal motility are characteristic, resulting in dysphagia. Emotional instability, hypertension, and inadequate lacrimation are part of the

RELATED CONGENITAL SYSTEMIC DISORDERS OF THE ESOPHAGUS
Familial dysautonomia (Riley–Day syndrome)

FIGURE 65.
Chalasia of the esophagus. From A. S. Johnstone, Lesions of the esophagus of special radiological interest. Avery Jones, et al. Medical Trend Series in Gastroenterology, Butterworths, Woburn, England, 1952.

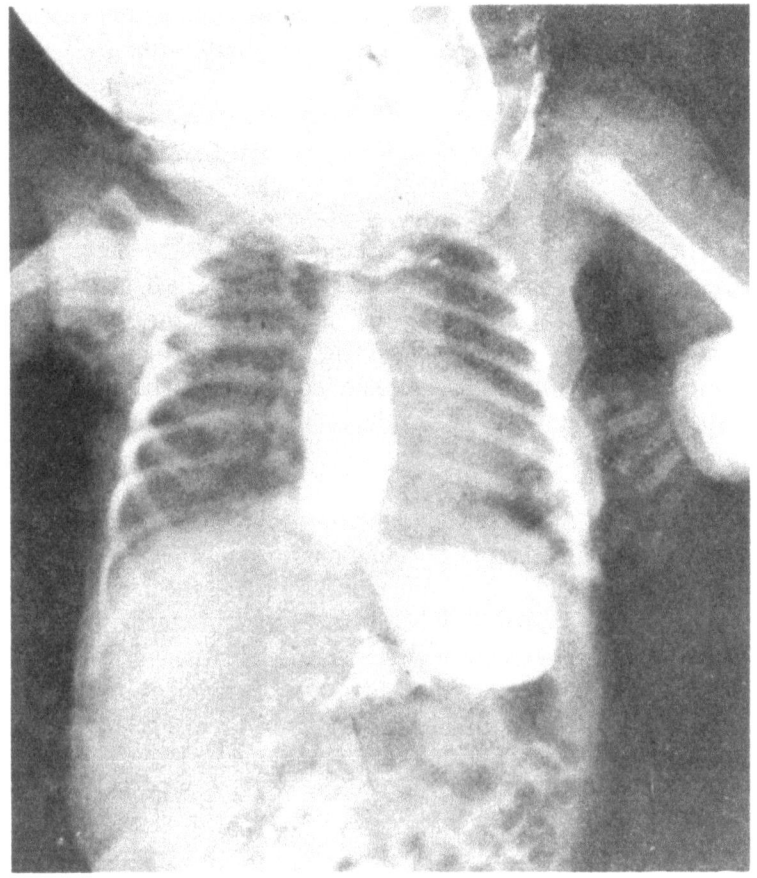

entity (158). Lung infections are common because of the frequency of aspiration of food during swallowing. The clinical diagnosis can be suspected upon the failure to identify the papillae of the tongue. The intradermal injection of histamine produces a reduced local reaction when compared with normal individuals.

On cineradiography, abnormally slow or totally absent peristalsis of the esophagus is noted. Esophageal atony with dilatation are accompanied by rapid emptying only in the erect position.

Oculopharyngeal muscular dystrophy

This hereditary familial disease shows histologic findings in affected muscles, typical of muscular dystrophy (254). The pharyngeal and striated esophageal muscles are involved, but the upper esophageal sphincter is spared. Progressive muscular paresis results in facial weakness, ptosis of the eyelids, and dysphagia in addition to other muscular dysfunctions. Fluoroscopic examination shows reduced or absent contractions of the constrictor muscles, resulting in stasis of food in the hypopharynx with aspiration into the lungs. Motility studies reveal weakness in motor function of both the pharynx and the upper end of the esophagus.

Micrognathia

This disorder of the autonomic nervous system is characterized by superimposed sensory abnormalities involving the swallowing mechanism (95). It produces delayed relaxation of the pharyngoesophageal sphincter and disturbed esophageal motility, resulting in aspiration of food into the lungs. The diagnosis can be made on physical examination and the radiologic examination of the skull and facial bones. The disorder is caused by immaturity of development.

Sjogren's syndrome

This disease, of unknown cause but of congenital or familial origin, is characterized by deficient laryngeal, salivary, and mucosal secretions. It manifests itself during the age of menopause of women, possibly because of an endocrine imbalance. Scleroderma-like changes of the skin, arthritis and dysphagia caused by excessive dryness, and atrophic changes of the mucosa of the orohypopharynx are characteristic. The radiologic findings are reminiscent of sideropenic anemia (see Chapter 6).

CHAPTER

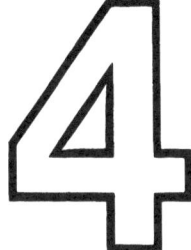

MECHANICAL FACTORS AFFECTING THE CONTOUR OF THE OROHYPOPHARYNX AND ESOPHAGUS

Because of the location of the esophagus in the posterior mediastinum, opacification of the esophagus can be utilized in the evaluation of many disorders and lesions of this region. In this chapter, the external and internal factors mechanically displacing, distorting, compressing, occluding, or rupturing the orohypopharynx and esophagus are discussed. The main external structures and spaces affecting the orohypopharynx are the retropharyngeal space, the thyroid and parathyroid glands, the trachea, and the cervical spine. The structures surrounding the esophagus in the posterior mediastinal space are the heart, aortic arch, thoracic aorta, pleura and lungs, mediastinal lymph nodes, and thoracic spine. Intrinsic abnormalities that are discussed here are foreign bodies, perforations, erosions, and lacerations.

EXTERNAL FACTORS
Retropharyngeal abscess

In infants up to 6 months of age, the thickness of the retropharyngeal soft tissues varies considerably with crying, phonation, and swallowing. In children, the thickness of the retropharyngeal space is normally about one-third the anterioposterior diameter of the body of the fourth cervical vertebra (168)—a useful index in determining the presence and even the size of any retropharyngeal mass.

The most common cause of a retropharyngeal abscess in infants and children is a lymphadenitis secondary to an acute tonsillitis. Other acute or chronic inflammatory causes, such as an undetected perforation from a foreign body of a tuberculous cervical adenitis and retropharyngeal abscess, may be noted anterior to the retrovertebral space when its origin is pharyngeal. The mass is usually painful and in the acute stage can increase considerably in size within a relatively short time. Forward displacement of the larynx, trachea, and epiglottis is common, delineated with a barium swallow when the presence of a fistulous tract is excluded. If the abscess ruptures into the prevertebral space, spread into the mediastinum with resultant mediastinitis may be apparent. In infants, swelling in the prevertebral area must be differentiated from congenital cervical hygroma and in older children from lymphosarcoma (see Chapter 7).

In the adult, an abscess in the prevertebral area is either acute or chronic. It may be secondary to lymphadenitis, although less frequently than in childhood (Fig. 66). A chronic process may be caused by tuberculous or by brucellar or pyogenic spondylitis of the cervical spine. The cervical retropharyngeal stripe is blurred or displaced anteriorly by a paraspinal abscess and destructive changes of the cervical spine are noted. A barium swallow outlines a soft tissue mass located

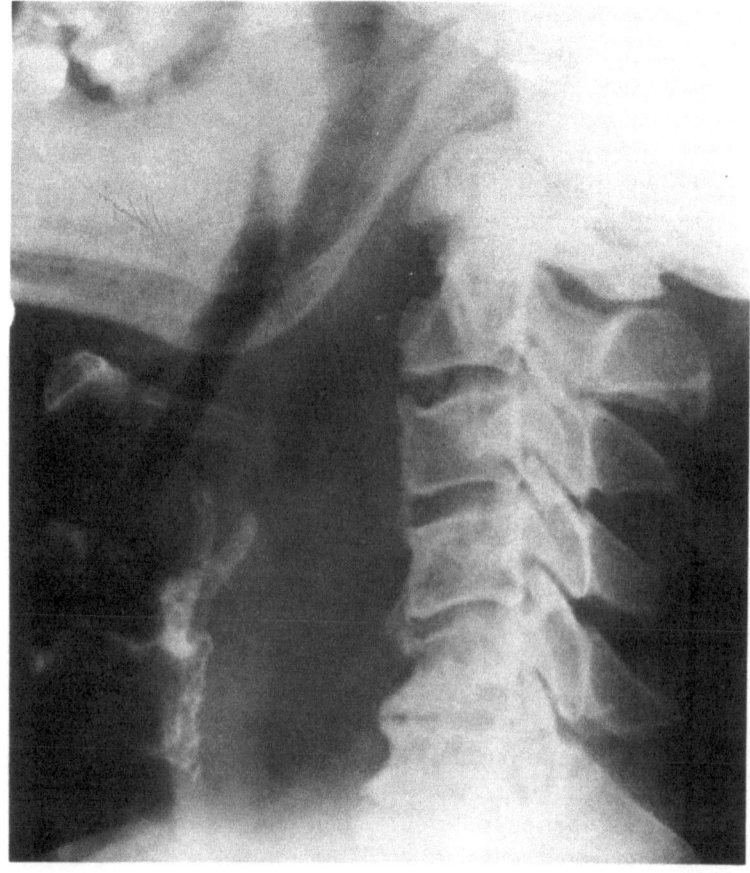

FIGURE 66.
Retropharyngeal abscess.

posteriorly. Calcified lymph nodes may accompany tuberculous spondylitis.

On occasion, a perforated pharyngeal diverticulum may be the cause of a retropharyngeal abscess. On radiologic examination, with barium, part of the diverticulum may be opacified. Fistulous tracts and air in the retropharyngeal space are usually present.

A retropharyngeal abscess in the adult must be distinguished from a neoplasm. The latter, except for dysphagia, is often clinically silent and radiologically indistinguishable from an infective abscess. A retropharyngeal parathyroid adenoma may also simulate a retropharyngeal abscess (see section on parathyroid tumors).

The thyroid gland enlargement

Compression and displacement of the cervical esophagus may be caused by a thyroid gland enlarged by thyrotoxicosis, benign nodular struma, or a malignant neoplasm. The normal thyroid does not displace or compress the cervical esophagus or trachea. The thyroid is located in the region of the pharyngoesophageal sphincter, above the thoracic inlet. However, a diseased gland may enlarge uniformly, expanding in all directions, or enlargement may be asymetrical if only one lobe is affected. The posterior lobes of the gland extend backward on enlargement, partly surrounding both the trachea and esophagus, or may grow posteriorly between the trachea and esophagus. The thyroid may also extend substernally and intrathoracically. Calcification may be observed in the thyroid in a number of disorders, e.g., thyroid adenoma.

Thyrotoxicosis

Thyrotoxicosis usually is associated with a uniform, symmetrical enlargement of the entire gland, resulting in a shallow compression of the trachea followed subsequently by compression of the esophagus. A lateral soft tissue roentgenogram and anteroposterior view of the cervical region usually demonstrates a soft tissue mass constricting the trachea (Fig. 67). Additional films should be obtained upon the ingestion of a barium bolus, to exclude compression and/or deviation of the cervical esophagus. Fluoroscopic examination, particularly during a barium swallow, is very helpful in detecting esophageal compression and in confirming the upward and downward movement of the soft tissue mass, synchronous with swallowing. Spasm of the pharyngoesophageal sphincter may be noted if toxic myopathy is present. Following thryoidectomy, regrowth of the gland can take place with recurrent enlargement, particularly in the retroesophageal area. On these occasions, a distinct anterior displacement of the cervical esophagus will be observed.

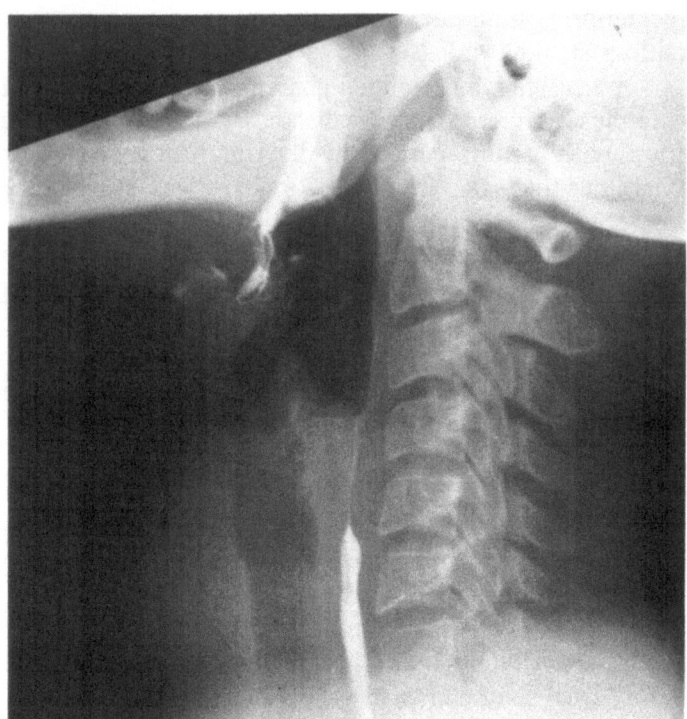

FIGURE 67.
Thyrotoxicosis. Note uniform enlargement of gland with compression of trachea and esophagus.

Benign nodular struma

Benign nodular struma is usually asymmetrical. The process grows in one direction either laterally, anteriorly (substernal), or posteriorly (intrathoracic). Lateral enlargement can readily be detected on physical examination. Anterior enlargement usually occurs above the level of the sternal notch but can extend substernally. Posterior enlargement extends around both the trachea and esophagus, resulting in displacement of both structures. Further growth posteriorly may occur between the trachea and esophagus below the level of the sphincter zone, even extending intrathoracically. Radiologic examination with opacification of the esophagus is very helpful in the diagnosis. In the presence of a posterior intrathoracic goiter, a soft tissue mass usually is noted on the right side in the superior mediastinum. On plain films, compression and right-sided displacement of the trachea is noted. Fluoroscopic examination and/or films obtained upon ingestion of a thick barium bolus will show anterior displacement of the upper thoracic esophagus, with bowing of both trachea and esophagus. The thoracic esophagus will be displaced posteriorly and the trachea anteriorly. The aortic arch may be depressed. A grid film of the superior mediastinum may delineate the reflection of the mediastinal pleura, below the level of the goiter. On fluoroscopy, the goiter is observed to move with swallowing, although this feature

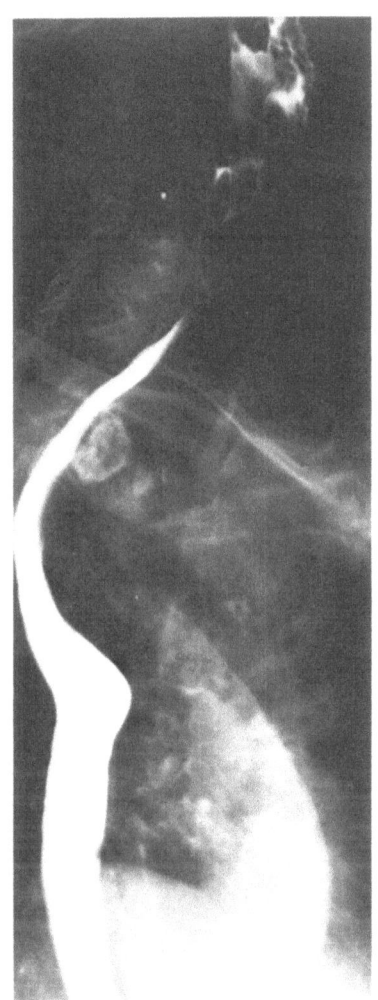

also may be simulated by an enterogenous cyst. Obstruction of the superior vena cava with resultant venous engorgement may also be present. A goiter must be differentiated from aneurysm of the innominate artery or aortic arch, neurogenic tumor, teratoid lesion, thymic mass, enlarged metastatis nodes from a bronchogenic carcinoma, or even a primary bronchogenic carcinoma itself. An intrathoracic goiter, however, is usually observed at a higher level in the mediastinum than with these lesions just mentioned, and the smooth localized displacement or compression of the opacified esophagus is quite distinctive of a goiter (Fig. 68) (217). The presence of a calcified mass in the area of the thyroid is helpful in making the diagnosis of a benign adenoma (Fig. 69).

Malignant Neoplasm

Malignant changes of the thyroid gland may be difficult to detect. On films, the presence of pin-sized, clumped calcification suggests the presence of psammoma bodies, associated with papillary carcinoma. On fluoroscopic examination, rigidity, fixation, and irregularity of the soft tissue mass of an enlarged,

FIGURE 68.
Intrathoracic goiter with displacement of the cervical and upper thoracic esophagus to the right. Note the presence also of a small calcified adenoma.

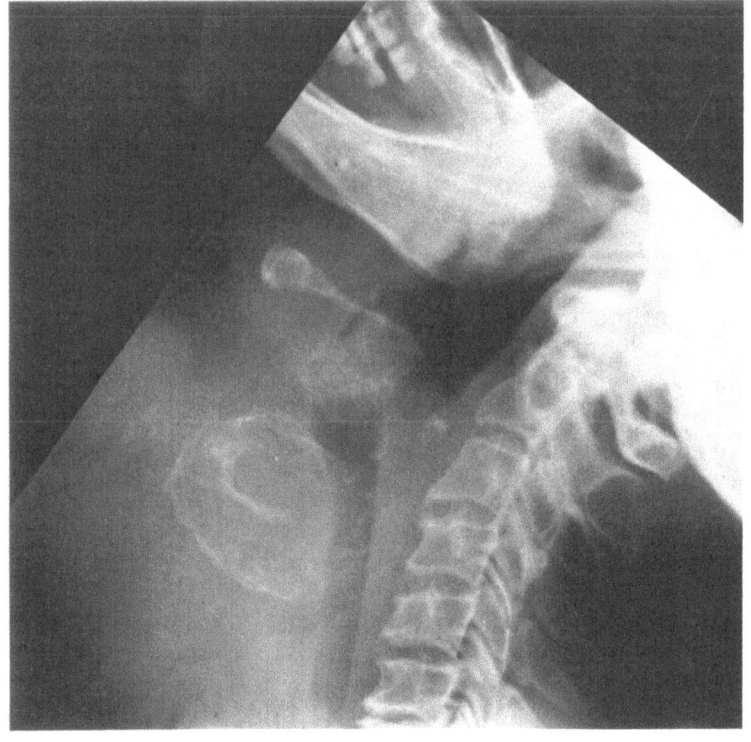

FIGURE 69.
Calcified thyrod struma.

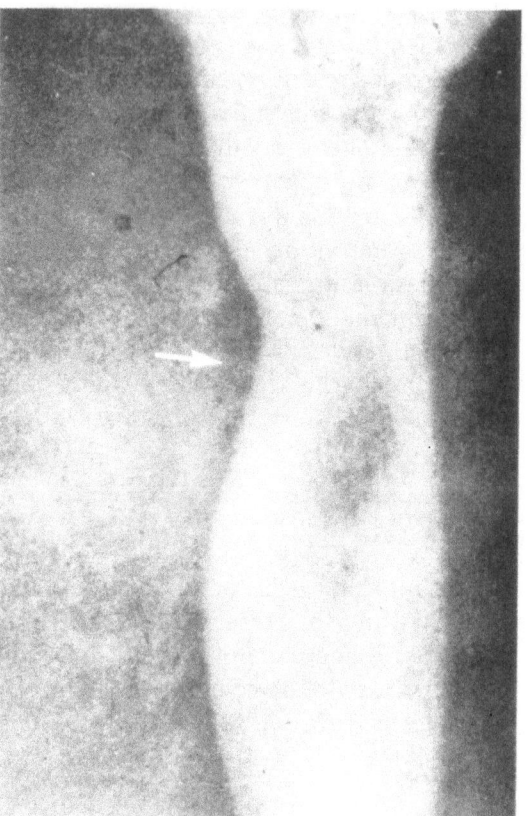

FIGURE 70.
Hyperthyroid tumor. Note esophageal indentation at arrow. From Stevens, A. C., and Jackson, G. E. Localization of parathyroid adenomas by esophageal roentgenology. AM. J. Roentgenol., 99:234, 1967.

asymmetrical thyroid gland suggest malignancy. Considerable compression and even partial obstruction of the cervical esophagus may be present (Fig. 7). Angiography and tomography as well as cervical pneumography may aid in the differential diagnosis (136). Radioactive iodine scan is helpful.

Parathyroid tumors

The parathyroid glands may enlarge secondary to hyperplasia or neoplasm. These masses are usually located in the cervical region and are situated posterior to the thyroid gland. They are usually unilateral and small so that compression is not demonstrated. In the presence of unequivocal clinical evidence of hyperparathyroidism the radiologist plays an important role in localizing the parathyroid tumor. Cineradiographic studies are helpful. The cervical esophagus is deviated slightly in the anterioposterior views with a prominent cresent-like pressure defect of the esophageal wall between C-7 and T-2 and loss of its normal distensibility (232) (Fig. 70). Small thyroid adenomas may show similar findings. These are much more commonly calcified, in contrast to rarely occurring calcification of parathyroid tumors. Pneumomediastinography is helpful but angiography has assumed an important role in localizing a parathyroid tumor.

Changes of the cervical and thoracic spine affecting the hypopharynx, pharynx, and esophagus

Cervical spine

Spondylosis deformans (degenerative disease of the spine) may demonstrate excessive osteophyte formation which can produce indentations and considerable encroachment on the posterior wall of the pharynx and cervical esophagus (Fig. 71). Endoscopy in such instance may result in pharyngeal or esophageal tears, particularly if a rigid endoscope is used. In degenerative disease of the spine, the posterior esophageal membranes and fascial sheets may become fused by fibrous adhesions, affecting the musculature of the hypopharynx and cervical esophagus, and resulting in the formation of small localized traction diverticula. Such adhesions may also produce abnormalities of the swallowing mechanism and dysphagia, especially when the sphincter zone is involved. Fluoroscopic examination after a barium swallow is very helpful in determining the degree of fixation of the cervical esophagus affected by the changes of spondylosis deformans. Abnormal fixation with deviation of the pharyngoesophagus to right or left may occur (Fig. 72). A cervicothoracic scoliosis also causes displacement and abnormal angulation of the cervical and upper thoracic vertebrae, secondarily affecting the pharyngoesophageal sphincter. (Fig. 73). Rheumatoid arthritis produces shortening of the neck caused by involvement of the intervertebral small joints and narrowing of the intervertebral disk, resulting in an apparent downward shift of the upper sphincter zone.

Thoracic spine

Scoliosis, kyphosis, or kyphoscoliosis results in curvatures of the spine and displacement of the esophagus, thoracic aorta, and mediastinal structures. The thoracic aorta is fixed to the thoracic spine because of the intercostal arteries, causing the aorta to follow the spinal curvatures. The esophagus usually accompanies the descending aorta with which it is intimately connected. Depending on the presence or absence of adhesions produced by aortitis, other inflammatory causes, or the aging process, the esophagus, aside from following the aorta and spinal curvatures (Fig. 74A), may remain as a straight tube apparently suspended in the mediastinum (Fig. 74B). When the esophagus accompanies the spine and aorta, it may become redundant and exhibit abnormal kinks and deviations contributed by the effects of the other mediastinal structures (Fig. 75).

In the presence of a kyphoscoliosis and a rigid atheromatous thoracic aorta, the esophagus may be displaced into the posterior portion of the lower left hemithorax, producing a sharp angulation of its distal end. The aorta is then identified in the right anterior oblique position "en face," as a spheroid soft tissue mass or as a calcified density above the diaphragm, dis-

FIGURE 71.
Spondylosis of the cervical spine with esophageal compression.

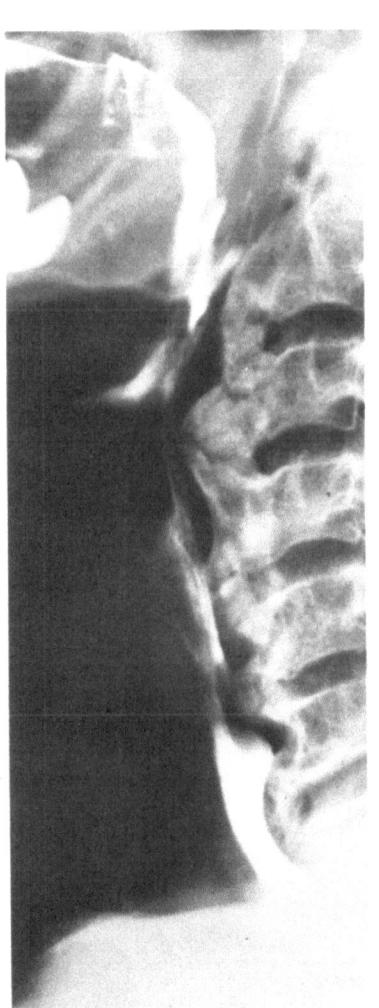

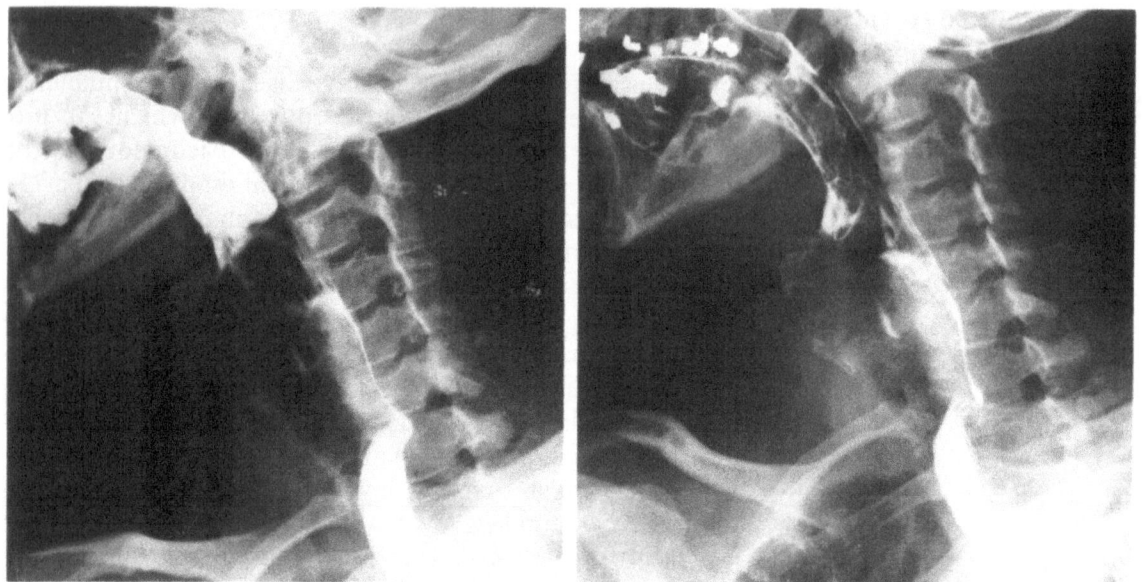

FIG. 72(A)   (B)

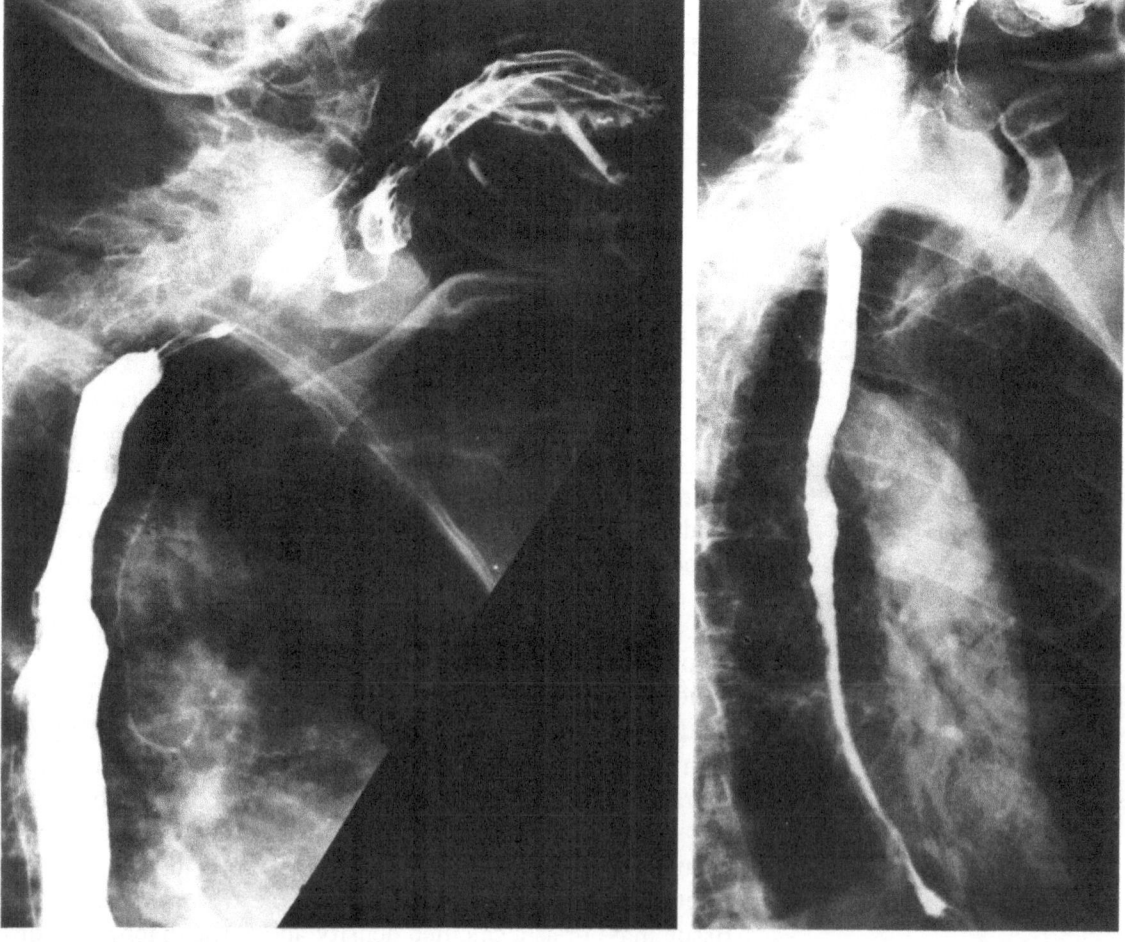

FIG. 73(A)   (B)

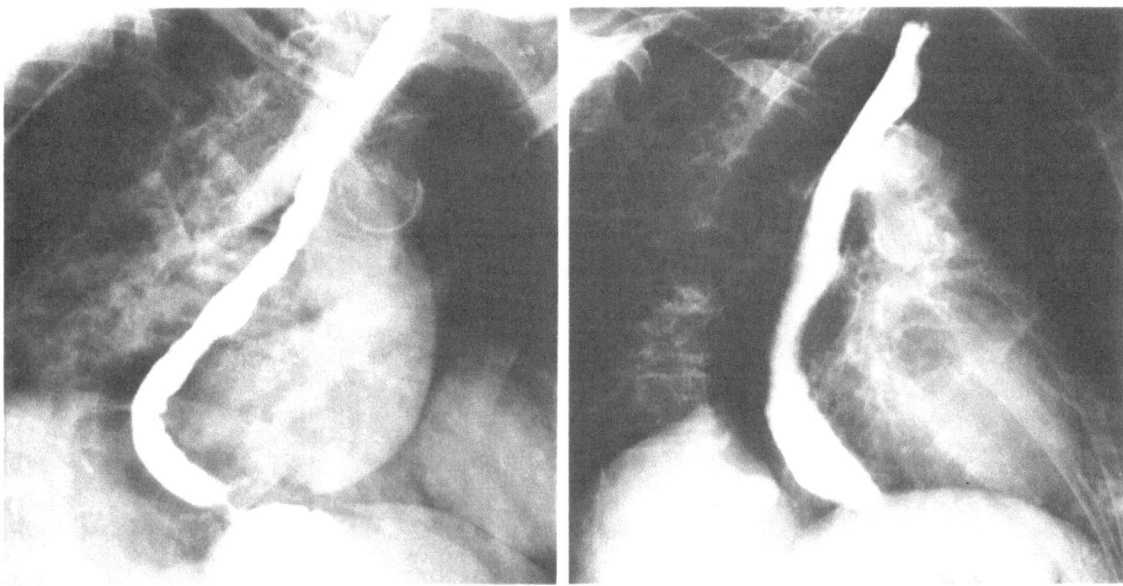

FIG. 74(A)   **(B)**

FIGURE 72.
Idiopathic and asymptomatic deviation of the cervical esophagus.
(A) At the beginning of a second barium swallow, (B) following the
second barium swallow.

FIGURE 73.
Cervico-thoracic scoliosis resulting in abnormal angulation of the
cervical esophagus. (A) Contracted upper esophageal sphincter is
also present. (B) Pulmonary emphysema is also present.

FIGURE 74.
Kyphoscoliosis of the thoracic spine. In the presence of (A) a
redundant esophagus following the contour of the spine, (B) a
short esophagus apparently "suspended in air."

FIGURE 75.
Lateral scoliosis with marked deviation. Irritability of the
mid-esophagus is present.

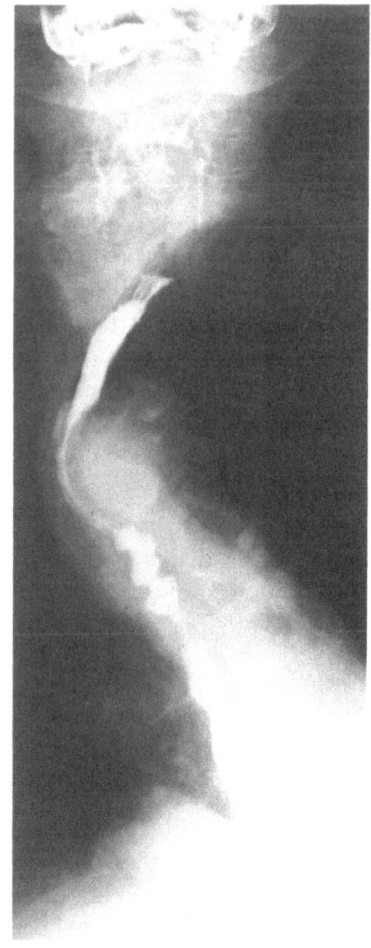

FIG. 75

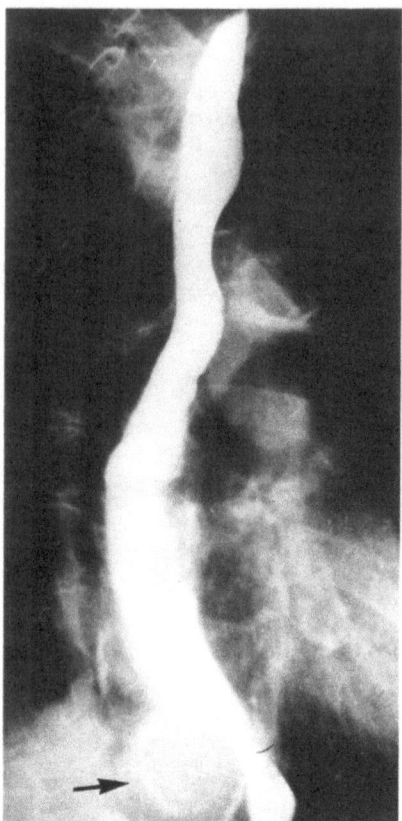 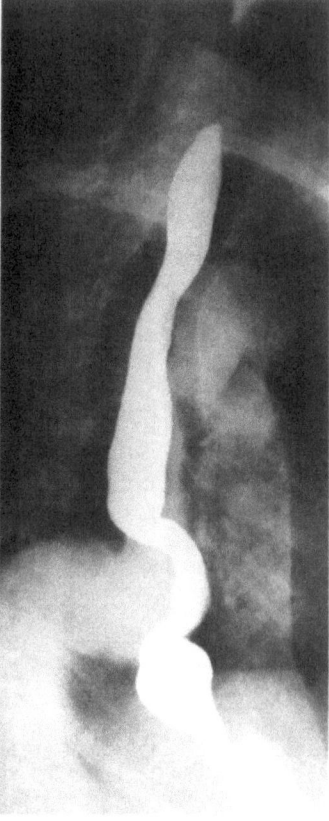

(A) **(B)**

FIGURE 76.
Tortuosity of the lower thoracic aorta with compression and deviation of the lower esophagus. (A and B) Various degrees of obliquitity of the chest. In (A) the partly calcified lower thoracic aorta is seen "en face" and resembles an aneurysm (at arrow).

placing the esophagus laterally (Fig. 76). In the presence of shortening of the esophagus and laxity of the phrenoesophageal membrane, which is common in elderly individuals, a sliding-type hiatal hernia is usually observed.

In infective lesions of the spine, especially tuberculosis associated with a paraspinal abscess, the esophagus becomes fixed in position contiguous with the spinal disorder. Erosions into the esophagus may result even with formation of an esophageal fistula. Extramedullary hematopoesis or a fractured vertebral body resulting in a paravertebral hematoma may compress or displace the esophagus. Degenerative changes of the thoracic spine (spondylosis deformans) may also be responsible for esophageal indentations (Fig. 77).

Cardiovascular lesions

In infants and children an enlarged cardiac silhouette on a chest film usually indicates the presence of a congenital heart disorder, although rheumatic heart disease may also be present. In the adult, cardiomegaly generally suggests acquires heart disease. The cardiomegaly may include enlargement of only a single cardiac chamber, a combination of chambers or enlargement of the entire heart. The barium esophagogram is a valuable adjunct in detecting individual chamber enlargement (e.g., left atrium), thus aiding greatly in the differential diagnosis of the various cardiac disorders (74).

Cardiac chamber enlargement (Diagram 9)

LEFT ATRIUM The left atrium is located posteriorly, being in close contact with the middle third of the esophagus. No deviation or compression of the esophagus is created by a normal left atrium. In early enlargement of the left atrium the anterior wall of the opacified esophagus is observed to be minimally indented. This indentation can escape observation in the standard right anterior oblique position, frequently obtained to detect left atrial enlargement (213). The presence of left atrial enlargement, however, may be diagnosed more accurately in an upright left lateral chest film, exposed in deep inspiration (114). With progressive enlargement, an additional posterior displacement of this portion of the esophagus occurs with obliteration of the normal space between the esophagus and

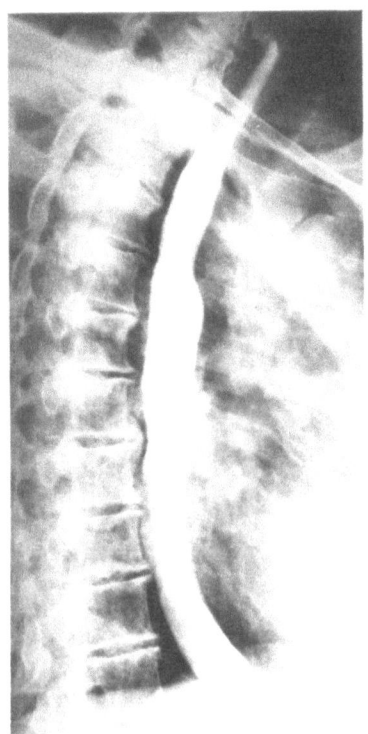

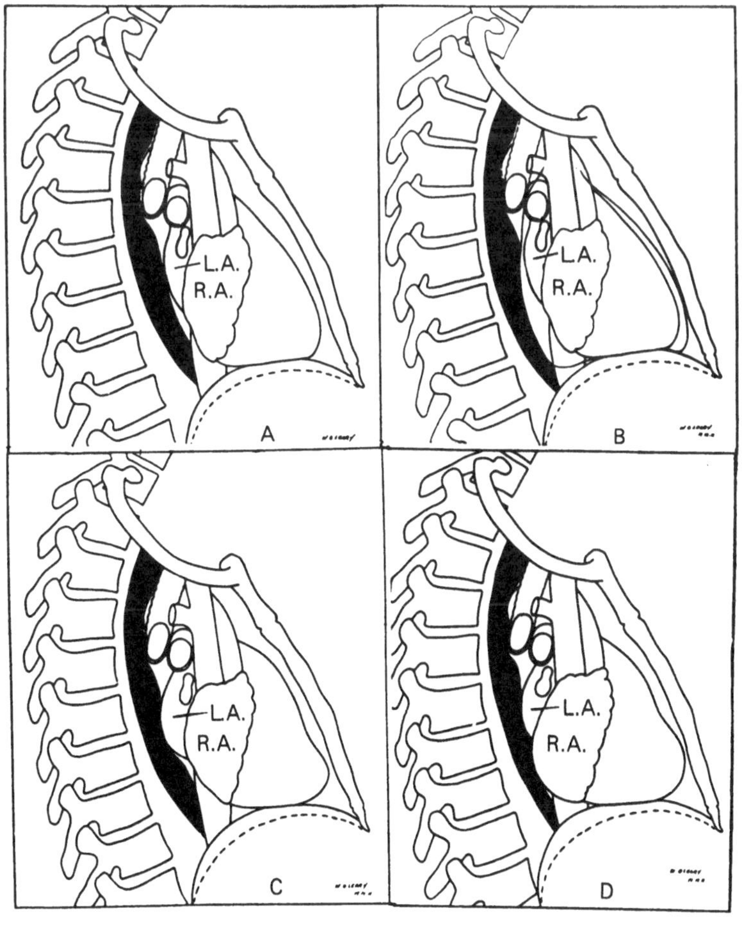

FIGURE 77.
Spondylosis changes of the thoracic spine indenting the opacified esophagus.

DIAGRAM 9.
Esophagograms showing compression of enlarged cardiac chambers and pericardial effusion. (A) Normal, (B) Pericardial effusion, (C) enlarged left atrium, (D) enlarged left and right atria (heart failure). From Levene, G., and Kaufman, S. Roentgen diagnosis of pericardial effusion. Am. J. Roentgenol., 57:380, 1951.

spine. With further enlargement, more marked displacement of this segment of the esophagus to the right occurs, with widening of the angle between the right and left main bronchus. These features are best observed in an overpenetrated posteroanterior film of the chest with a barium-opacified esophagus (Fig. 78).

A fluoroscopic sign has been described (43) which may facilitate the diagnosis of mitral insufficiency. This is referred to as the posterior wedging sign. Following a barium swallow the esophagus is noted to be displaced to the right and the descending aorta to the left during ventricular systole in instances of mitral insufficiency. These findings result from the wedging action of a dilated left atrium.

Occasionally the esophagus is displaced to the left because of aortic, esophageal adhesions or a mobile esophagus. Right atrial enlargement may produce a similar appearance.

RIGHT ATRIUM The right atrium has no direct contact with the normal esophagus, although it is located posteriorly. A dilated

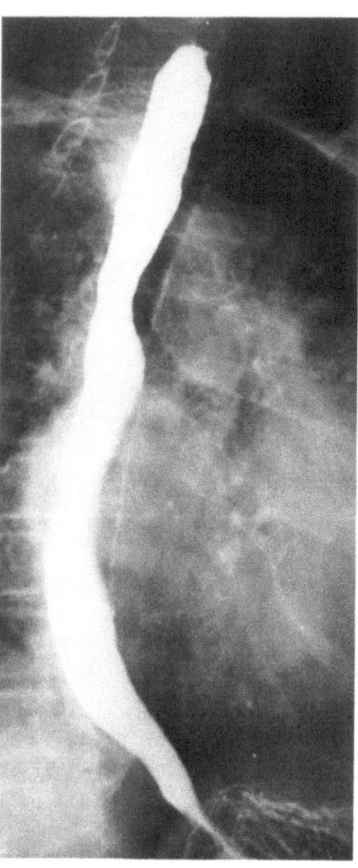

FIGURE 78.
Enlarged left atrium displacing and compressing the lower third of the esophagus.

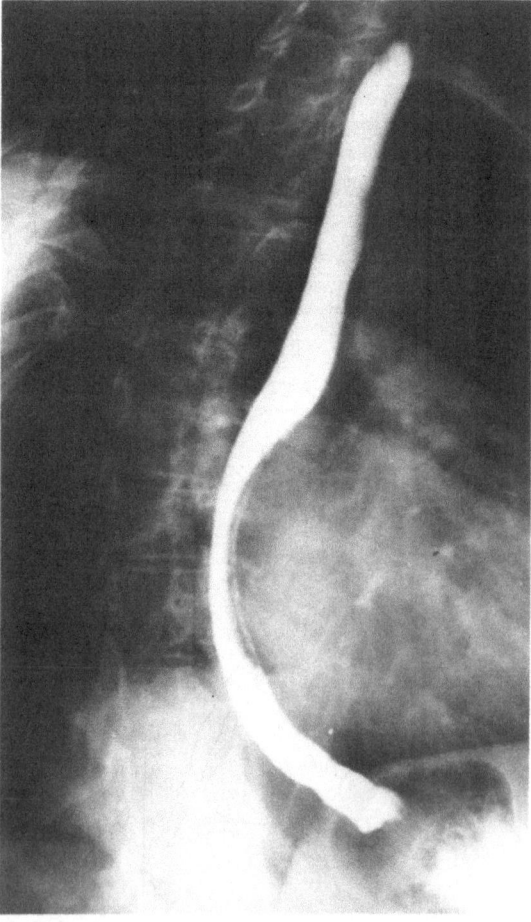

FIGURE 79.
Enlarged left and right atria in congestive heart failure with reverse "3" in lower esophageal impression.

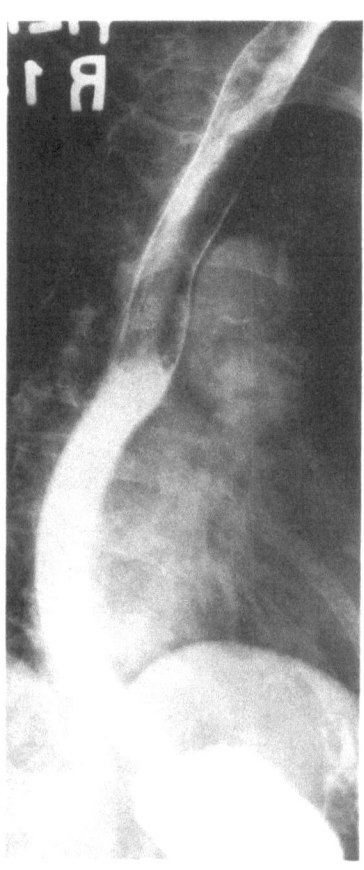

FIGURE 80.
Enlarged left ventricle.

right atrium, often caused by tricuspid valvular disease, may result in compression and displacement of the lower third of the esophagus to the left—an abnormality best demonstrated in the posteroanterior and left anterior oblique views with an opacified esophagus. The esophagus is not displaced posteriorly by an enlarged right atrium as occurs in left atrial enlargement.

LEFT AND RIGHT ATRIUM Enlargement of both the right and left atrium will deviate the esophagus posteriorly and to the right, producing a reverse "3" impression on the opacified esophagus in its middle third. The upper impression is caused by the left atrium and the lower impression by the right atrium (141) (Diagram 9C, and Fig. 79).

Left-sided indentation of the mid-esophagus may be caused by compression from a tortuous aortic arch. This indentation starts usually at a higher level than that caused by enlargement of the left atrium and the cardiac silhouette may be normal. Because such patients usually are in an older age group, the aortic arch often shows calcification in its wall. (See section on aortic arch.)

LEFT VENTRICLE An enlarged left ventricle usually affects the lower third of the esophagus. The esophagus is in contact anteriorly with a small portion of the normal left ventricle, lying anterior and to the right of the descending aorta. The esophagus then turns sharply to the left to enter the stomach, leaving clear space between the spine and the esophagus above the diaphragm.

When the left ventricle enlarges, commonly observed in hypertensive and arteriosclerotic heart disease, the esophagus is noted to be in contact with the heart border down to the diaphragm, with disappearance of the normally clear lower retrocardiac space (Fig. 80). This clear space is not obliterated by an enlarged left atrium.

GENERALIZED CARDIAC ENLARGEMENT Generalized cardiac enlargement may occur in heart failure and in the presence of a variety of systemic disorders and specific cardiomyopathies. Here the opacified lower third of the esophagus may be indented and displaced, without the characteristic findings of specific chamber enlargement.

A variety of congenital and acquired heart and vascular lesions may result in abnormal esophagograms, but their differential diagnosis is beyond the scope of this book.

PERICARDIAL EFFUSION Pericardial effusion produces compression and deviation of the opacified esophagus. In the plain chest film, straightening of the left cardiac border, the presence of acute cardiophrenic angles, and elongation of the cardiac silhouette are characteristic. Esophagograms show compression and displacement of the esophagus at a lower level than that produced by an enlarged left atrium. In addition, the presence of diminished cardiac pulsations and absence of pulmonary vascular congestive changes are helpful in establishing the diagnosis, which may be substantiated by ultrasound studies, angioradiography, or the use of carbon dioxide. (Diagram 9-B).

Degenerative and involutional changes of the aortic arch affect the normal esophageal indentation. In infants, an aortic impression is generally absent or relatively inconspicuous normally because of incomplete development. However, with increasing age, the aortic indentation becomes increasingly prominent. At the level of the fourth thoracic vertebra, the aortic arch passes inferiorly and posteriorly along the left side of the trachea and esophagus to the vertebral column, where it becomes the descending aorta.

The aortic arch and thoracic aorta

FIG. 81   FIG. 82

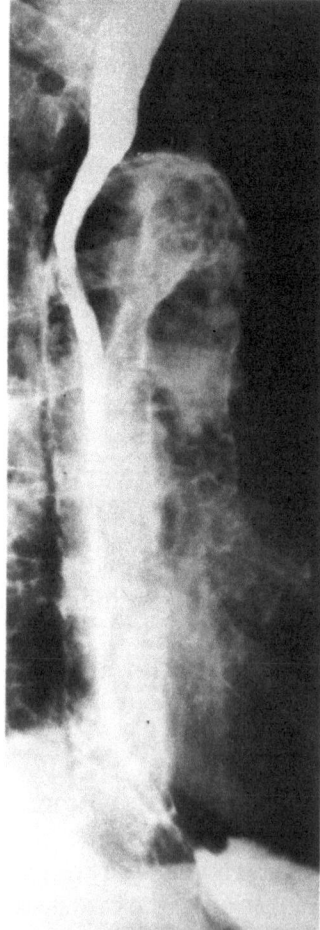 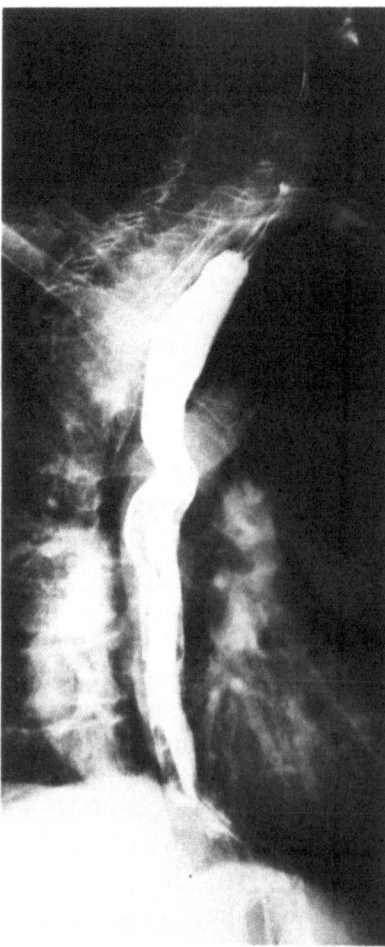

FIGURE 81.
Calcified thoracic aortic arch and descending aorta with compression of esophagus (ball and socket effect).

FIGURE 82.
Tortuous middle thoracic aorta producing a pseudo-vascular ring impression on opacified esophagus.

A partially obliterated esophageal impression caused by the aorta in the adult may be the result of aneurysm, fusiform dilatation of the aorta, an elongated pulmonary artery, an uncoiled aortic arch, mitral disease, a mediastinal mass, spinal deformity, and other pathologic pulmonary or mediastinal diseases. An accentuated aortic arch, which is quite commonly calcified in older individuals and is caused chiefly by atheromatous and degenerative changes, creates the classic "ball and socket" appearance, as the aortic knob indents the opacified esophagus (Fig. 81). The decending thoracic aorta usually becomes uncoiled, elongated, tortuous, and more rigid, depending on the degree and extent of calcific deposits in its wall. Compression of the mid-esophagus in such instances mimic the presence of a vascular ring (Fig. 82). The descending aorta in advanced cases may resemble an inverted "S" and can indent the esophagus posteriorly, even narrowing its lower third, causing dilatation above (Fig. 83). Severe atheromatous changes of the aorta typically produce a rigid tube which may compress the esophagus and produce dysphagia (dysphatia aortica) (22). In the elderly patient, associated motor disturbances also may be present.

Aneurysms

Aneurysms are caused by a number of disorders, notably syphilis and arteriosclerosis. Syphilis often involves the ascending aorta because of the underlying aortitis. Saccular or fusiform dilatation of the ascending arch may produce compression or deviation of the esophagus. Aneurysms of syphilitic origin also occur in the transverse and descending segments of the thoracic aorta, where they may attain a large size (Fig. 84). An aneurysm may produce a solitary or multiple compressions and even cause obstruction of the esophagus, if large enough. An aneurysm actually may erode into the esophagus, resulting in esophageal perforation (see section on esophageal erosion). An aneurysm of the transverse arch plainly causes esophageal deviation to the right and posteriorly, in contrast to vascular rings which produce an anterior compression. An elongated aortic arch may also displace the esophagus to the left and posteriorly; this must not be confused with the displacement, caused by an enlarged left atrium, that is observed at a lower level.

Just superior to the diaphragm, the esophagus lies in front of the aorta and is closely attached to it so that any tortuosity or aneurysmal dilatation produces an anterior and left-sided displacement of the distal end of the esophagus. A saccular aneurysm in this area may produce complete obstruction and resemble a mediastinal tumor. An aneurysm may or may not pulsate, depending on the thickness of the wall and the presence or absence of blood clot (Fig. 85).

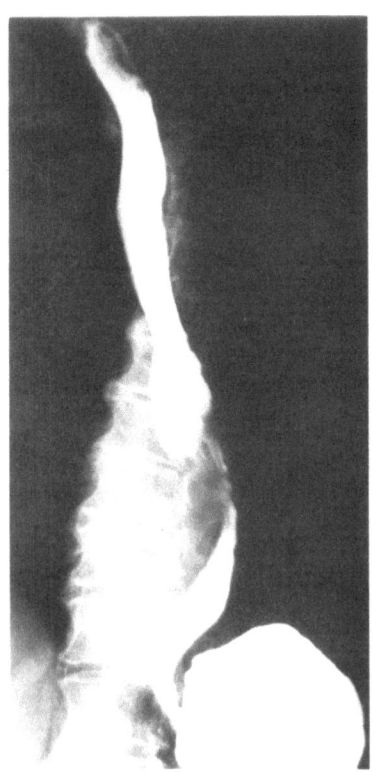

FIGURE 83.
Tortuous descending aorta producing the inverted "S" sign caused by compression and deviation of the esophagus.

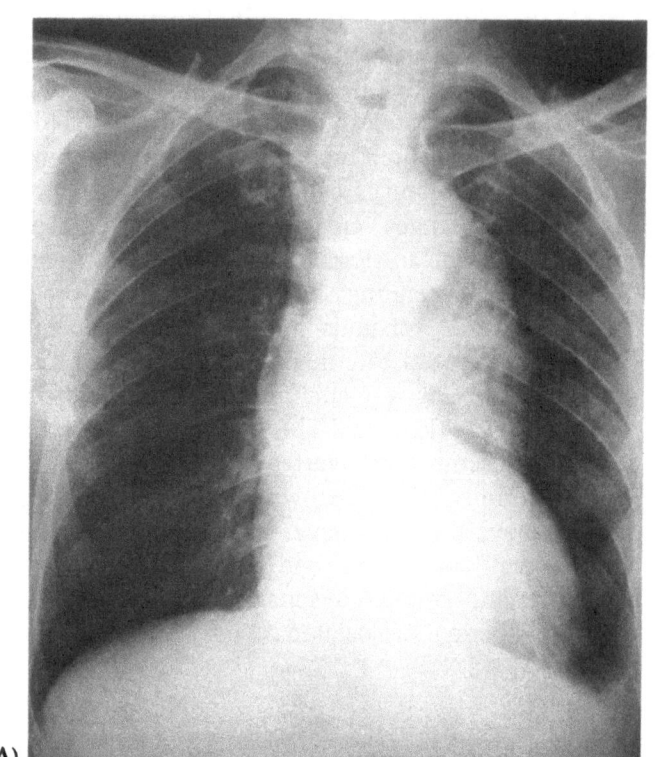

FIGURE 84.
Luetic aneurysm of the thoracic aorta. (A) Chest film, (B) esophagogram, frontal view, (C) esophagogram, lateral view, showing displacement and compression of the esophagus.

(A)

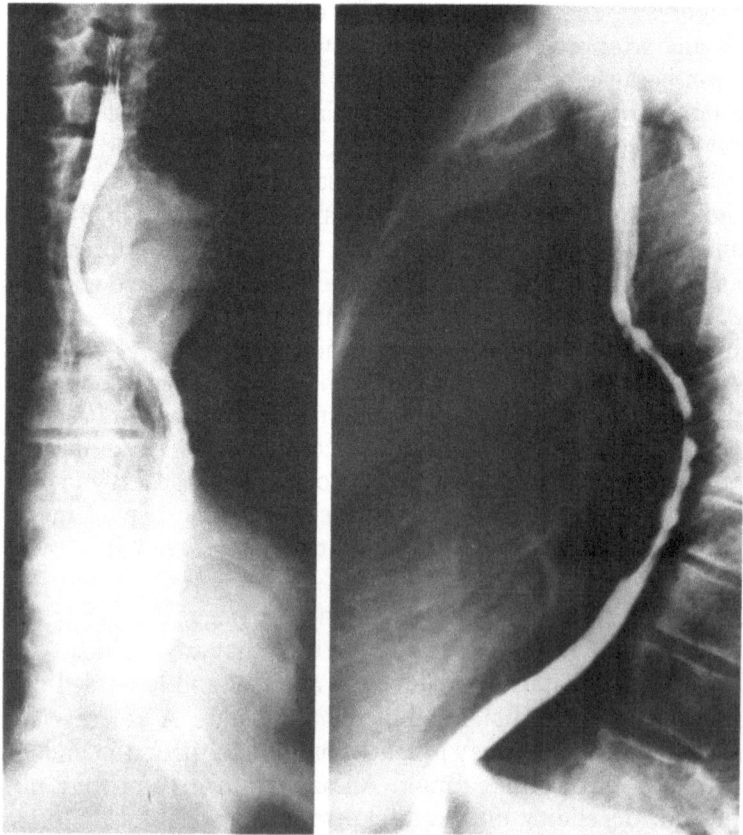

(B)

(C)

FIGURE 85.
Saccular aneurysm with considerable compression and displacement of lower esophagus.

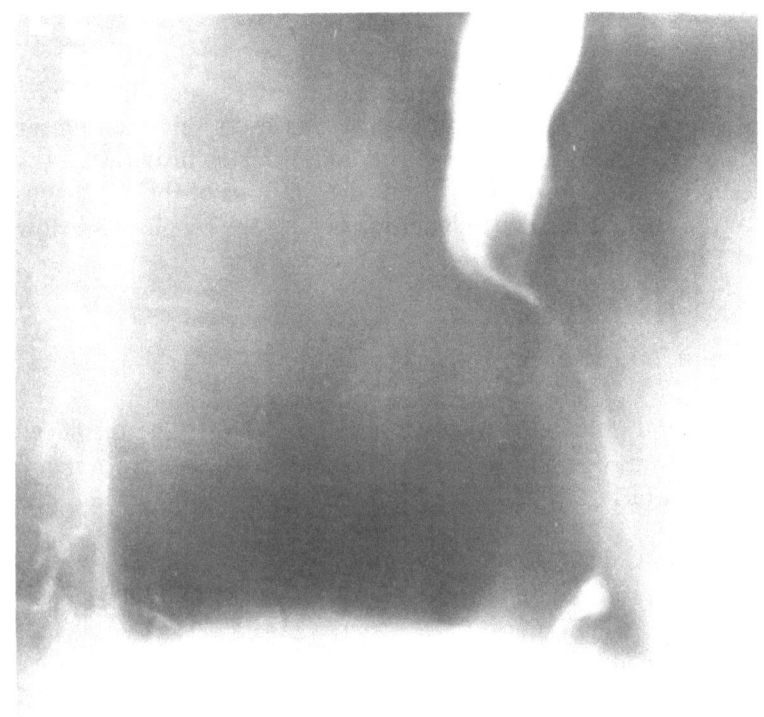

Arteriosclerotic aneurysms occur more commonly in the abdominal than in the thoracic aorta. Arteriosclerotic aneurysms generally are smaller than syphilitic aneurysms and aortitis is absent. Aneurysms in the transverse arch of the aorta and the descending portion of the thoracic aorta bulging posteriorly may result in extensive erosion of the anterior surfaces of the adjacent vertebral bodies (Oppenheimer's sign).

Other less commonly encountered causes of aneurysms of the thoracic aorta exist. Poststenotic aneurysms are usually congenital, being associated with coarctation of the aorta. Mycotic or other infective aneurysms are usually small and are associated with a localized aortitis. Post traumatic aneurysms often occur in the area of the left subclavian artery. Such aneurysms often calcify in later stages. A hematoma at the site of trauma may simulate an aneurysm on occasion.

Dissecting aneurysms may compress or displace the esophagus. The tear in the wall of the aorta in dissections most commonly occurs in the ascending aorta, often extending down into the abdominal aorta. The tear in a dissecting aneurysm may communicate with the pericardial sac, the pleural cavity or the mediastinum.

Aortitis

Aortitis is produced by a number of diseases, including syphilis, rheumatic fever, septicemia, scarlet fever, and meningitis. The aorta is usually dilated and adhesions form between the esophagus and aorta, fixing the adjacent area of the esophagus to the aorta. Irregular indentations along the esophagus below the level of the aortic arch are observed.

Pleural effusion

Pleural and lung abnormalities

In pleural effusion the opacified esophagus may be displaced either to the right or to the left, depending on the location and amount of fluid.

Pleuropulmonary adhesions

In pleuropulmonary adhesions, especially from chronic pulmonary tuberculosis, the upper thoracic esophageal segment (and trachea) is usually pulled to the right by fibrotic bands, often producing a sharp angulation and, occasionally, even serrated irregularities of the lateral border of the adjacent esophageal segment (Fig. 86).

Pleural adhesions

Pleural adhesions and organized pleural effusions may affect the lower esophageal segment when present on the left side, preventing normal distensibility and slowing the rate of emptying. Occasionally, fixation of a segment of the esophagus occurs and pseudodiverticular formation of the esophagus may even result. If an hiatal hernia is present, pleural fibrotic changes may result in incarceration of the hernia, also producing abnormal contours of the herniated segment of stomach.

Atelectasis

Atelectasis can produce abnormal displacement of the esophagus on the side of the collapsed lung or pulmonary segment. In instances of total collapse, the mediastinal structures are displaced to the ipsilateral side.

Pneumothorax

In pneumothorax, displacement of the esophagus to the contra-

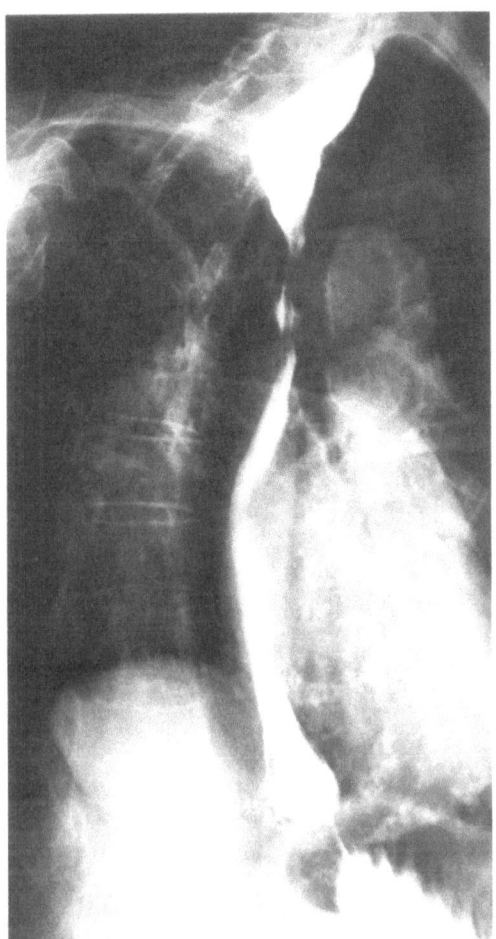

(A)

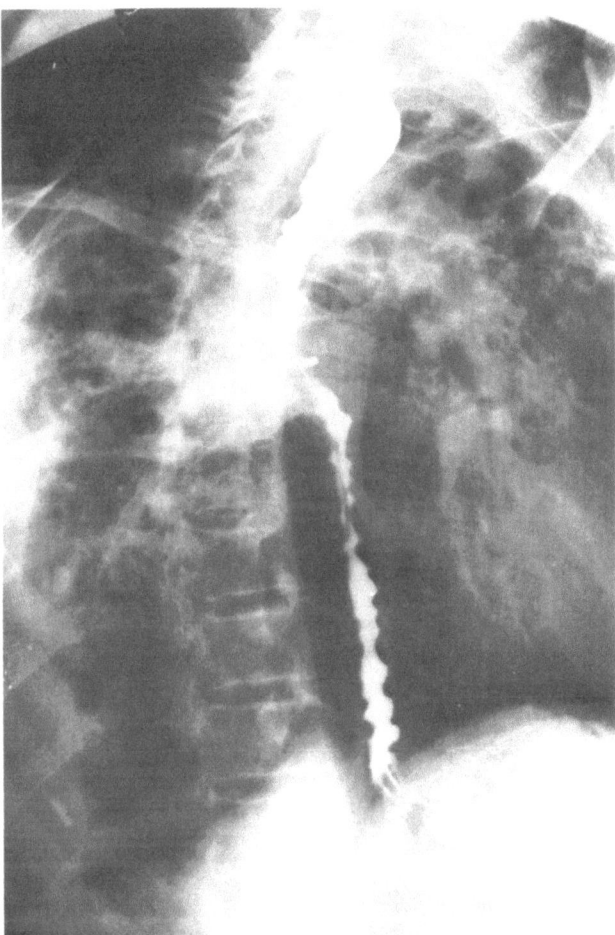

(B)

FIGURE 86.

(A) Pulmonary fibrosis, right apex, resulting in angulation of the upper esophagus. (B) Chronic pulmonary tuberculosis. Fibrotic changes affecting contour and displacement of the esophagus. Also note presence of diffuse spasm of the esophagus.

lateral side is common, but the extent of the deviation depends on the pressure of air in the pleural cavity.

Pulmonary emphysema

In pulmonary emphysema the overaerated lungs tend to restrict the distensibility of the esophagus during swallowing, thus impeding the normal rate of the passage of barium. The normal bronchial esophageal impression is more pronounced, particularly in the elderly patient (Figs. 87 and 88).

Acquired tracheal and bronchoesophageal fistulae

Acquired tracheal and bronchoesophageal fistulae are complications caused by a number of disorders. The etiologic factors include neoplasms, infection, and trauma. Neoplasms may be of esophageal or mediastinal origin. Erosion may occur into a bronchus (or esophagus). Infection (and inflammation) of mediastinal nodes, usually caused by tuberculosis, histoplasmo-

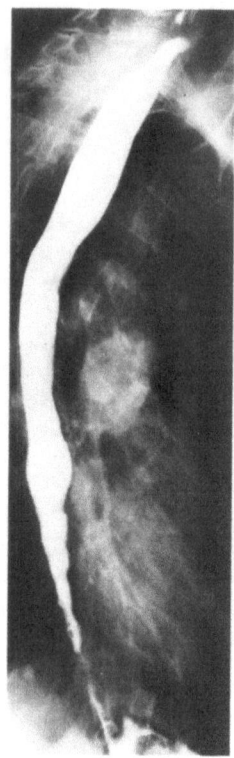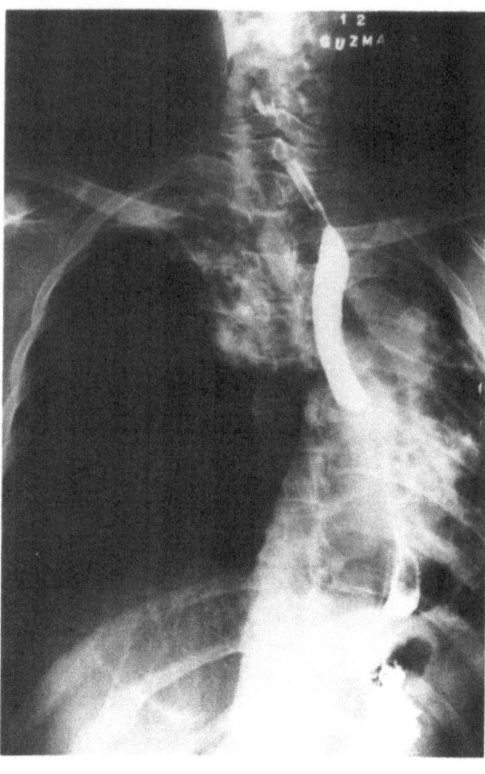

FIGURE 87.
Chronic pulmonary emphysema. Note compression of lower esophagus and constriction of both sphincters.

FIGURE 88.
Atelectasis, compensatory emphysema, and fibrosis with displacement of the esophagus.

FIG. 87   FIG. 88

sis, and sarcoid, may produce involvement of the esophagus, trachea, or main bronchi causing indentations and even erosions and development of fistulae. An esophageal diverticulum may rupture or erode into the wall of the trachea or bronchi. Foreign bodies, instrumentation, surgical procedures, caustic burns, crushing, and penetrating injuries may also produce fistulous tracts between the esophagus and the bronchial tree. The examination following ingestion of a thin barium mixture during fluoroscopic examination usually demonstrates the fistulous tract (Figs. 89 and 90).

In young adults with frequent, recurring pulmonary infections, a small, congenital bronchoesophageal fistula, previously undetected, may be present. In older patients who develop pulmonary complications, e.g., pneumonia, following chest surgery, a fistulous tract should be suspected.

Mediastinal adenopathy

Mediastinal masses

Mediastinal adenopathy is the most common cause of mediastinal masses. The main mediastinal glands are grouped into the paratracheal, parabronchial, hilar, and bifurcation nodes (81a). However, not all these glands, if enlarged, may show esophageal involvement on radiologic examination. Enlarged carinal

FIGURE 89.
Tracheoesophageal fistula secondary to a high esophageal lesion.

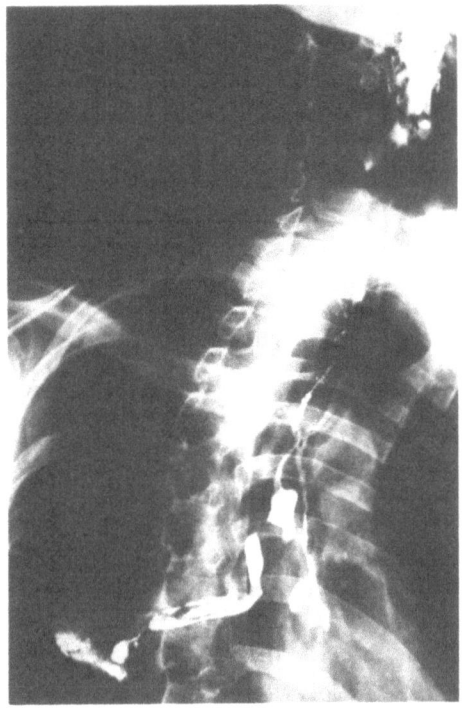

FIGURE 90.
Bronchoesophageal fistula in presence of traction diverticula of the esophagus secondary to an advanced case of *achalasis* in a relatively young patient. (A) RAO esophagogram, (B) Chest film showing residual barium in the diverticula and fistulous tracts.

(A) 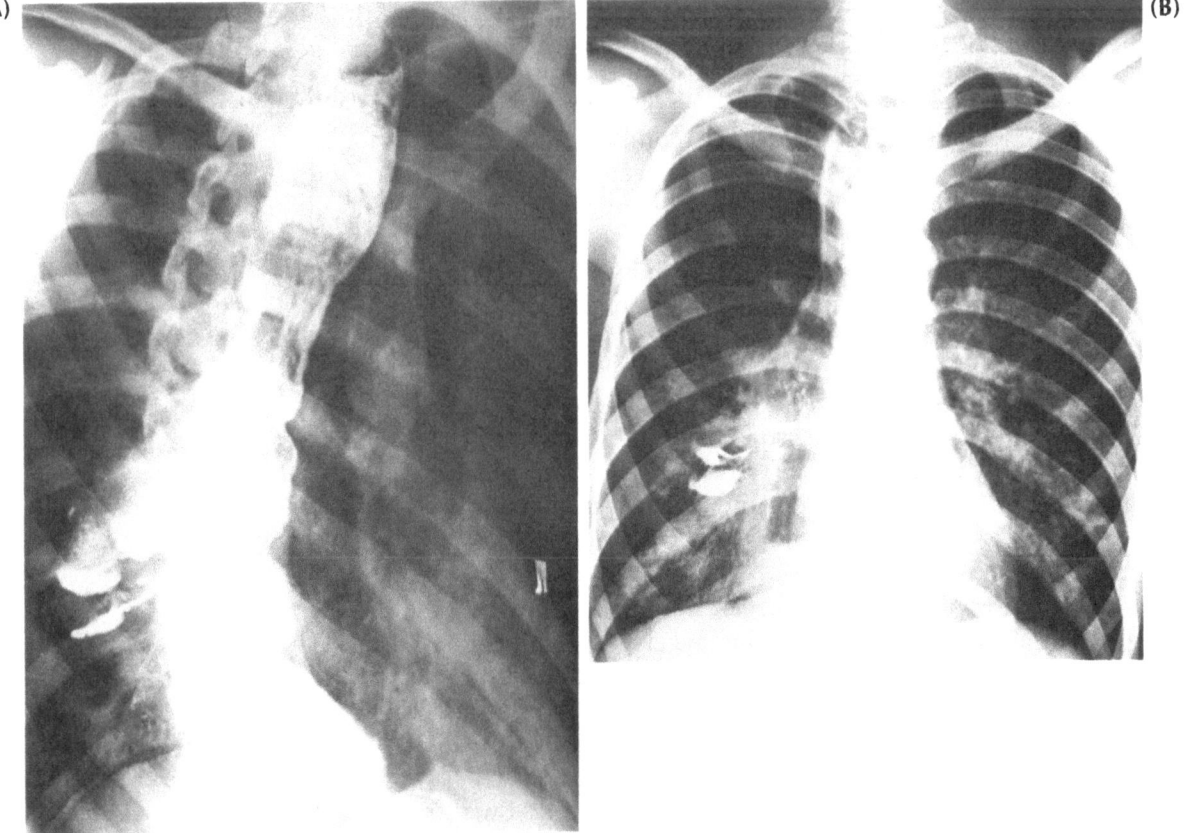 (B)

or bifurcation nodes are not identified on plain chest films but can be observed to compress or displace the opacified esophagus anteriorly and to the right below the level of the tracheal bifurcation, particularly in lateral and anterior oblique views. Widening of the carinal angle also may be noted but must be differentiated from an enlarged left atrium, where the esophageal displacement is mostly to the right and posterior. Enlarged carinal nodes, in addition to causing semilunar indentations of the wall of the esophagus, produce irregularity and rigidity below the level of the bronchus.

Enlarged lymph nodes can be caused by lymphoma, metastic disease (Fig. 91), infective agents, and chronic granuloma. Lymphoma, particularly Hodgkin's disease, constitutes a common cause of enlarged lymph nodes. Multiple lymph nodes, usually in the anterior mediastinum and less commonly in the mid-mediastinum, are involved in lymphoma. On occasion, a large solitary mass of nodes produces displacement and compression of the esophagus. On radiologic examination, enlarged nodes characteristically produce semilunar indentations of the esophagus that may simulate benign intramural lesions (see Chapter 7). However, such nodal indentations do not move with the esophagus as do intramural esophageal lesions.

Enlarged *metastatic nodes* are a frequent cause of mediastinal nodal enlargement and may occur at various levels (164) (Fig. 92). Metastatic nodes chiefly are observed in the interbronchial segments, whereas inflammatory nodes are located primarily at the level of the tracheal bifurcation. Metastatic hilar nodes commonly have their focus of origin in carcinoma of the bronchus, gastrointestinal tract, prostate, and kidney.

Metastatic nodes caused by bronchogenic carcinoma affecting the esophagus are usually located in the middle mediastinal compartment and may compress the esophagus by direct extension (Fig. 249, Chapter 8). The primary lesion may be so small as to be unnoticed except for the appearance of enlarged hilar nodes (particularly in oat-cell carcinoma). Any of the main mediastinal nodes can be involved, with resultant displacement of the aortic knob or distortion of the left bronchial impression on the opacified esophagus.

Other mediastinal tumors affecting the paraesophageal nodes are located mainly in the mid or posterior mediastinum. Such enlarged lymph nodes can be caused by granulomas, such as tuberculosis, histoplasmosis, or sarcoid. These nodes often not only compress the esophagus but actually invade the esophageal wall, producing erosions and esophagobronchial fistulae. The distinction from a primary lesion of the esophagus may be difficult. On occasion, granulomatous, even calcified mediastinal nodes may be observed in the anterior mediastinum without effect on the esophagus (Fig. 93).

A localized tubercular granulomatous nodal mass without pulmonary involvement is uncommon. It usually presents as a

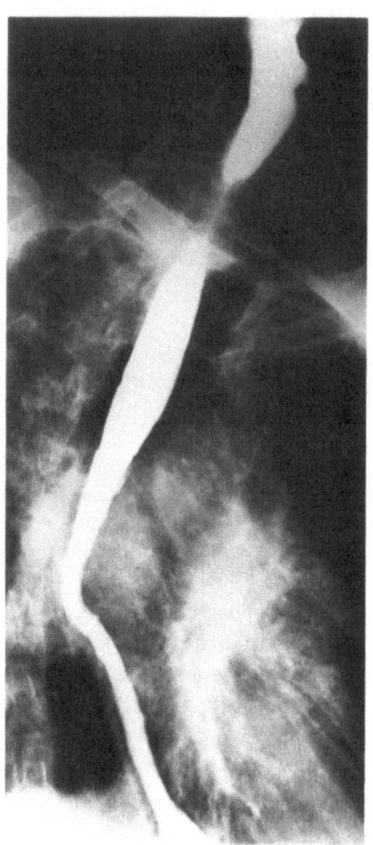

FIGURE 91.
Metastatic enlargement of mediastinal lymph nodes from a laryngeal carcinoma.

loculated mediastinal mass displacing and compressing the esophagus. The accompanying fibrosing mediastinitis results in fixation of the segment of the affected esophagus involved.

Neurogenic neoplasms

Neurogenic neoplasms most often are present in the posterior mediastinum. Three main varieties exist: those of peripheral

(A)   (B)

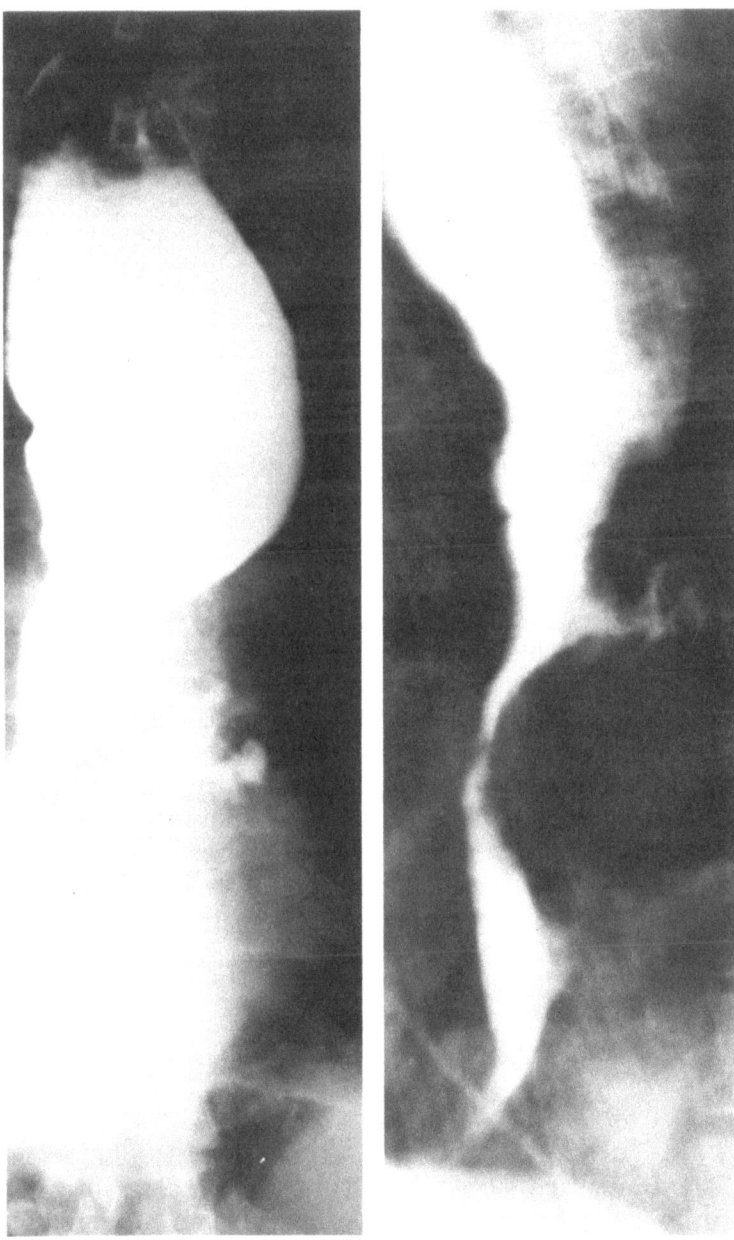

FIGURE 92.
Metastatic enlargement of mediastinal nodes from a carcinoma of the adrenal, showing marked obstruction and compression of the esophagus Bronchoesophageal fistula is also present. (A) Frontal view, (B) oblique view.

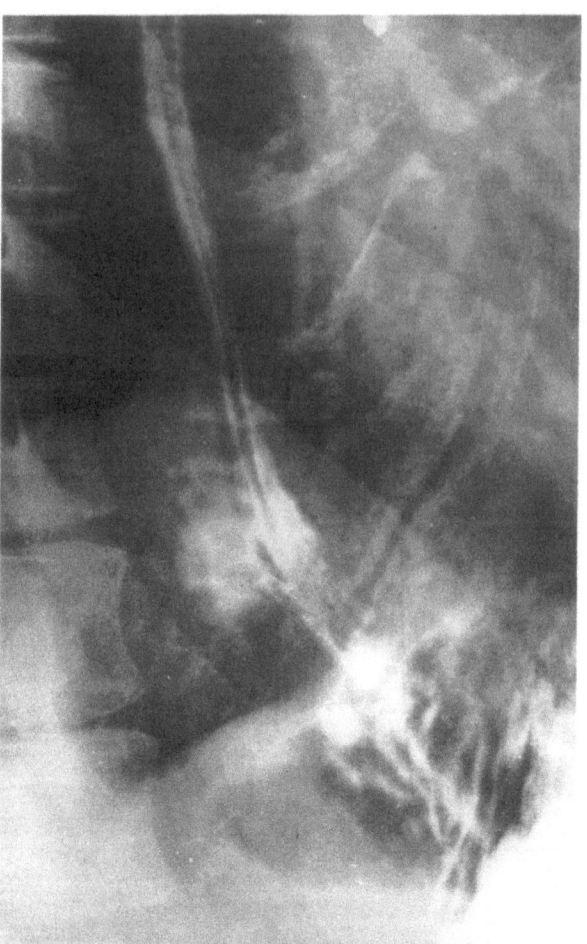

FIGURE 93.
Large calcified mediatinal lymph nodes with no involvement of the esophagus.

nerve origin, such as neurofibromas (also associated with von Recklinghausen's disease), those of sympathetic nerve origin, e.g., ganglioneuromas; and those of paraganglion cell origin, e.g., pheochromocytoma. The last two named are more common in children with a malignant potential. On radiologic examination in all three types, a well-circumscribed, spheroid homogenous density characteristically is observed in the paravertebral area, with evidence of erosion of posterior ribs and occasionally the thoracic vertebrae, with compression and/or displacement of the esophagus. Ganglioneuromas tend to be more elongated than neurofibromas. Meningocoele and neuroenteric and gastroenteric cysts have been discussed in Chapter 3 and must be distinguished from the mediastinal masses described above.

Mediastinitis may be acute or chronic. The acute form is usually secondary to extension of an inflammatory process

Mediastinitis

from the hypopharynx, lungs, pleura, pericardium, or from an esophageal perforation. Esophageal perforation may be caused by a primary carcinoma of the esophagus, foreign bodies, esophagoscopy, esophageal biopsy, or spontaneous esophageal rupture. The radiologic findings vary with the location and nature of the underlying causes. These are discussed in section on esophageal perforations but, in general, obstruction and compression of the esophagus occurs and widening of the mediastinum is noted. Special diagnostic procedures may be necessary for an accurate diagnosis.

Chronic mediastinitis is often secondary to granulomatous lesions, such as tuberculosis, histoplasmosis, or sarcoidosis. These result ultimately in fibrosing changes, with fixation and narrowing of the esophagus. Traction diverticula, especially in the mid-esophagus, may be present.

Fibrosclerosis

Fibrosing mediastinitis is a disorder of unknown etiology that may be part of a systemic process. Fibrosclerotic changes can also be secondary to an acute spondylitis. In the cervical region the fascial spaces are obliterated by adhesions resulting in involvement of the hypopharynx and the development of dysphagia. Fibrosclerosis can be the end result of a chronic granulomatous infection. As a result of a chronic granulomatous process, it is multifocal and possibly associated with orbital pseudotumors and Reidel's thyroiditis (87). Extensive hypertrophic changes of the cervical vertebra may also be present, producing direct compression of the hypopharynx and/or cervical esophagus with anterior displacement of the larynx and hypopharyngeal pseudo-diverticula and irregularities of the posterior pharyngeal wall. Fibrosclerosis can be indistinguishable from a chronic mediastinitis.

External trauma

Penetrating injuries (e.g., stab wounds) or blunt trauma (e.g., auto accident) may result in mediastinal hemorrhage from a major vessel, producing a uniform, symmetrical widening of the mediastinum or a localized mass (hematoma) that compresses and restricts the normal distensibility of the esophagus. A spontaneous, localized mediastinal hematoma secondary to hemophilia or other blood coagulating disorders produces similar radiologic features, characterized by a localized area of restricted mobility and distensability of the esophagus without direct involvement or distortion of the esophageal wall and mucosal pattern.

INTERNAL FACTORS
Foreign Bodies

Ingestion of foreign bodies is not unusual in infants and children. These may be opaque or nonopaque. The most frequently encountered are coins, safety pins, buttons, bobby pins, clips, etc.

In adults, the ingestion of foreign bodies is usually accidental. Such patients involuntarily swallow, pork, chicken, or fish bones; large boluses of meat; false dentures; or bulk laxatives.

In infants and children, these foreign bodies are most commonly arrested in the hypopharynx above the level of the contracted sphincter zone. This is especially true of coins. An anteroposterior film of the chest readily indicates whether the coin is located in the esophagus or in the larynx by its position. If seen "en face," the coin is in the hypopharynx or esophagus; if projected in its broadest diameter it usually is in the trachea. Sharp objects may be lodged in the sphincter zone area, especially when a spastic contraction has been produced by the foreign object.

In adults, a large bolus of meat may be lodged in the hypopharyngeal area, compressing the larynx and resulting in an acute respiratory crisis. This is particularly likely to happen in older edentulous patients or in patients with poor dentures who fail to chew their food properly. If the bolus of meat passes beyond the upper sphincter it may become lodged at the thoracic inlet, above the areas of compression of the aortic arch, or above the level of the lower sphincter (Figs. 94 and 95). Vegetable skins, celery, and hydroscopic bulk laxatives also may be lodged above the lower sphincter.

If the foreign body is opaque, usually no problem exists in its localization radiologically. A lateral view of the neck should be obtained, in addition to views of the chest. Also, in trying to

FIGURE 94.
Foreign bodies. (A) Pork chop bone at thoracic inlet, (B) meat bolus above level of aortic arch.

(A)   **(B)**

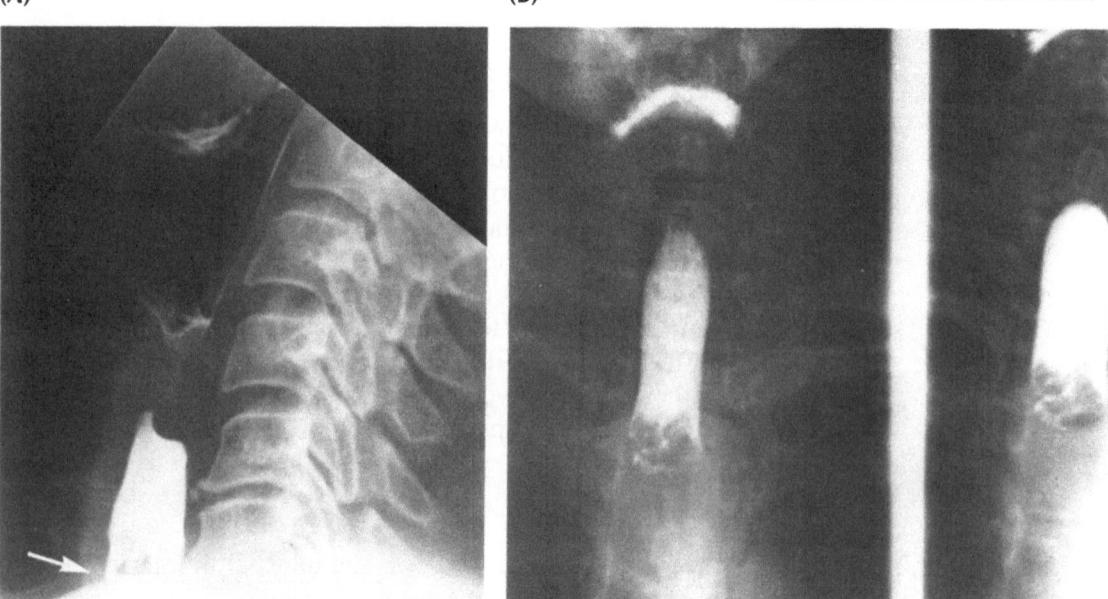

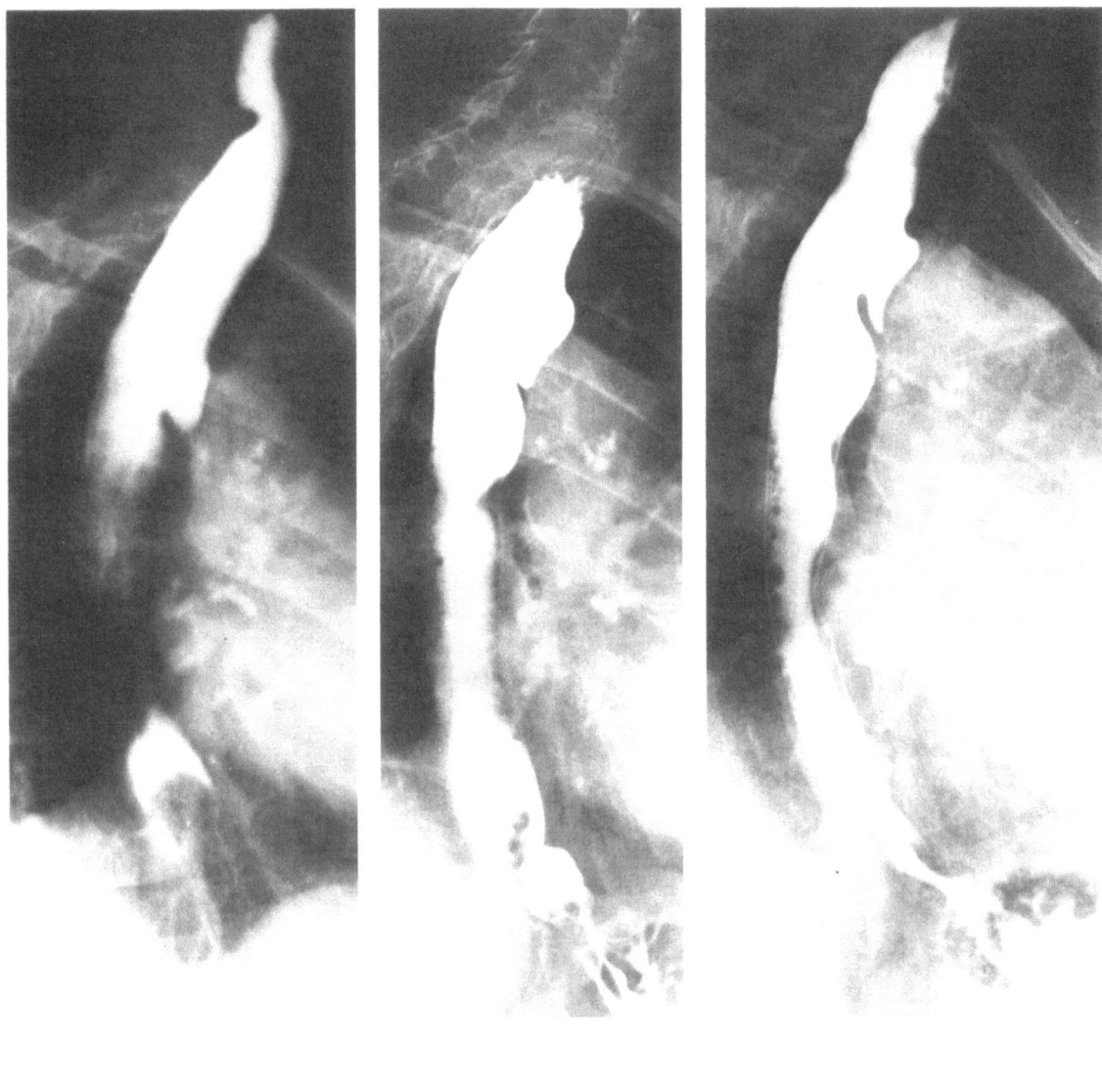

(A) (B) (C)

FIGURE 95.
Foreign bodies. (A) Turkey bolus above level of lower sphincter in an 86-year-old female. (B) Steak bolus in same location in the same patient 2 years later. Note presence of traction diverticulum of the upper end of esophagus. (C) Note presence of ring in lower end of esophagus after passage of second bolus several days later.

detect a fish bone or any unusually opaque object which may be lodged in the upper sphincter, a film should be obtained at the height of the swallowing act in order to elevate the sphincter for full visualization. If the foreign body is not opaque various studies should be attempted, including fluoroscopic examination with ingestion of an opaque aqueous contrast substance or preferably an opaque tablet or capsule. Unsuspected foreign bodies may be responsible for unexplained stridor or frequent attacks of pneumonia (224).

For nonopaque foreign bodies of the hypopharynx and cervical esophagus, a cotton pledget soaked in aqueous contrast medium is swallowed in the hope that the pledget may be "impeded" by the foreign body (see Chapter 1) (Fig. 96).

An impacted bolus of meat in the lower end of the esophagus is usually located above the lower sphincter. On radiologic examination following a barium swallow, obstruction to the passage of the barium is noted with the appearance of a filling defect, which appears fixed and irregular and resembles a neoplasm. The history of acute dysphagia while eating meat is helpful in establishing the diagnosis. Hydroscopic bulk laxative substances, when retained in the esophagus above the level of the lower sphincter, expand and produce a mass with a spongy, partly opaque material resulting in obstruction. The passage of foreign bodies through the esophagus may also be impeded at sites of previous obstructions, surgical repairs, or webs and rings. Figure 97 shows a ball bearing above an area of a previously repaired tracheobronchial fistula in a child.

In psychotic patients, chronic alcoholics, and even occasionally normal individuals, ingested foreign bodies may be silent and remain in the esophagus above areas of normal physiologic constrictions or strictures, webs, rings, or neoplasms. In turn, such foreign bodies may be responsible for abnormal motility, localized esophagitis, or foreign body granulomas.

An intramural esophageal abscess may occur secondary to a tear in the mucosal wall produced by a foreign body. On radiologic examination, the appearance is that of an intramural cavity without a fistulous tract. A double barreled esophagus with a connecting channel above may be noted (143) (Fig. 98). This finding must be differentiated from a congenital duplication,

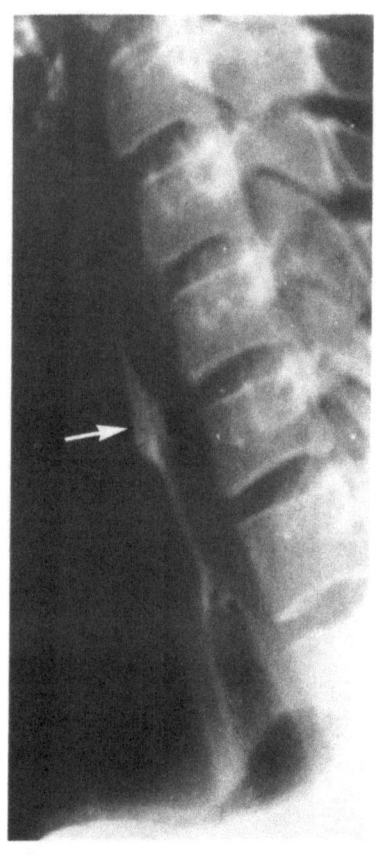

FIGURE 96.
Cotton pledget impregnated with aqueous contrast material held up at site of a nonopaque foreign body (arrow).

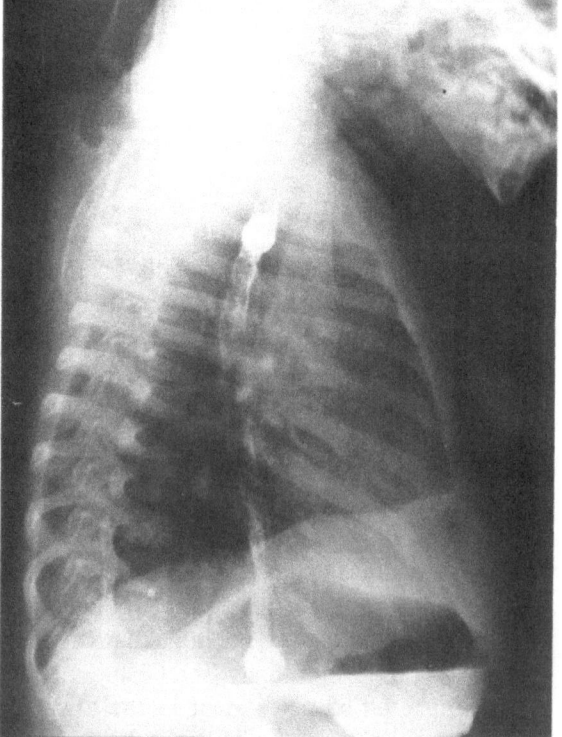

FIGURE 97.
Foreign body (ball bearing) stopped at level of a previously repaired tracheobronchial fistula in a child.

FIGURE 98.
Intramural abscess secondary to trauma from a foreign body showing a double barreled esophagus. From Lichter, I., and Barrie, J., Intramural esophageal abscess. Br. J. Surg., *52*:185, John Wright & Sons, Ltd., Bristol, England.

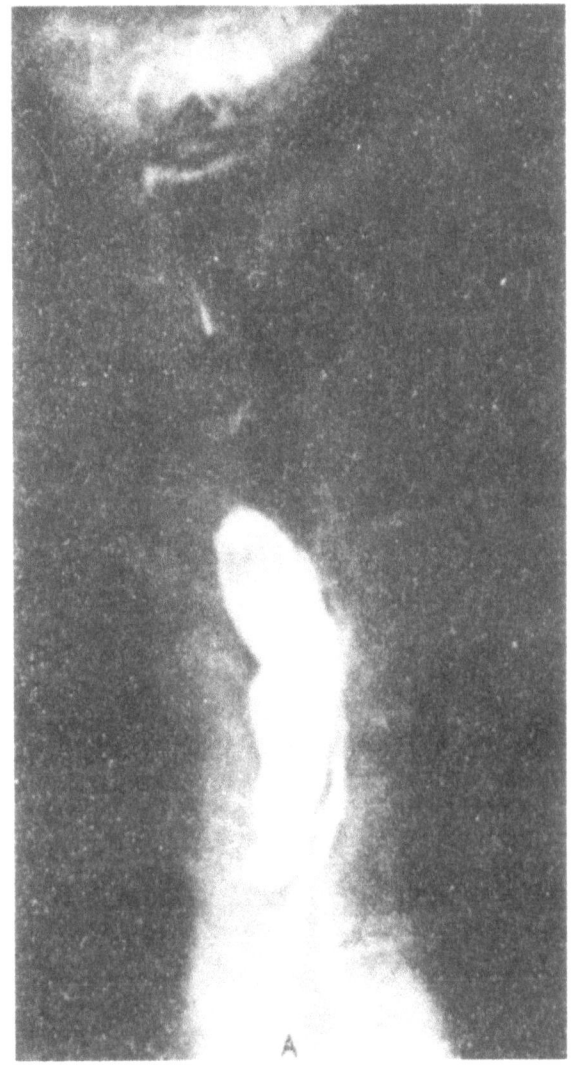

where the connecting channel is usually at the lower level and no history of direct trauma to the esophagus mucosa is elicited.

Esophageal perforations, erosions, and ruptures

Esophageal perforations in a normal esophagus result from direct trauma (e.g., during instrumentation) or by an ingested sharp foreign body. Esophageal erosions through the esophageal wall also produce perforations, but these are usually secondary to a preexisting disease process. Esophageal ruptures usually represent an abrupt process secondary to a sudden increase in the intraluminal pressure. Esophageal rupture can also be caused by external trauma, such as a severe abdominal blow. The rupture can occur in a normal esophagus or in a preexisting condition, such as a peptic ulcer, esophageal diverticulum, or hiatal hernia. A spontaneous esophageal rupture can be the result of severe vomiting, retching, or straining, in either a normal or a diseased esophagus.

Perforations

Esophageal perforations in the hypopharyngeal area are primarily caused by ingestion of sharp foreign bodies and are most prevalent in children. Rigidity of the cervical spine with extensive cervical degenerative vertebral changes can facilitate esophageal perforation in the adult during esophageal endoscopy. A bubble of gas is first noted in the soft tissues outside of the hypopharyngeal wall, at the site of the perforation, on a plain lateral film of the cervical region. Thickening of the retropharyngeal soft tissues is next noted, with forward displacement of the larynx and/or trachea. If the perforation is con-

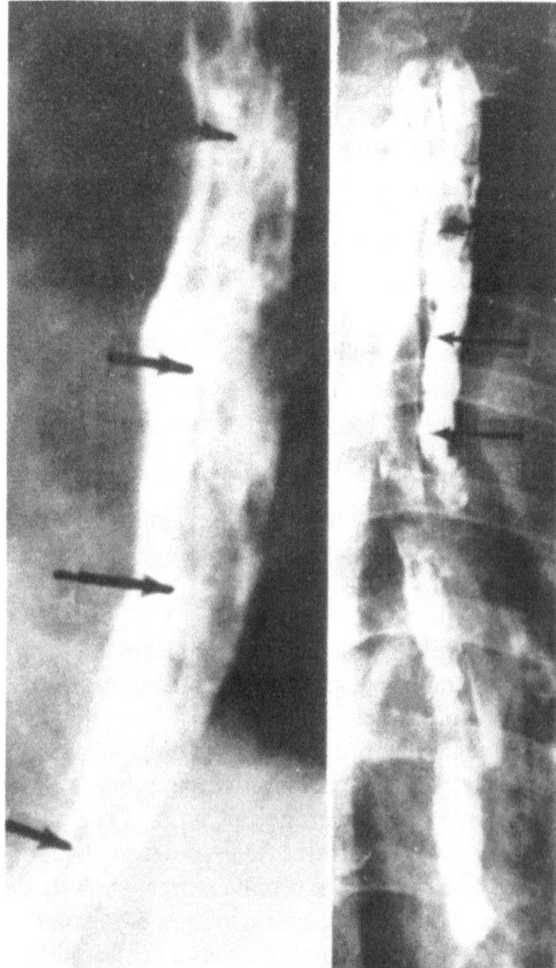

FIGURE 99.
The mucosal stripe sign secondary to incomplete esophageal rupture (at arrows). From Lowman, R., et al. The roentgen aspects of intramural dissection of the esophagus. Radiology, 93:1329, Dec. 1969. Radiologic Society of North America, Easton, Pa.

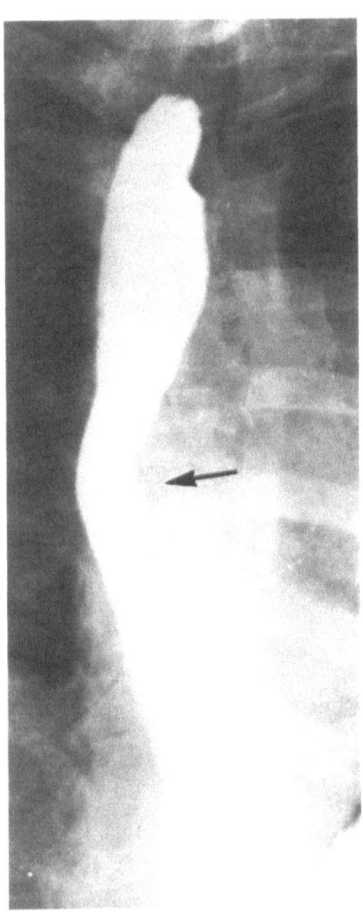

FIGURE 100.

Esophageal erosion with rupture of the esophagus secondary to a syphlitic aneurysm. Site of erosion (at arrow).

tained within the retropharyngeal space, a localized abscess forms. If the perforation extends into the prevertebral space, the infection can spread inferiorly into the mediastinum and produce an acute mediastinitis. Some degree of subcutaneous and mediastinal emphysema is usually present. A contrast swallow may reveal the presence of the perforation site. Where frank perforation is suspected an aqueous contrast medium is preferable, because it is readily resorbed outside the lumen. Before endoscopy is attempted, therefore, the hypopharyngeal area should always be examined roentgenologically and fluoroscopically with a barium swallow to exclude any diverticula. The roentgenologic findings of perforations will be the same as just described.

Instrumentation can produce not only actual perforations but also mucosal and/or submucosal tears. These can be detected during opacification studies of the esophagus. Such tears are visualized on barium swallow as extraluminal parallel channels of barium or irregularities in the mucosal pattern of the wall of the hypopharynx with intramural extension of the medium. These tears are most common in the hypopharyngeal area, above the esophageal sphincter. The sphincter itself may be in spastic contraction during the examination, producing a temporary obstruction. Repeated attempts at passing an endoscope can produce such tears, especially when there is fixation of the hypopharyngeal wall by fiberosclerosis or chronic spondylitis.

Incomplete rupture of the esophagus following instrumental trauma may also produce intramural seepage of barium following a barium swallow, with the appearance of a double lumen separated by a translucent stripe, referred to as the "mucosal stripe sign" (153). The lumen itself becomes cleared of barium, with the extraluminal, intramural barium retained excessively long within the esophageal wall (Fig. 99). Spontaneous recovery usually takes place.

Erosions

Esophageal erosions with perforation can be the result of injury to the esophagus, following the ingestion of alkali or acid solutions eroding the wall of the esophagus. Undetected foreign bodies, especially in children, may also produce esophageal erosions. Such erosions with sudden rupture into the esophagus producing massive hemorrhage may also occur in patients with an adherent luetic or arteriosclerotic aneurysm. The rupture site may be partly occluded by blood clots. The site of rupture may occasionally be observed on radiologic examination following the ingestion of barium, as a localized, shallow irregularity at the site of the perforation (Fig. 100). Erosions into the esophagus also take place secondary to Pott's abscess of tuberculous spondylitis, suppurative paraesophageal nodes, or malignant lymphomas. Perforations also may be caused by primary esophageal neoplasms (Fig. 101). The presence of a fistulous tract demonstrated radiologically may be diagnostic.

Ruptures

Spontaneous rupture of a normal esophagus may be caused by severe vomiting with a full distended stomach, most commonly following an alcoholic bout. This entity is known as the "Boerhaave's syndrome." The perforation is caused by the sudden elevation of intraluminal esophageal pressure associated with a tear usually on the left side of the esophagus and above the level of the contracted lower sphincter. This portion of the lower end of the esophagus has been shown experimentally to have the weakest wall. Spontaneous rupture of the esophagus, however, can also occur at different sites in the presence of a diseased esophagus, stricture, diverticulum, or hiatal hernia.

(A)   (B)

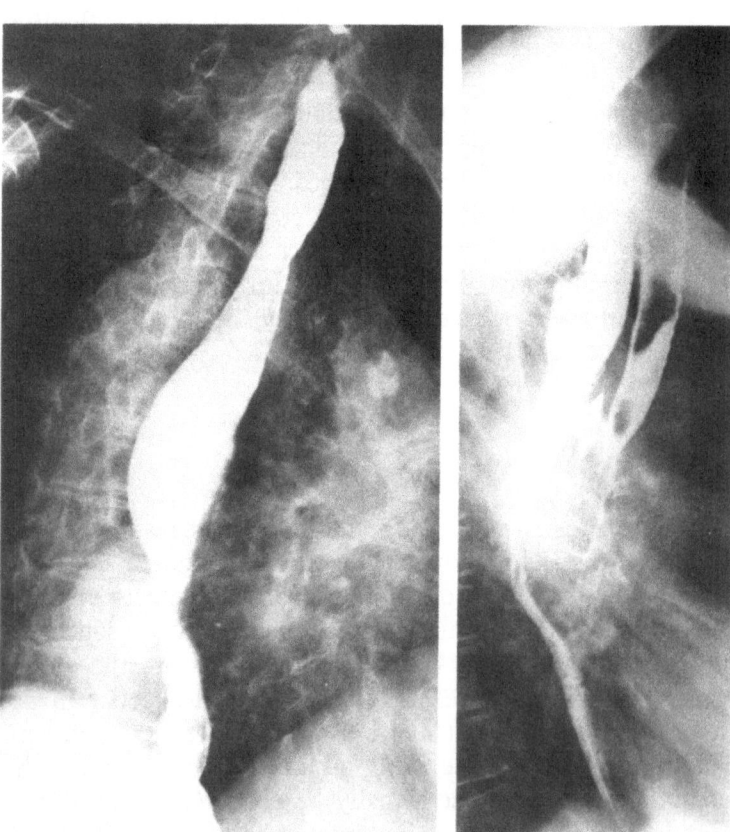

FIGURE 101.
Perforated esophagus at site of primary malignant disease. (A and B) Two different patients.

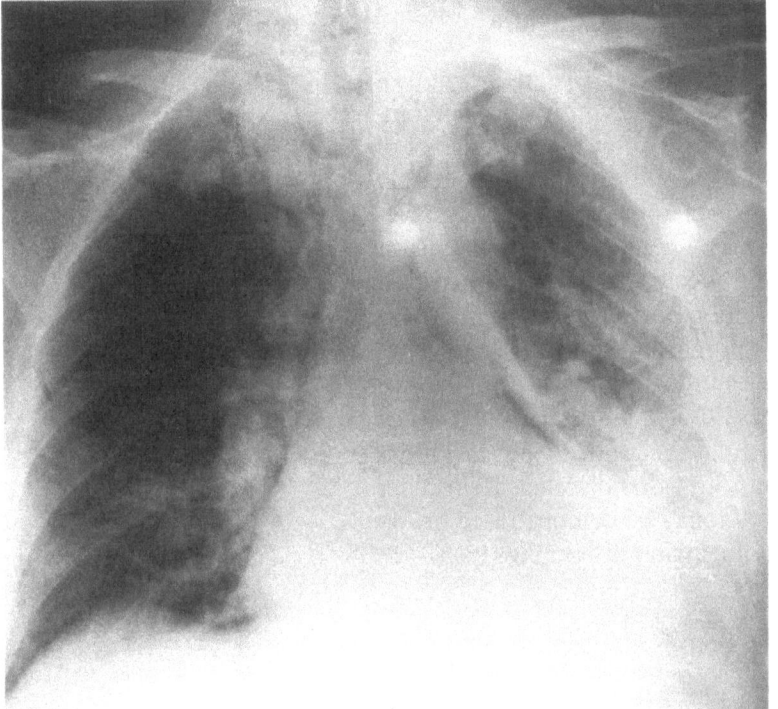

(A)

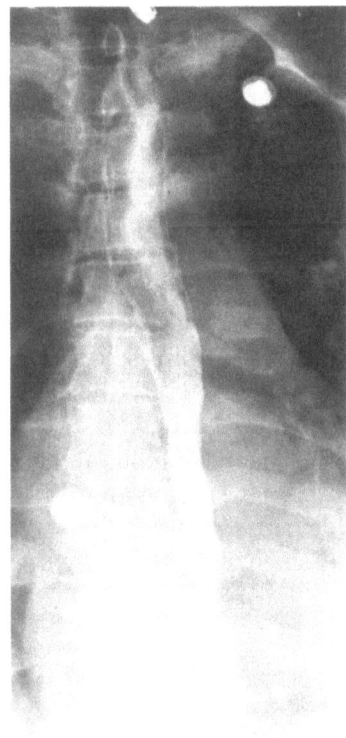

FIGURE 102.
Boerhaave's syndrome. Spontaneous esophageal rupture. (A) Chest film, (B) esophagogram showing site of rupture. Lower end of esophagus on the left side.

(B)

A sudden onset of severe chest pain during or immediately after a vomiting bout is the characteristic clinical manifestation of a spontaneous rupture of the esophagus. On radiologic examination of the chest, mediastinal and subcutaneous cervical emphysema and left-sided pleural effusion are observed frequently. A "V" sign, caused by air outlining the fascial pleural planes and diaphragmatic pleura, has been described (170). Hydropneumothorax is present if the tear is extensive. An aqueous contrast swallow will show extraluminal contrast in the chest cavity at the site of the rupture and in the mediastinum and/or interpleural space (Fig. 102).

A neonatal Boerhaave syndrome has also been reported (104). It differs from the adult type in that a tension pneumo- or hydropneumothorax is present. It occurs more frequent in females and more commonly on the right side. The right-sided predelection of the tear in infancy results from the position of the lower end of the esophagus; it is situated on the right side, whereas the aorta protects its left lateral wall. The precipitating cause, as in adults, is a sudden increase in esophageal luminal pressure.

Mallory–Weiss syndrome

Instead of a spontaneous rupture of the esophagus being produced during a severe bout of retching and vomiting, an incomplete tear of the esophageal mucosa may occur at the level of the gastroesophageal junction, followed almost immediately by hematemsis (5). This condition is more common in association with a sliding hiatal hernia, where a sudden distension of the herniated stomach can occur against a contracted sphincter. The tear is usually a long mucosal laceration. Spontaneous healing takes place or a chronic ulcer may develop at the site of the tear (52). Radiologic examination at the time of the hemorrhage may show retained barium within the channel, produced by the tear at the gastroesophageal junction (Fig. 103). Later in the course of this disorder, if an ulcer develops at the site of the tear, it may be demonstrated on radiologic examination with the ingestion of barium.

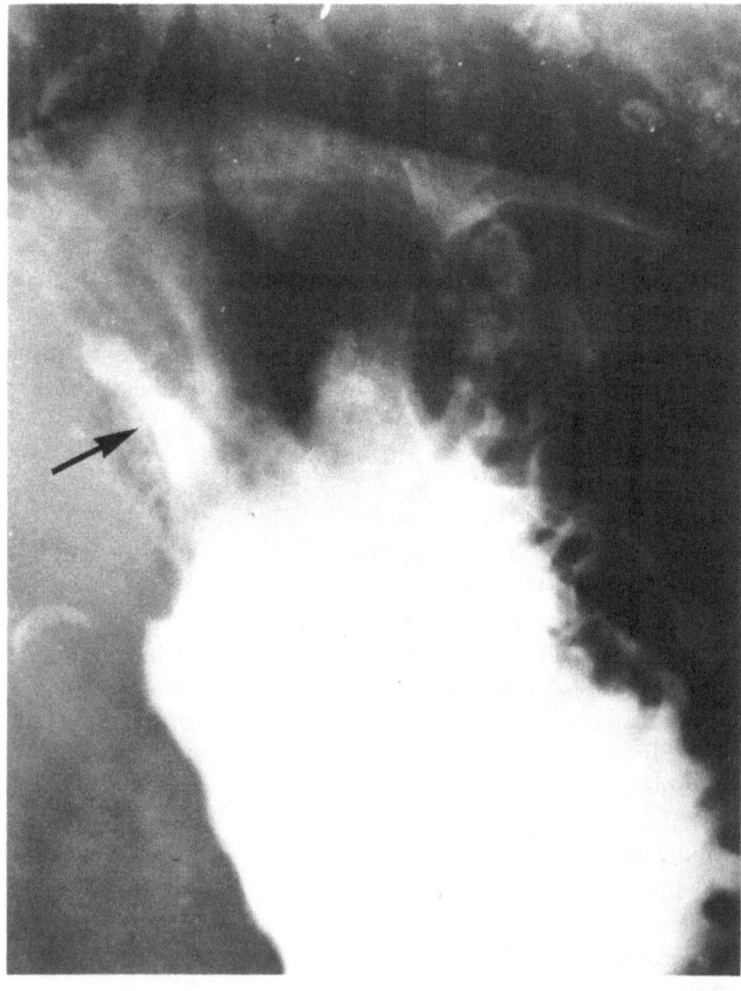

FIGURE 103.
Mallory–Weiss syndrome. Lacerated mucosa (arrow) at gastroesophageal junction.

CHAPTER

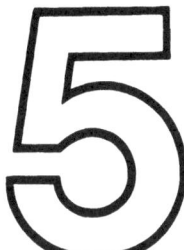

FUNCTIONAL, INVOLUTIONAL, AND DEGENERATIVE DISORDERS

FUNCTIONAL CHANGES

Functional changes or impaired peristaltic action of the upper gastrointestinal tract may occur with or without obvious organic abnormalities. These functional changes consist of abnormal motor manifestations that can be radiologically demonstrated in the absence of symptoms, that are detectable only on manometry with or without radiologic findings and symptoms; or that present with radiologic abnormal manometric findings and a clearly defined symptom complex. These functional alterations are usually transient, intermittent, and often recurrent but may become chronic and constant. These physiologic changes may also be caused by emotional, local, or systemic factors.

Psychic functional disturbances

In the absence of demonstrable organic findings, radiologically, endoscopically, or by manometric tests, when an usually sudden, severe attack of dysphagia occurs the disorder may be ascribed to severe emotional problems.

Globus hystericus

"Globus hystericus" is an emotional disturbance usually observed in young women, who complain of a "lump" in the throat interfering with normal swallowing. Endoscopy, manometry, and cinefluorography are normal. The condition usually recedes spontaneously, but treatment of the emotional factors may be helpful.

Functional dysphagia

Functional dysphagia is also a psychologic disorder precipitated by traumatic events. The patients chew their food carefully and for a long period, using the front teeth. Swallows are made gingerly because of the fear of choking. Severe malnutrition may result. No abnormal radiologic findings are apparent (71). Psychiatric treatment may be necessary.

Hysterical dysphagia

Hysterical dysphagia is a more severe and protracted entity with relatively constant radiologic findings. These include poor bolus formation, hesitant deglutition, asymmetrical swallowing, stasis of barium in the valleculae and pyriform sinuses, poor distensibility of the hypopharynx, lack of inversion of the epiglottis, and poor elevation of the larynx. These radiologic findings disappear spontaneously as the dysphagia subsides. This disorder has been ascribed to an emotional disturbance, although it may represent an early stage of sideropenic dysphagia (see Chapter 6)

Functional vomiting

Functional vomiting without nausea may be habitual, being occasionally observed in emotionally disturbed patients. This disorder resembles rumination or self-induced vomiting to gain relief from the epigastric distress of peptic ulcer or other gastric disturbances. Radiologic examination is noncontributory.

Neuromuscular disturbances

Functional disorders secondary to neuromuscular disturbances (60) can be ascribed to acute, chronic, or segmental spasm; vigorous achalasia; and "elevator" esophagus.

Acute spasm

Acute spasm of the sphincters, intermittent and inconstant in nature, may be secondary to emotional factors. However, it is also associated with local or remote reflex action as a result of other local or systemic organic abnormalities. At roentgenologic examination the contracted pharyngoesophageal sphincter is observed as a narrowed segment several centimeters long and deviated anteriorly (Fig. 104). The pharyngoesophageal sphincter in this disorder opens slowly at the approach of a bolus. A prominent cricopharyngeal impression has been described as being the contracted sphincter (214). We

FIGURE 104.
Spasm of the pharyngoesophageal sphincter (at arrow).

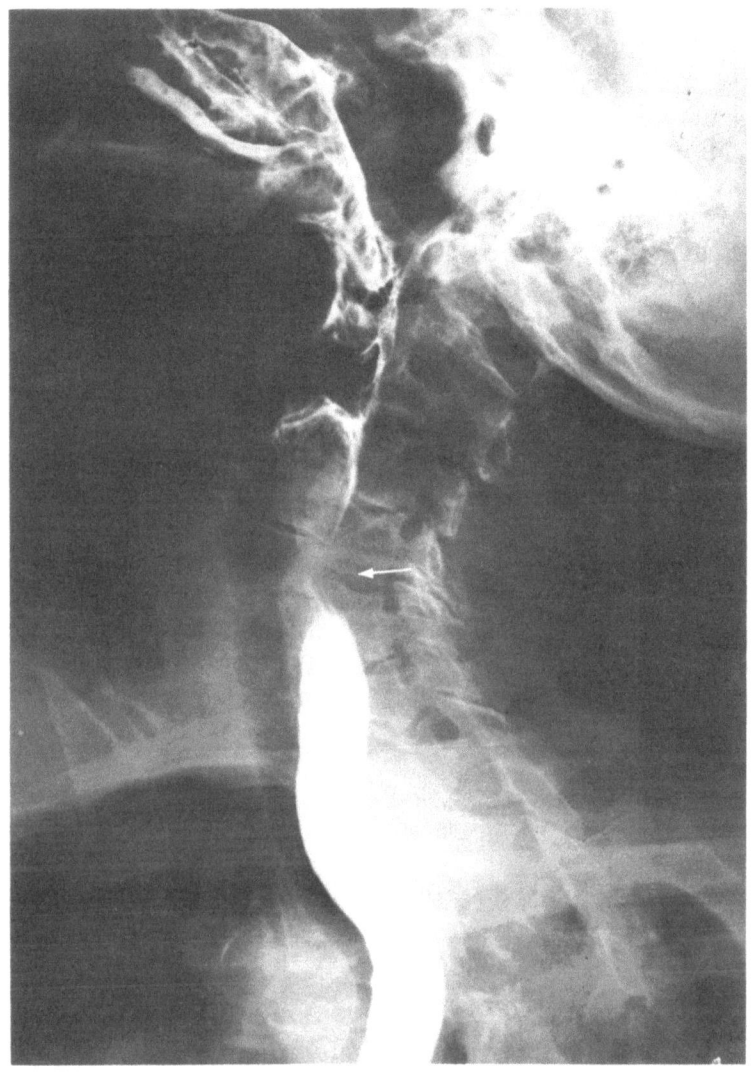

have observed a prominent cricopharyngeal muscle impression repeatedly in numerous individuals, in the absence of symptoms. However, if a patient complains of dysphagia and the only finding noted is a prominent cricopharyngeal impression, the possibility of hypertrophy of the transverse fibers of this muscle must be considered as the causative factor. If both the impression and a contracted sphincter are present, then the symptoms are most likely caused by a spastic sphincter. This concept can be supported when manometric studies show a high pressure level in the sphincter zone segment. Idiopathic spasm of the upper sphincter may be of psychologic origin in young and emotionally unstable individuals.

Similarly, acute spasm of the lower esophageal sphincter can be encountered with or without consistent changes in the upper sphincter. A filiform type of narrowing of the lower sphincter, usually located within or slightly above the esophageal hiatal canal, may be noted, with intermittent sluggish emptying of the esophagus (Fig. 105). Manometry confirms the presence of a hypertensive sphincter (47). Such spasm, however, is inconstant. It may recur, occasionally associated with symptoms of substernal pain, mild dysphagia, or discomfort. Again, such spasm may be secondary to emotional causes or reflex stimulation from local or remote sites. The symptoms in such instances are relieved by antispasmodics, such as probanthine or buscopan. Prolonged intubation of the esophagus may be responsible for persistant spasm of both sphincters as well as the regurgitation of acid gastric contents into the lower esophagus, with secondary severe inflammatory changes.

Simple spasm of the esophagus other than of the sphincters, is manifested on radiologic examination as localized areas of overactivity consisting of multiple ripples or contractions traveling rapidly along the esophagus. These contractions actually represent exaggerated secondary peristaltic waves. Temporary shortening of the esophagus during these contractions may occur at the same time, with or without an esophageal hiatal hernia (Fig. 106).

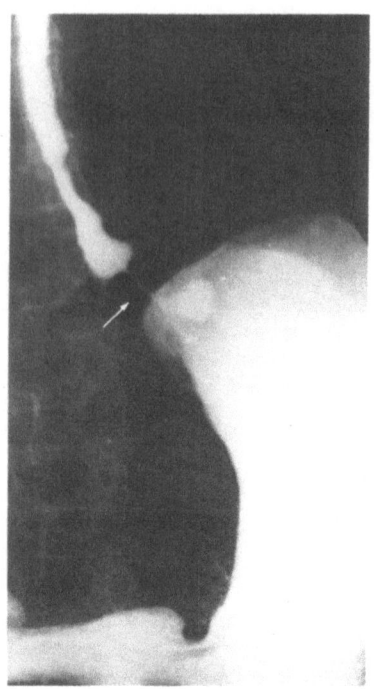

FIGURE 105.
Spasm of the lower esophageal sphincter (at arrow).

(A)   (B)

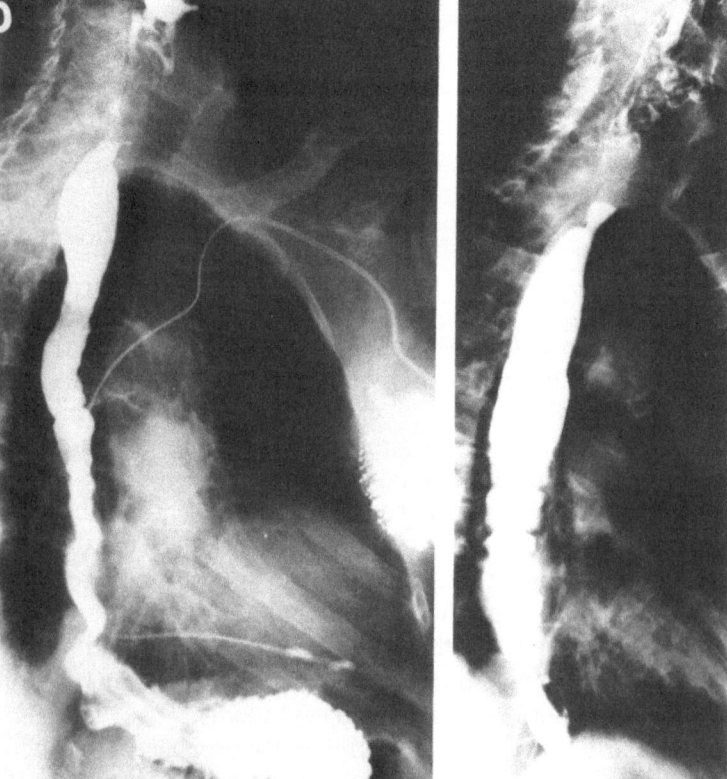

FIGURE 106.
Spasm of lower end of esophagus. (A) with foreshortening in presence of a pacemaker, and sliding hiatal hernia, (B) with shortening of the esophagus in the presence of a hiatal hernia in another patient.

Chronic spasm

Chronic spasm results from frequent attacks of acute spasm. In such instances, persistent high pressures are recorded in the sphincters even in the absence of esophageal dilatation or motor dysfunction, which often develop subsequently (Fig. 107). The chronic spasm eventually produces hypertrophic muscular changes in the esophagus, yet hypertrophy specifically of the upper and lower sphincters is rarely reported. Hypertrophy of the cricopharyngeal muscle above the contracted upper sphincter zone and of the circular muscular fibers of the lower esophagus does occur.

Diffuse spasm

Diffuse spasm (166) represents a neuromuscular disturbance chiefly involving the lower third of the esophagus. The disorder primarily is diagnosed in a radiologic examination. During the associated esophageal contractions substernal discomfort simulating cardiac pain may be experienced. Diffuse spasm is encountered often in young emotionally labile women, oc-

FIGURE 107.
Chronic spasm. Lower esophageal hypertensive sphincter at (A) first examination, (B) 2 years later.

(A) **(B)**

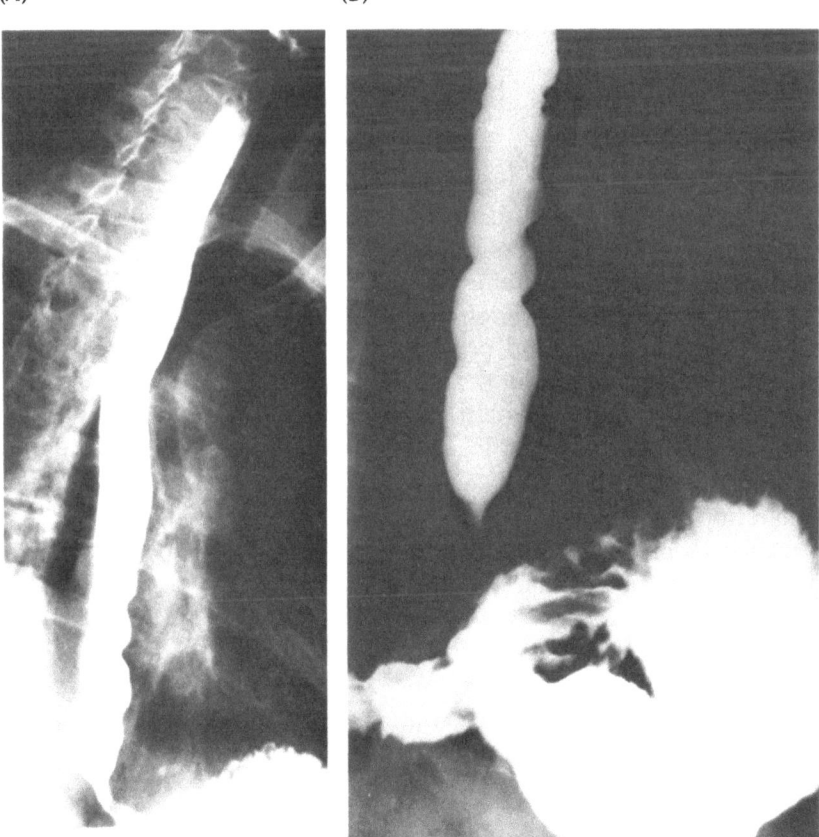

curring frequently in the presence of hiatal hernia and reflux esophagitis. Diffuse spasm of the esophagus simulates "curling" or the corkscrew esophagus (99) and is chiefly ascribed to degenerative changes in the esophageal wall.

Manometric studies are helpful in confirming the diagnosis of esophageal spasm. During manometry simultaneous, repetitive contractions of high amplitude involving the distal two-thirds of the esophagus (smooth muscle) are observed. These esophageal contractions are not responsive to the mecholyl test. A normal resting pressure is present in both the upper and lower sphincters, although pressure may be increased slightly in the lower sphincter.

On radiologic examination of individuals with diffuse esophageal spasm the primary peristaltic wave is suddenly replaced by segmental uncoordinated contractions involving the lower third of the esophagus. These abnormal waves are obliterated after ingestion of a subsequent bolus with the reappearance of normal peristaltic waves (Fig. 108).

A more severe or persistent form of diffuse spasm producing a pseudo-diverticular type of contractions is called segmental spasm, being responsible frequently for substernal pain (Figs. 109A,B and 110). In this disorder, the esophagus is not dilated, nor is obstruction observed. However, hypertrophy of the esophageal musculature eventually develops (see section on giant hypertrophy of the esophagus).

Vigorous achalasia

Vigorous achalasia (71) is described as a neuromuscular disorder having motor pattern features resembling both diffuse spasm and achalasia. Vigorous achalasia is a response to a poorly functioning lower esophageal sphincter. Manometric studies reveal a normal lower sphincter pressure with poor relaxation of the sphincter on swallowing. On radiologic examination, periods of severe, vigorous, irregular, segmental contractions of the lower esophagus occur; they are repetitive and may not be obliterated by peristaltic waves (Fig. 111). These contractions are accompanied by substernal discomfort. Usually some degree of obstruction and esophageal dilatation is noted, with occasional esophageal reflux. The presence of an hiatal hernia is not unusual, possibly accounting for imparied function of the lower sphincter.

The radiologist will encounter many varying degrees of lower esophageal spasm, as manifestations of motor dysfunction, with or without evident structural lesions. An accurate evaluation of such observations often is challenging. An underlying primary disorder, such as esophageal hiatal hernia, should be eliminated. The characteristics of the contractions in the context of the age of the patient and the symptoms

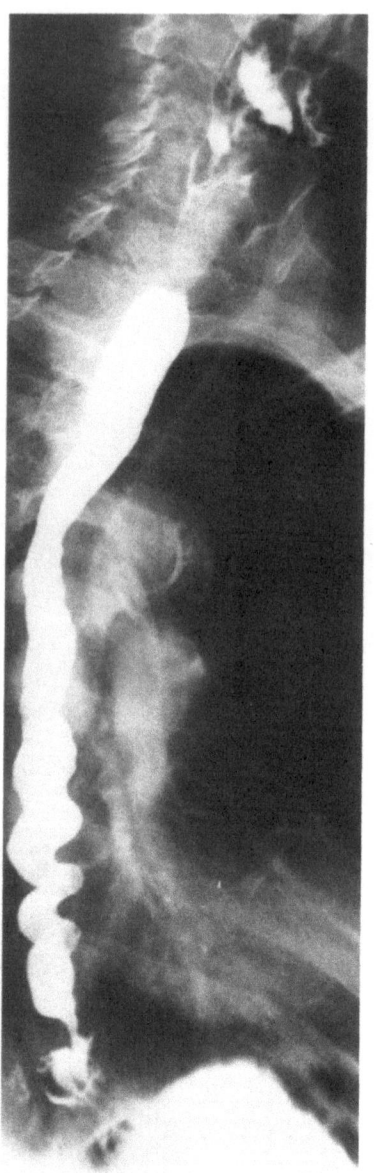

FIGURE 108.
Diffuse spasm in the presence of a sliding hiatal hernia and some degree of invagination.

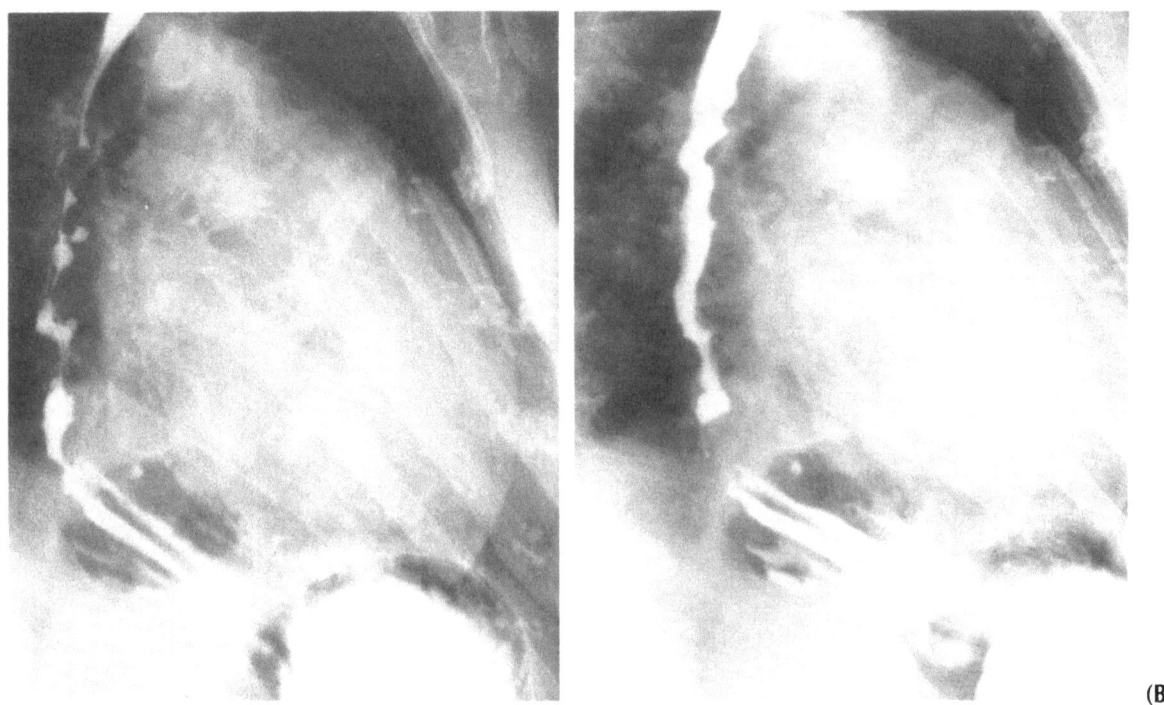

(A)

(B)

FIGURE 109.
Early segmental spasm. (A and B) Same patient. Note presence of pseudo-diverticula.

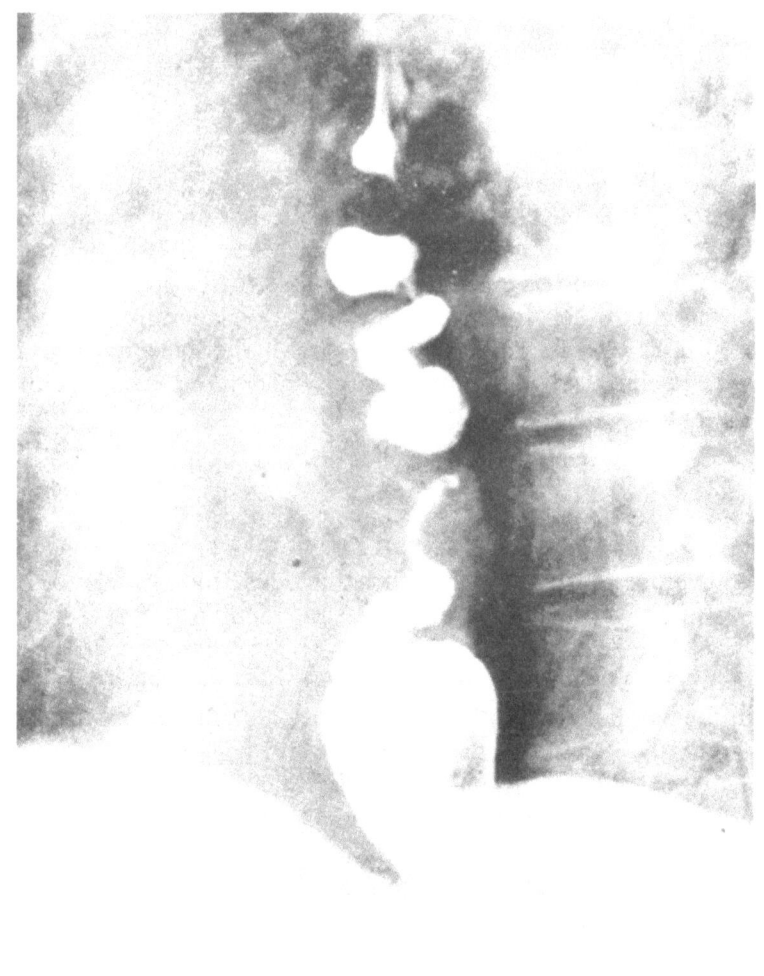

FIGURE 110.
Segmental spasms, advanced. From A. S. Johnstone, Lesions of the esophagus of special radiological interest. Avery Jones, ed. Medical Trend Series in Gastroenterology. Butterworth, Woburn, England, 1952.

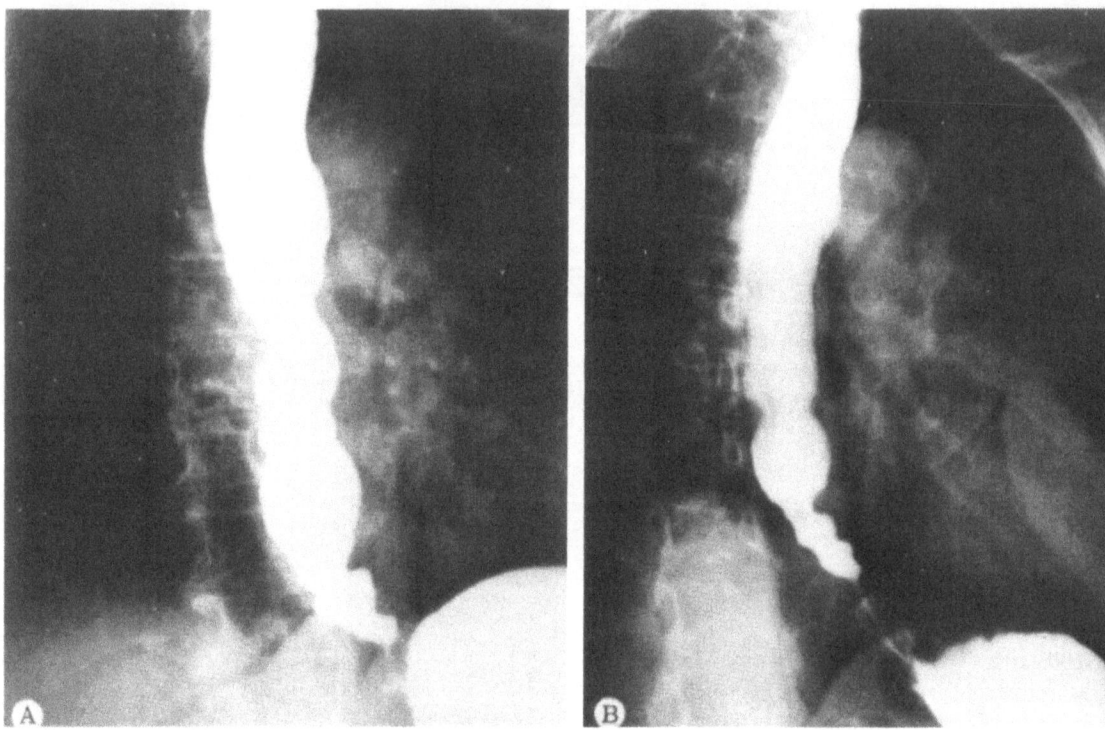

FIGURE 111.
Vigorous Achalasia. (A) Expiration, (B) inspiration. From Ellis, F. H., and Olsen, A. M. *Achalasia*, 1969. Courtesy W. B. Saunders Co., Philadelphia, Pa.

should be considered. The effect on the contractions of repeated ingestion of barium, their obliteration by peristaltic waves, and the presence or absence of primary peristaltic contractions should be considered. The radiologic demonstration of obstruction of the lower end of the esophagus and esophageal dilatation is important. The area of the lower sphincter zone itself must be evaluated carefully to determine whether it remains contracted or is patent.

Elevator esophagus

"Elevator esophagus" (65) is a term that refers to a distinct motor dysfunction of the lower esophagus in elderly patients, associated with a serious local or distant organic disease, usually a malignancy. Fluoroscopic examination, in the upright position immediately following the ingestion of a barium mixture and especially after the first few swallows, reveals a frenzied and distinctly abnormal up and down motion of the fluid level of barium within the lower esophagus. The appearance resembles an erratic elevator. This fluoroscopic pattern disappears when the patient is examined in the prone or supine position. The cause of the disorder is thought to be secondary to an impaired neuromuscular mechanism with disturbed peristalsis of local or reflex origin. It is reminiscent of diffuse esophageal spasm.

The disorder is often a clue to the presence of a serious organic lesion.

INVOLUTIONAL CHANGES

Involutional changes occur in the process of aging of the body tissues, resulting in thinning of muscles and ligaments and a general loss of muscle tone. Such changes are manifested in the esophagus muscle tone, with a downward shift of the larynx and upper sphincter and diminished tone of both upper and lower esophageal sphincters. Laxity of fascial attachments of the sphincter zone causes upward displacement of the lower sphincter, resulting in an increased incidence of esophageal hiatal hernia and redundancy of the entire esophagus (Fig. 112).

FIGURE 112.
Involutional changes: redundancy of the esophagus.

FIGURE 113.
Involutional changes: hypopharyngeal atonia in a 90-year-old patient.

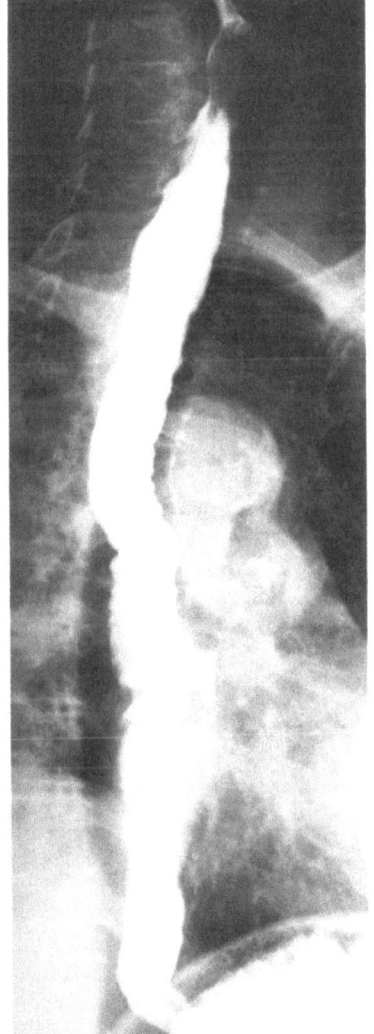

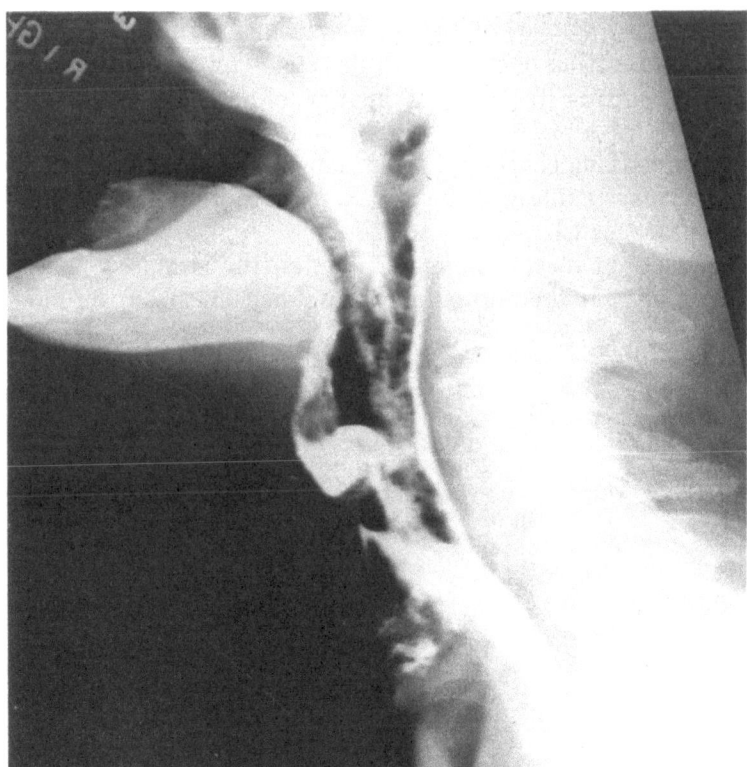

Muscular relaxation in the orohypopharyngeal area because of diminished tone results not only in the inferior shift of the larynx and upper sphincter but also in weaker peristaltic contractions (Fig. 113). As a result, the swallowing process is retarded, beginning in the mouth, where the tongue sections off smaller sized boluses with more frequent swallowing attempts. On radiologic examination, the hypopharynx is observed to be dilated and the pharyngoesophageal junction is prominent, resulting in stasis above the level of the sphincter zone. Pseudo-diverticula of the hypopharynx develops, simulating small true hypopharyngeal diverticula. Because of the muscular atonia an increased incidence of true diverticula in this area has been noted.

The normal efficiency of the sphincters is also impaired as a result of excessive swallowing of air, belching, pyrosis, and regurgitation. Esophageal reflux is frequent but may not be as serious in older as in younger individuals because of the diminishing gastric acidity accompanying advancing age. Redundancy of the esophagus also produces more frequent invaginations and prolapse of the mucosa at its lower end, possibly contributing to a mild degree of physiologic esophageal volvulus (see section on volvulus).

Hiatal insufficiency and hernia

Hiatal insufficiency and hernia may be considered secondary to involutional changes. The sliding variety of hernia appears to occur in association with relaxation of the normal attachments of the lower end of the esophagus, resulting in the upward migration of the lower sphincter. This change accounts for the greater frequency of this type of hernia in elderly individuals with or without symptoms. In infancy and childhood an underlying congenital abnormality is frequently a cause of hernia, particularly in the presence of a short esophagus (branchioesophagus).

Based on recent anatomic findings, the phrenoesophageal membrane is the normal anchoring mechanism of the lower

DIAG. 10

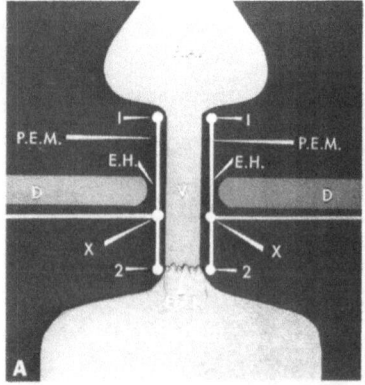
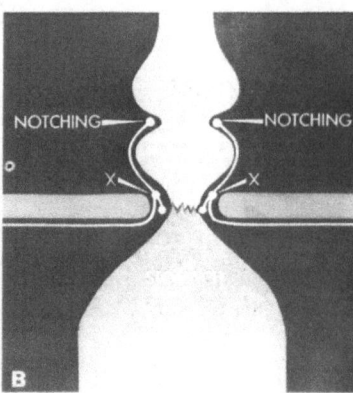
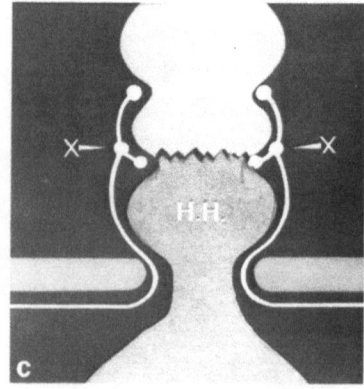

FIGURE 114

Hiatal insufficiency. Arrow at upper attachment of phrenoesophageal membrane. From Zaino, C., et al. *The Lower Esophageal Vestibular Complex,* 1963. Courtesy Charles C Thomas, Publisher, Springfield, Illinois.

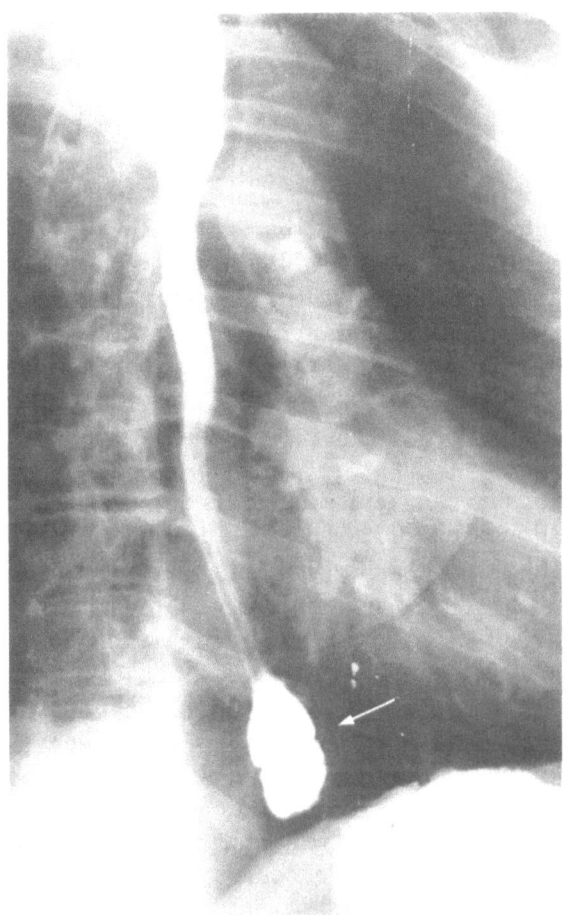

DIAGRAM 10

Anatomic changes involving the lower esophageal sphincter in the presence of hiatal insufficiency and hernia. (A) Normal anatomy, (B) hiatal insufficiency, (C) hiatal hernia. PEM, phrenoesophageal membrane; #1, upper attachment of the PEM; #2, lower attachment of the PEM; EH, Esophageal hiatus; D, diaphragm; X, point of division between the ascending limbs of the PEM; EPL, epithelial line (gastroesophageal junction). From Zaino, C., et al. *The Lower Esophageal Vestibular Complex,* 1963. Courtesy Charles C Thomas, Publisher, Springfield, Illinois.

sphincteric segment, being located within the hiatal canal (Diagram 10-A). Abnormal upward migration of the sphincter zone, increasing in frequency with advancing years, is the first step in the development of a hiatal hernia in adults. This upward migration is referred to as hiatal insufficiency (Diagram 10-B). The underlying factors are a lax muscular tone of the diaphragm and esophagus, thinning of the surrounding membranes, loss of the subdiaphragmatic fat surrounding the esophageal hiatus, and changes involving the upper abdominal structures which favor an increase in intraabdominal pressure and a decrease in intrathoracic pressure (Fig. 114).

With progressive upward migration of the sphincter, a hiatal hernia becomes inevitable (Diagram 10-C). The most common involutional type of hiatal hernia is the sliding variety, which is characterized, initially, by the upward pull of the gastro-esophageal junction with resultant funneling and obliteration of the cardiac incisura (Fig. 115). With progressive widening of the esophageal hiatus, part of the fundus may slip into the hiatus and migrate upward with the addition of a paraesophageal component which may be confused with a diverticulum (Fig. 116). Most sliding esophageal hiatal hernias are asymptomatic.

Esophageal hiatal hernias are more likely to produce symptoms and complications in younger patients, where they often are related to underlying congenital causes. The paraesophageal or rolling type of hiatal hernia is caused by the presence of an unusually large esophageal hiatus that permits part of the stomach to wedge itself above the hiatus (usually on the left side), without upward migration of the gastroesophageal junction. In the presence of a patent infracardiac bursa on the right side a degree of herniation of the gastric cardia may occur within this residual sac, resulting in a small paraesophageal hiatal hernia on the right (Fig. 117) (see Chapter 3).

Occasionally this type of herniation occurs through a defect in the esophageal musculature adjacent to the esophagus and actually represents a paraesophageal hernia and not a paraesophageal hiatal hernia. Such hernias bear the eponym of Sweet (Fig. 118) (238). As the hernia increases in size, however, the few strands of diaphragmatic muscle separating it from the esophagus may tear so that a sizeable portion of the fundus is observed to be lodged next to the esophagus above the diaphragm. The esophageal hiatus in such instances is noted to be unusually large. The sliding and the paraesophageal types are noted as the two basic varieties of hiatal hernia, although minor variations of each type are encountered depending on the age of the patient and the primary causative factor.

The radiologic diagnosis of hiatal insufficiency or esophageal hiatal hernia is relatively simple (268). However, it may be difficult to duplicate the radiologic changes on repeat studies, particularly if the hernia is truly small, although infrequently such hernias can only be demonstrated in one position (Fig. 119). Because of this, if the presence or abscense of an esophageal hiatal hernia becomes essential in the differential diagnosis of substernal cardiogenic pain, multiple radiologic examinations may be necessary, with films obtained in various positions and in all phases of respiration (Fig. 120). The use of such special maneuvers as the Trendelenburg position mainly are considered to be unnecessary, but cineradiographic studies and, of course, fluoroscopic observation of the advancing primary bolus as it enters the gastric cardia are of considerable importance. Although the anatomicoradiologic landmarks may be obscured by abnormal contractions, the visualization and localization of the lower sphincter zone segment is the key to the diagnosis (Fig. 121). This sphincter zone is best delineated radiologically as a contracted segment, several centimeters long, being repetitively demonstrated, recurring in the same area and uniformally showing the same length and caliber. As the sphincter zone contracts, following repeated primary and secondary peristaltic waves, identification is

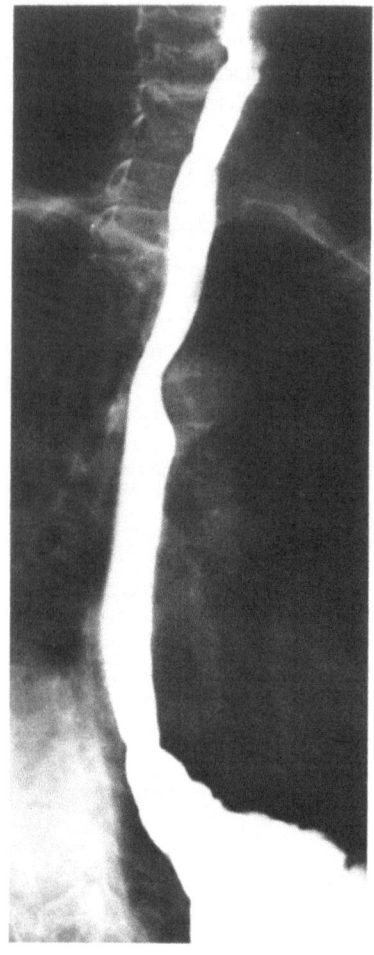

FIGURE 115.
Sliding-type hiatal hernia with funneling.

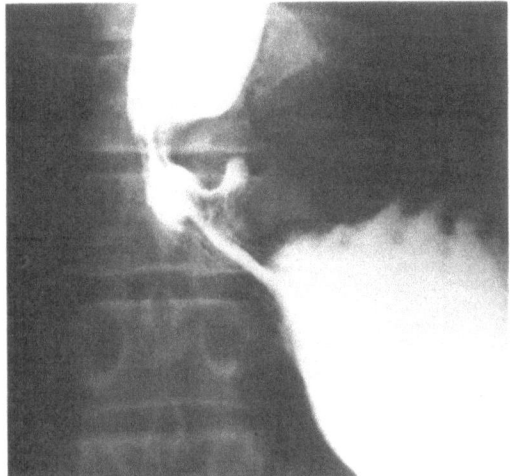

(A)

FIGURE 116.
Sliding-type hiatal hernia with a paraesophageal component resembling a diverticulum (A–C). (B) and (C) represents a different patient. Note presence of peptic esophagitis of the sphincter zone in (B) and (C).

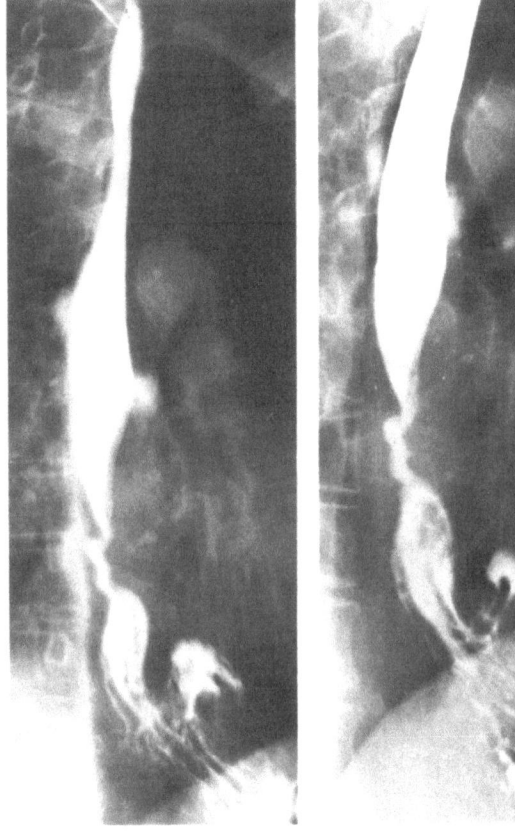

(B)   (C)

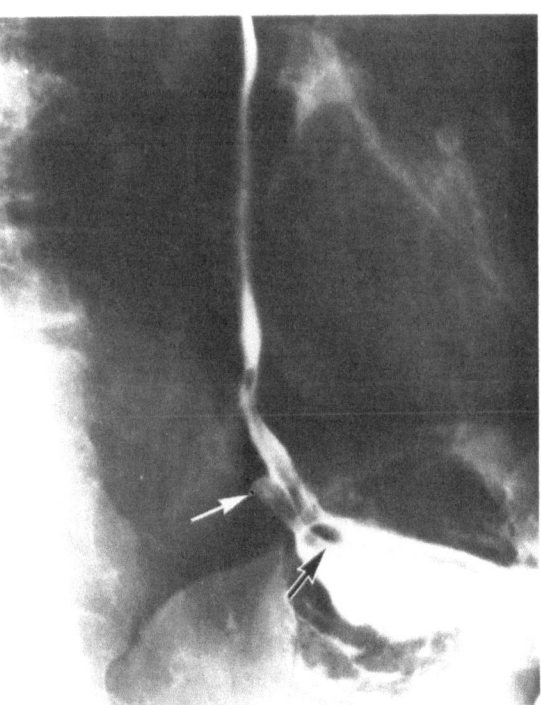

FIGURE 117.
Paraesophageal hiatal hernia (upper arrow). Gastroesophageal junction at lower arrows.

FIGURE 118.
Sweet-type paraesophageal hernia. (A and B) There is also a sliding-type hiatal hernia present. (C and D) Different patient; note two separate channels (at arrows).

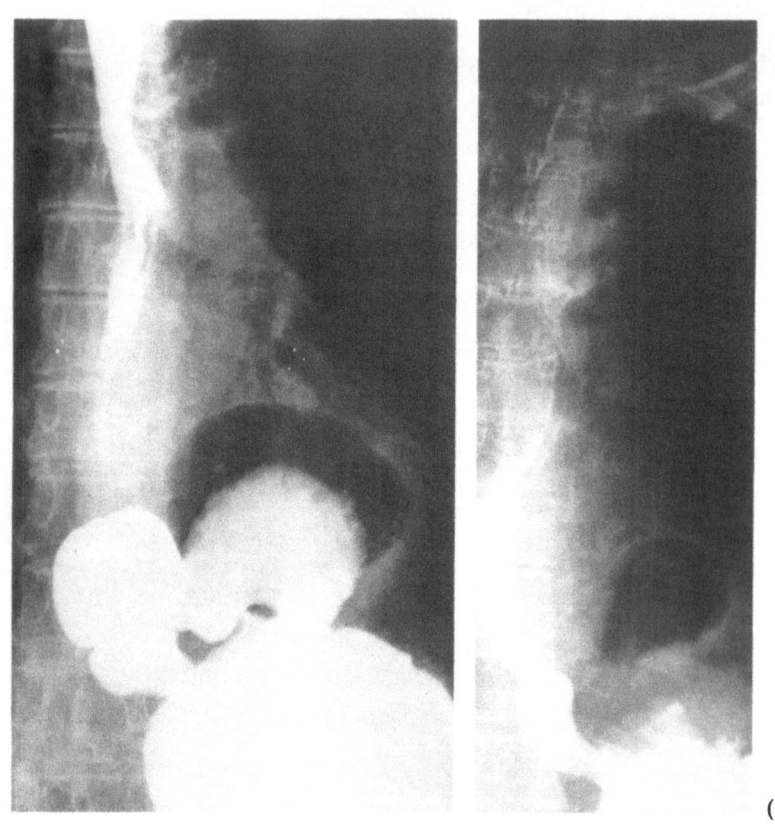

(A)

(B)

(C)

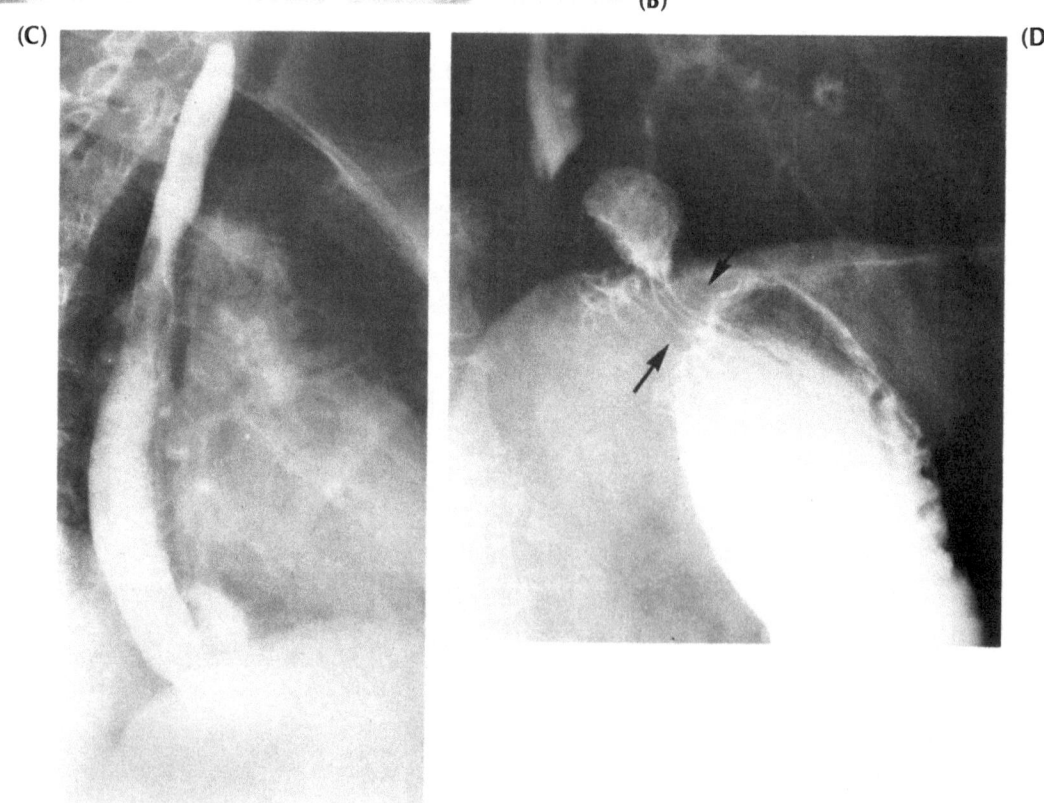

(D)

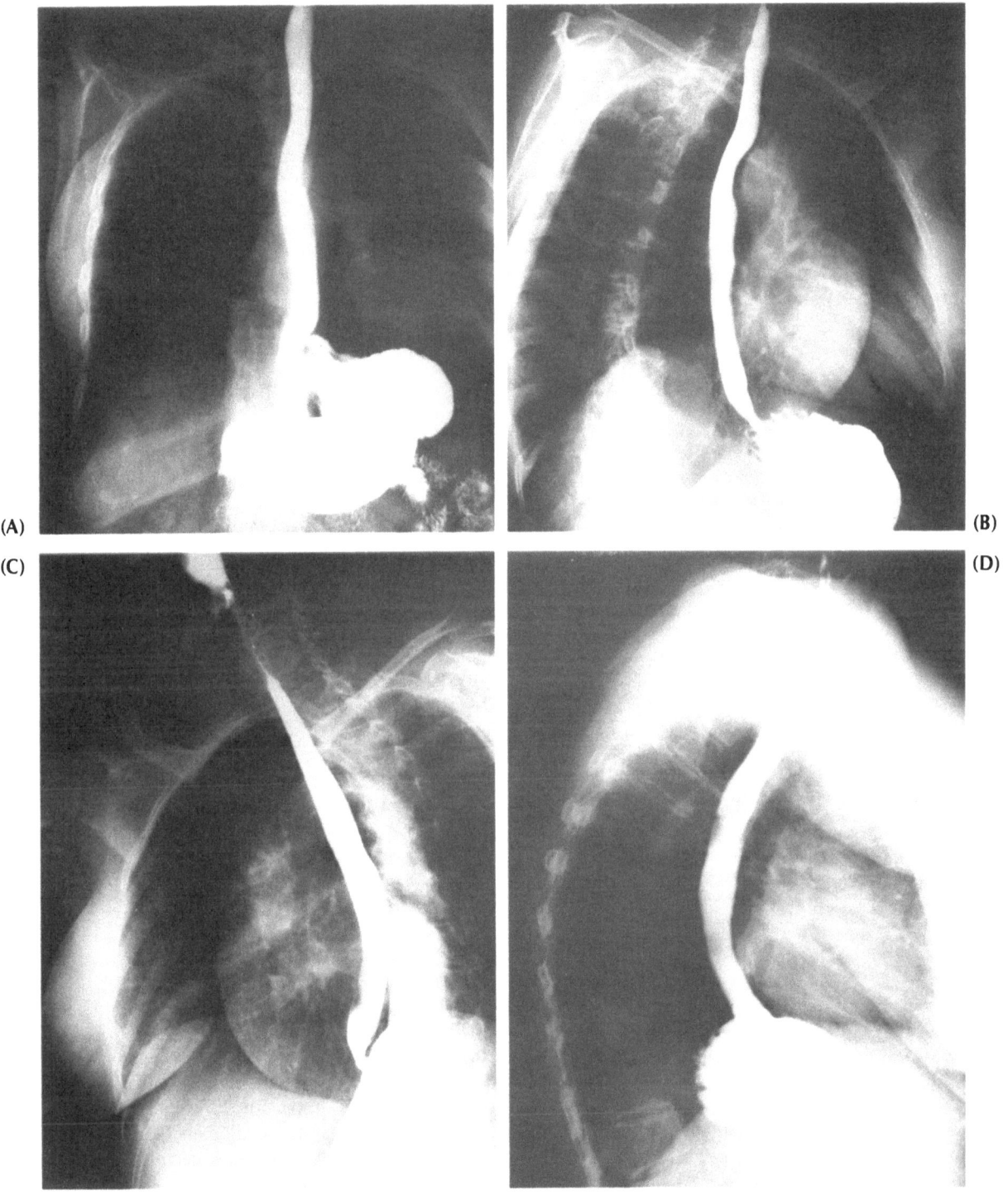

FIGURE 119.
Esophagograms in the supine position. (A) Frontal view, (B) left anterior oblique view, (C) right anterior oblique view, (D) lateral view. *Hiatal hernia* seen only in the frontal view.

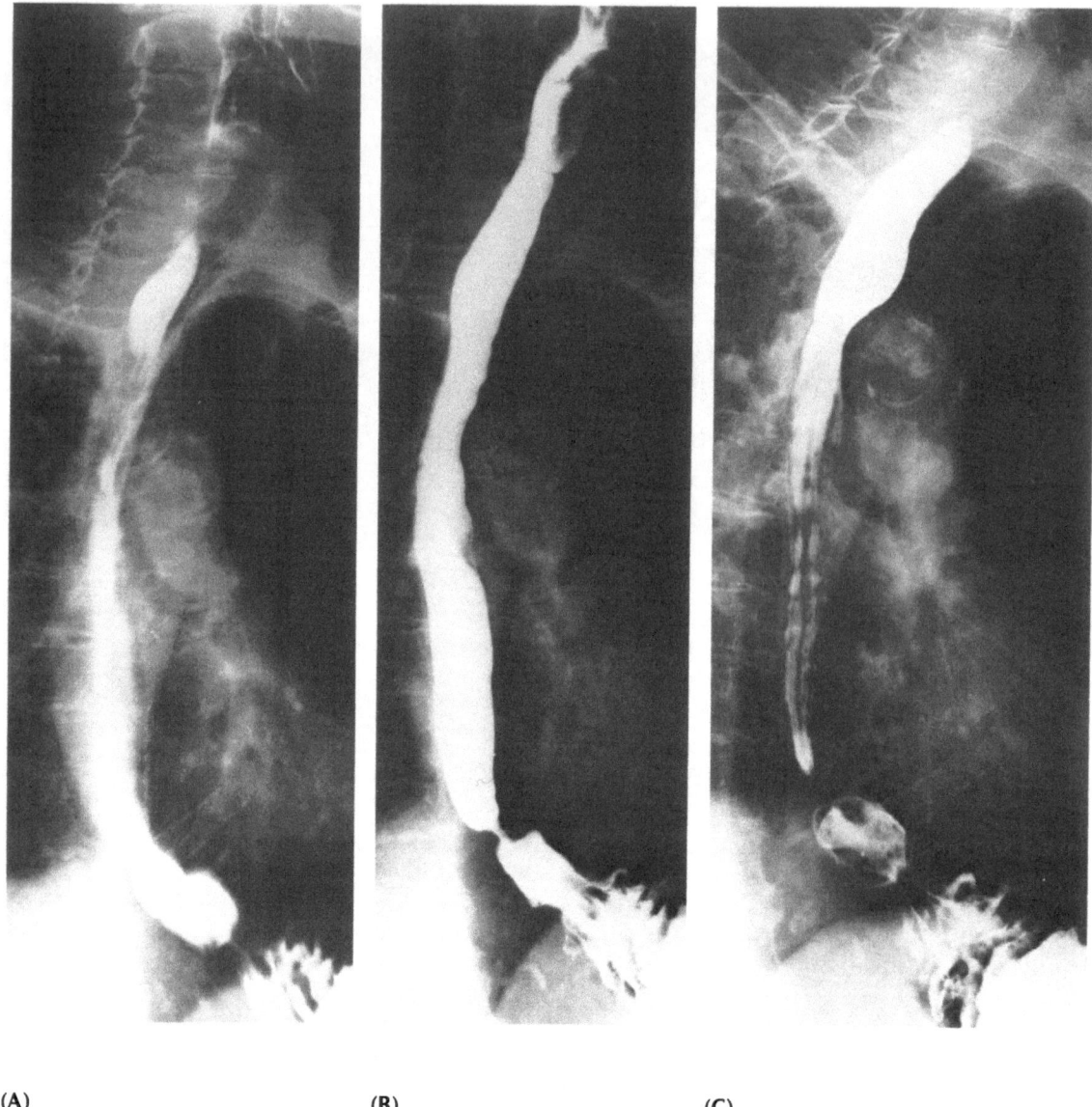

(A)   (B)   (C)

enhanced (Fig. 122). This segment also may be defined in its distended phase, when it is more difficult to detect (Fig. 123). If the contracted sphincter lies above the dome of the posterior segment of the diaphragm on full inspiration, particularly in the presence of a persistent phrenic ampulla (two dilated pockets above the diaphragm), it may be anticipated that an upward migration of the sphincter segment has taken place and that an hiatal insufficiency is present. If, in addition, a small knuckle of gastric cardia is identified below the contracted segment of the sphincter and above the diaphragm containing residual barium on a number of subsequent films (with three dilated pockets) then the diagnosis of a sliding-type hiatal hernia can be made (Diagram 10-C). The empty zone below

FIGURE 120.
Esophagograms in the right anterior oblique position. (A) Inspiration, (B) expiration, (C) at rest. Hiatal hernia best seen in (C). Note presence of a dilated lower sphincter in (A) and a contracted sphincter in (B) and (C).

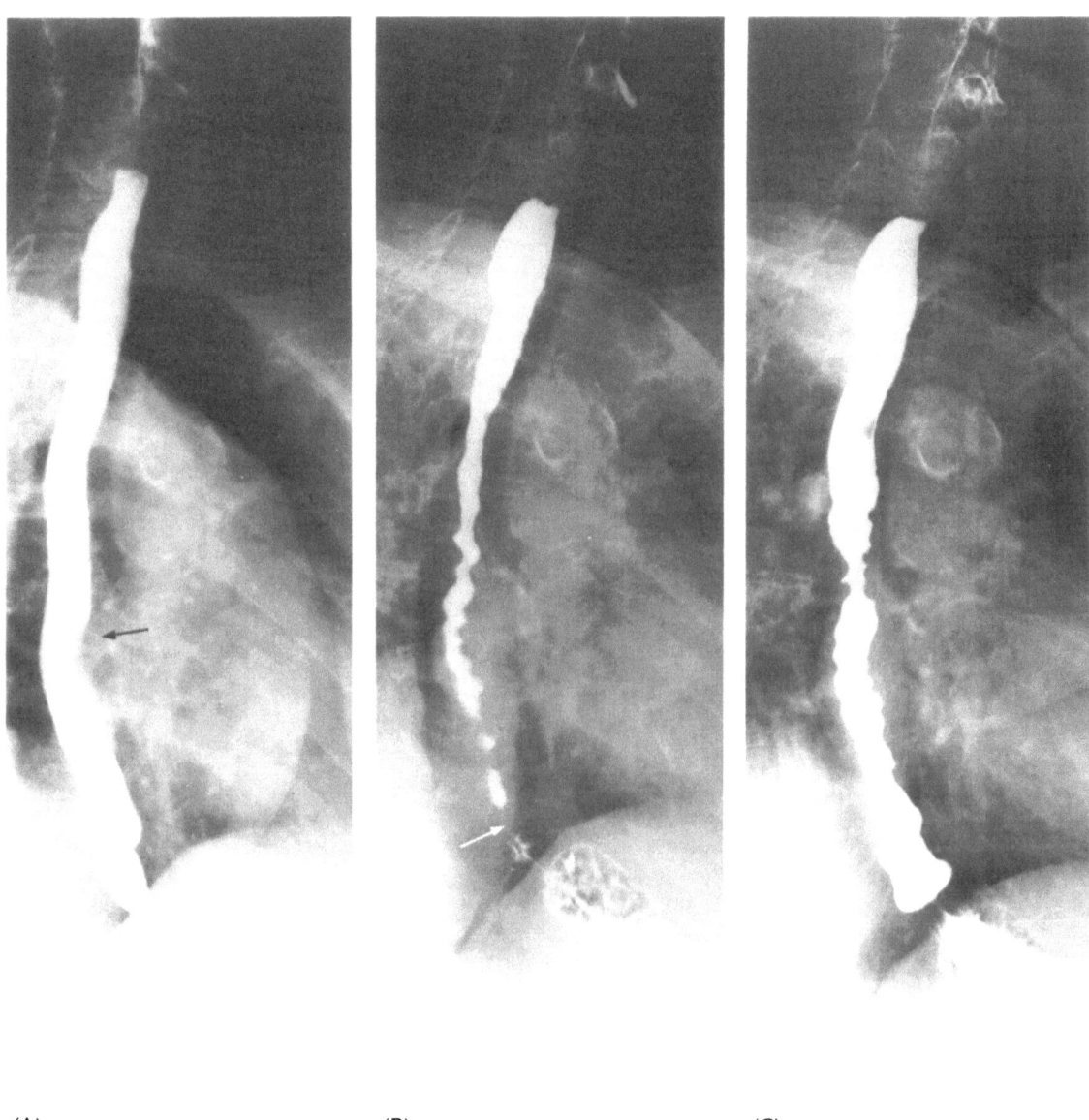

(A) (B) (C)

FIGURE 121.
Irritable esophagus in the presence of a small sliding hiatal hernia and an enlarged mediastinal lymph node. (A–C) All of the same patient in the RAO position. Arrow in (A) an inconsistent impression is present secondary to an enlarged mediastinal gland. Arrow in (B) shows position of contracted lower sphincter.

this level or additional narrowing of the cardia and/or fundus represents the portion of stomach within the hiatal canal (as seen in Fig. 123).

The effects on the lower esophageal segment by the phrenoesophageal membrane, in hiatal insufficiency, is noted at the attachment of the upper level of the sphincter zone (see Diagram 10-B). This results in notching at the site, caused by buckling of the mucosal membrane. With further upward migration and the development of a hiatal hernia, the pull is chiefly on the attachment at the lower level of the sphincter zone (gastroesophageal junction). Notching is thus produced at the lower level, with a gradual disappearance of the notches at the upper level. This notching at the gastroesophageal junction

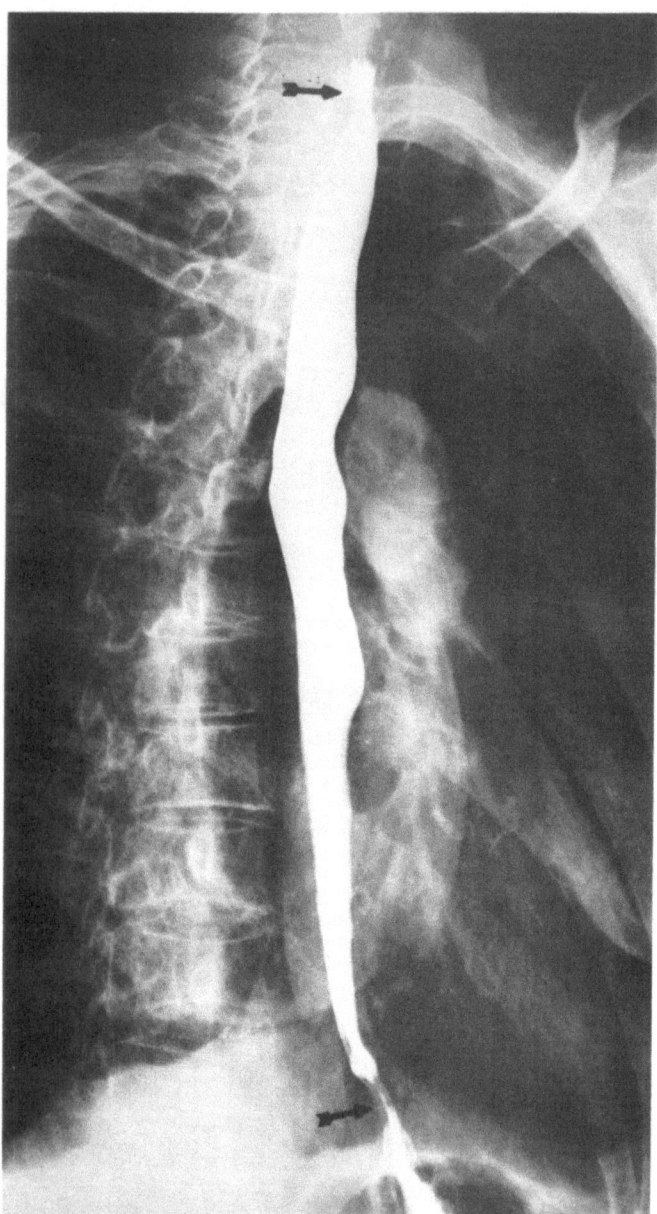

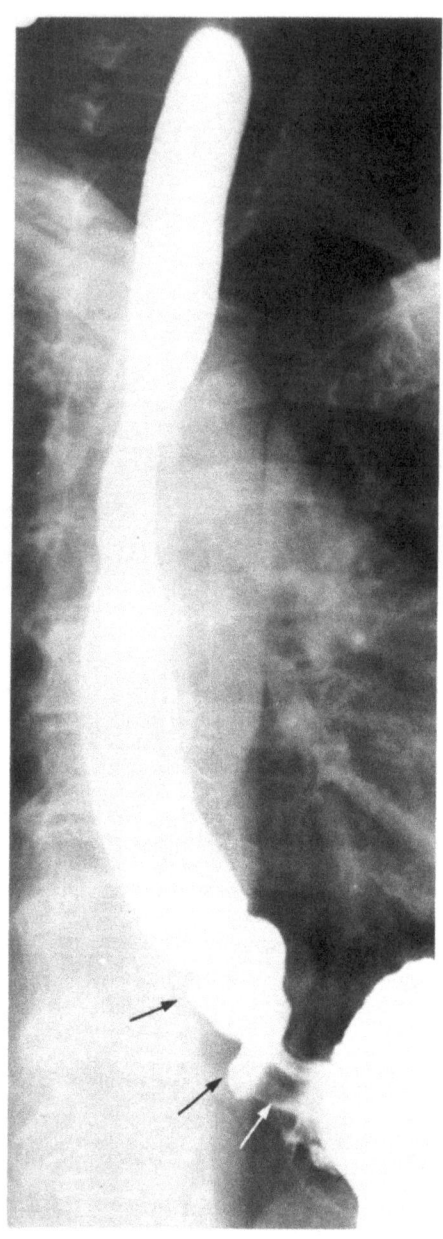

FIG. 122

FIG. 123

is caused also by a persistant mucosal fold, which may become a permanent ring demarcating the gastroesophageal junction and a sliding hiatal hernia (Fig. 124) (see Chapter 7).

The size of a hiatal hernia may be surprisingly large in the elderly, in the absence of any specific symptoms (Fig. 125). Large hernias may be identified on routine chest films appearing as large soft tissue masses with fluid levels observed through the heart. In very large hernias, the entire stomach may lie in the chest. A segment of the colon may also be present in the hernia.

FIGURE 122
Contracted sphincters (at arrows) in the presence of a small sliding-type hiatal hernia. Pulmonary emphysema is also present.

FIGURE 123
Hiatal channel compression (lower arrow) in the presence of a small sliding hiatal hernia (middle arrow). Note dilated lower sphincter (upper arrow).

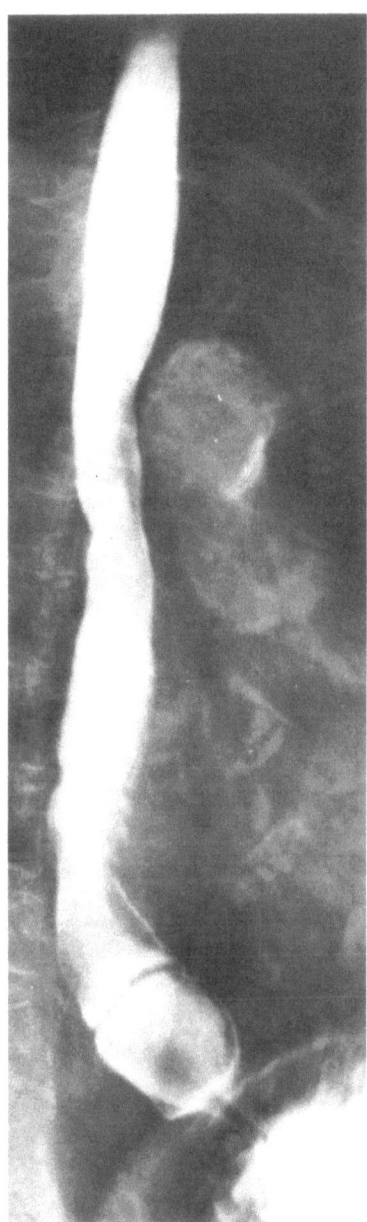

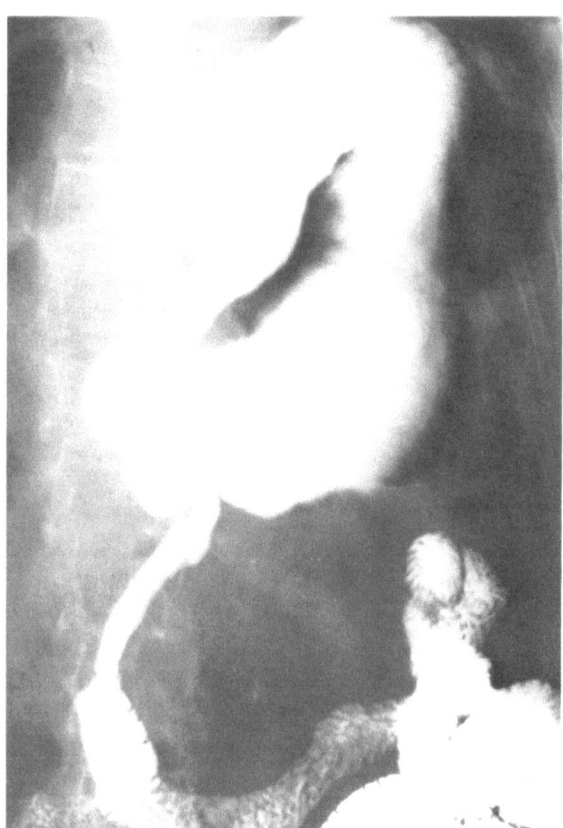

FIG. 125(A)

(B)

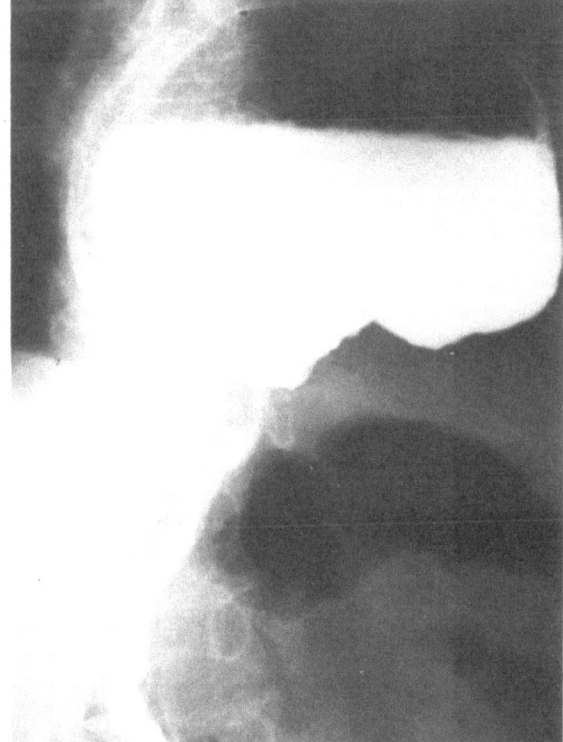

FIGURE 124.
Ring at gastroesophageal junction in presence of a sliding hiatal hernia.

FIGURE 125.
Thoracic stomach. (A) Supine, slightly oblique position; (B) erect, anteroposterior position.

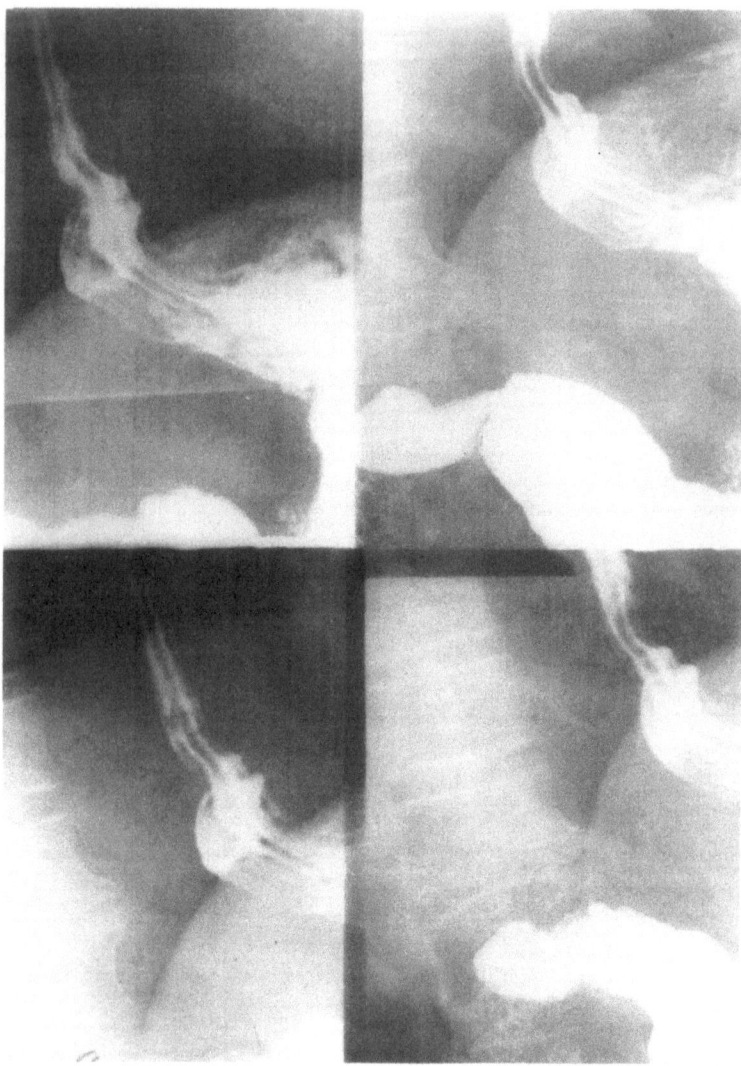

FIGURE 126.
Double ring shadows of a paraesophageal hiatal hernia. Polygraph views in inspiration and expiration. From Zaino, C., et al. *The Lower Esophageal Vestibular Complex,* 1963. Courtesy Charles C Thomas, Publisher, Springfield, Illinois.

Paraesophageal hiatal hernias are much less frequent than the classic sliding variety. In such cases, the sphincter zone is in its normal position. The cardiac incisure, which is part of the cardia or fundus of the stomach above the diaphragm on the left side, becomes smaller and may eventually become completely obliterated as the stomach "rolls" above the diaphragm. In the early stage the appearance of a "double ring" configuration is diagnostic. This double ring is produced by a partly dilated lower sphincter superimposed on a distended knuckle of gastric fundus, filled with air and/or barium (Fig. 126). Various degrees of rotation may be needed to confirm the presence of the "double ring" because it may be confused with an invaginated esophagus within a hernial pocket or an epiphrenic diverticulum. The diagnosis is simplified when the hernia is reducible and the invagination or diverticulum then disappears. Further study may be necessary if the ring persists. Stasis of air and/or barium in the herniated pocket is caused by the lateral pressure of the esophagus on the connection portion of the herniated stomach within the hiatal tunnel. Retrograde filling of this pocket, as observed at fluoroscopy, confirms the diagnosis. The size and shape of an epiphrenic diverticulum are more constant than of a infraesophageal hernia and the demonstration of the neck of the diverticulum extending from the esophagus above the diaphragm establishes the diagnosis (see Chapter 7). Fluoroscopy and films in multiple positions may be necessary to establish the diagnosis of a paraesophageal hernia (Fig. 127).

In the elderly, loss of esophageal tone often results in a sliding hiatal hernia (Fig. 128-A). If the esophageal hiatus is abnormally large the development of a sliding hiatal hernia with a paraesophageal component is common (Fig. 128B). With a good muscular tone or even exaggerated tone, a sliding hiatal hernia with a short esophagus may occur (Fig. 128C).

Considerable variations exist in the motor manifestations of the esophagus in association with a hiatal hernia. It may be that these motor changes depend on the presence of complicating factors and the degree of underlying neuromuscular imbalance, secondary to degenerative changes. In borderline cases manometric studies often are helpful in confirming the radiologic diagnosis.

Pyrosis

Pyrosis, or acid eructation, is a frequent gastrointestinal complaint that is probably precipitated by involutional changes. Other underlying causes, such as abnormal motor activity or gastroesophageal reflux, may exist. However, these etiologic factors may be difficult to detect (206). Various foods affect the basic pressure gradient of the lower sphincter and may also be responsible for initiating reflux (9). Yet pyrosis may be present without evident cause. Even the demonstration of esophageal reflux may not be related to pyrosis, because of the frequency of occurrence of esophageal hiatal hernia. Because of the loss of tone in the lower sphincter secondary to involutional changes, pyrosis is more frequently encountered in the elderly patients.

Gastroesophageal reflux

Gastroesophageal reflux (the free regurgitation of gastric contents into the lower end of the esophagus) (201) may be asymptomatic or can be accompanied by pyrosis. It need not be related to the ingestion of food. Gastroesophageal reflux, on occasion, is responsible for extensive esophageal inflammatory changes and even pulmonary complications.

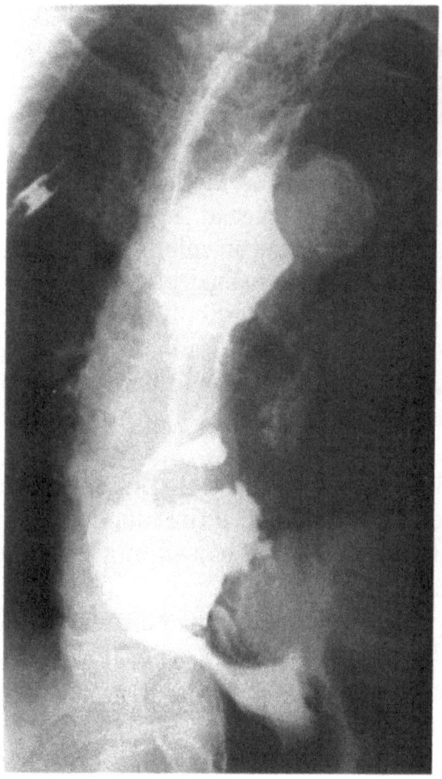

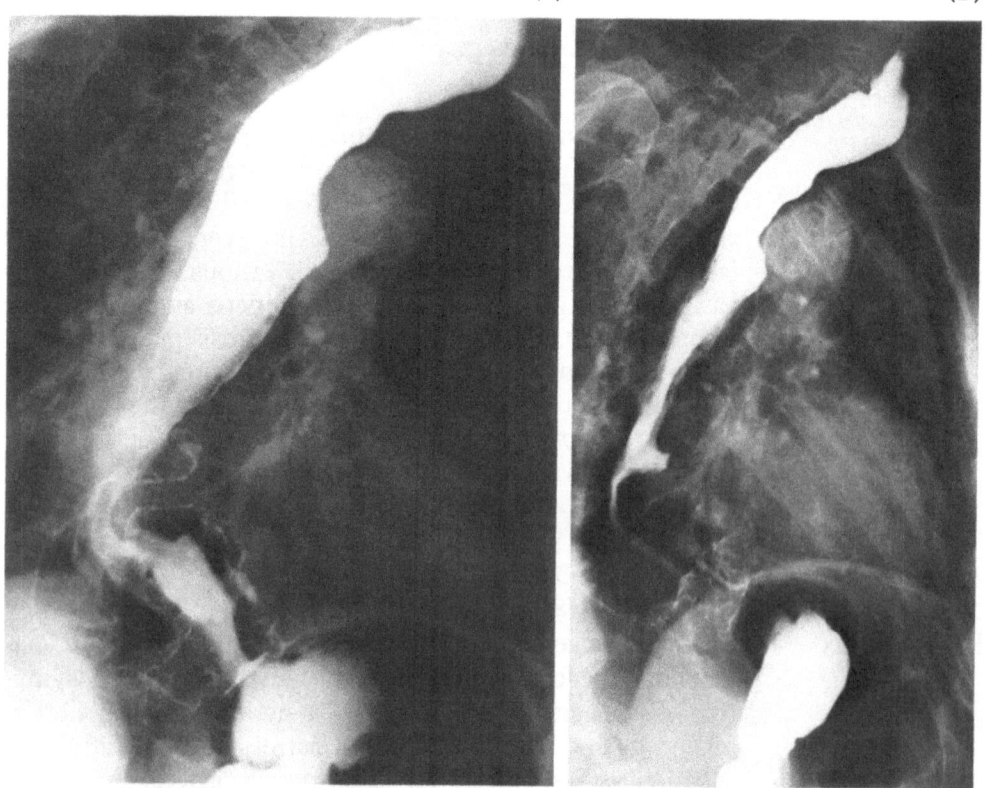

FIG. 127(A)   (C)   (B)   (D)

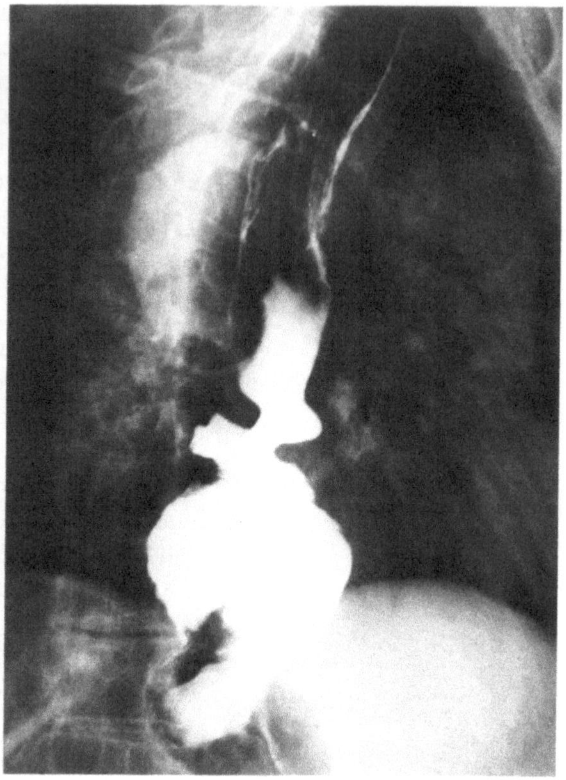

FIGURE 127.
Large paraesophageal hiatal
hernia. (A and B) Supine views,
(C and D) prone views. Hiatal
hernia seen best in these latter
views. There is also a traction
diverticulum in the lower
esophagus.

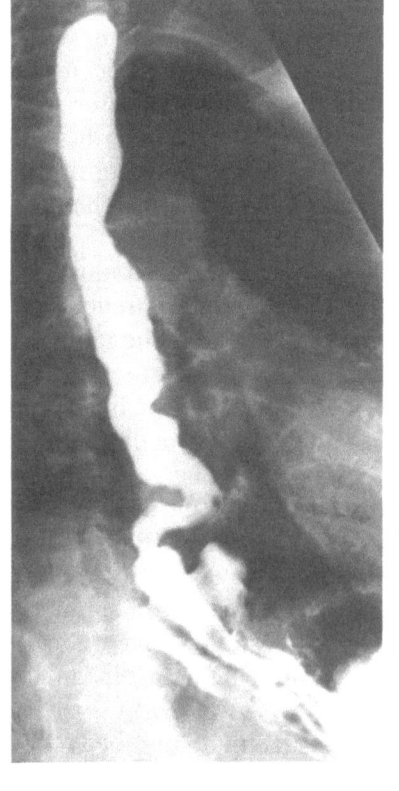
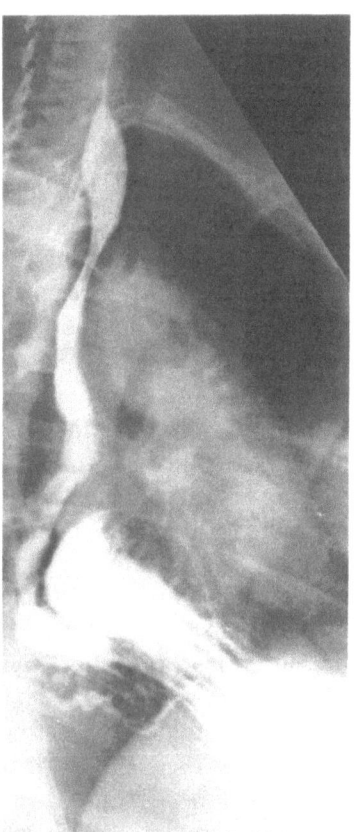

(A)
(C)

(B)

FIGURE 128.
Types of a sliding hiatal hernia.
(A) Redundant esophagus with
central sliding of the hernia; (B)
redundant esophagus with a
paraesophageal component; (C)
short esophagus. From Zaino,
C., et al. *The Lower Esophageal
Vestibular Complex,* 1963.
Courtesy Charles C Thomas,
Publisher, Springfield, Illinois.

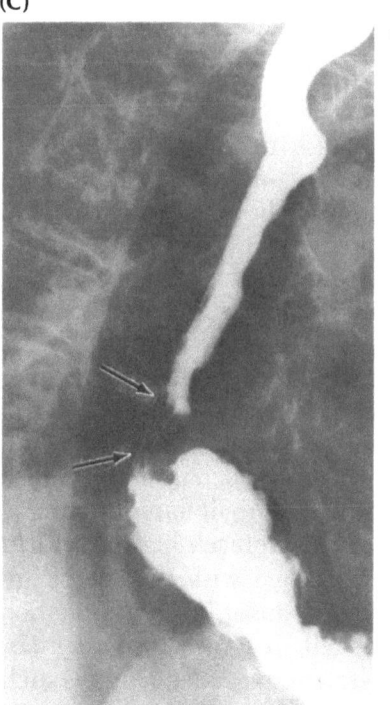

The subject of gastroesophageal reflux is being included in this section on involutional changes because it is most frequently observed in the elderly in association with decreased intraluminal pressure in the lower esophageal sphincter.

In this connection, the "three-factors theory" ascribes the following factors as the major determinants in affecting the pressure in the lower esophageal sphincter: mechanical, neurogenic, and hormonal.

The mechanical factors consist of the specialized muscular structure of the sphincter and its surrounding phrenoesophageal membrane. The neurogenic factors involve the reflex arc and the reciprocal innervation control of the sphincter function. The hormonal factors relate chiefly to gastrin, which affects the muscular tone of the sphincter. Normally, a functioning balance of these factors exists, allowing variability in sphincter pressure in accord with the physiologic status of the patient, e.g., swallowing or resting. The basic resting pressure is fairly constant with little variation for any given individual.

Although many causes of increased or decreased sphincter pressure exist, of importance are those etiologic factors contributing to a lowering of the pressure, resulting in an increased frequency of gastroesophageal reflux. Because these causes may affect any of the regulating factors, a number of disorders may be associated with reflux. Determining the essential cause may be difficult and may require extensive studies in addition to a radiologic examination.

The most common cause of sphincteric pressure change is hiatal insufficiency and/or hernia, which is classified under the involutional disorders. Surgical procedures affecting the sphincter zone and its attachments constitute an important cause. Any condition which increases intraabdominal pressure (e.g., pregnancy or ascites) may be responsible for reflux. Complete loss of sphincter tone, as in chalasia, is a significant cause of free regurgitation. Neurogenic degenerative changes affecting the reflex pathways to the sphincter can permit reflux during periods of abnormal motility. Excessive smoking and certain foods also relax the sphincter tone and facilitate reflux. A variety of drugs can also increase or decrease the sphincter pressure.

The standard radiologic examination does not always demonstrate reflux definitively. The technical details are described in Chapter 1. Examination in the prone right anterior oblique or Trendelenburg positions after the stomach has been filled with a thin barium mixture, associated with the use of dry swallows or the water syphon test, is most likely the method of choice. Because such studies fail to satisfactorily demonstrate reflux in a few instances, its determination requires such additional studies as manometry before surgical correction is attempted (see Chapter 8).

Redundancy, prolapse, invagination, and volvulus

Redundancy

Redundancy of the esophagus is not unusual in elderly individuals because of the loss of tone and relaxation and elongation of the longitudinal fibers of the esophagus. This redundancy is present with or without hiatal insufficiency or hernia and it may account for a number of minor changes, such as the occasional occurrence of physiologic volvulus, kinking, or abnormal displacement of the lower esophagus.

Prolapse

Prolapse of the gastric mucosa into the lower esophagus occurs but is rare (77). On radiologic examination this abnormality is characterized by a mushroom-type of filling defect, with delayed passage of barium at the gastroesophageal junction. Prolapse is identified best in the prone right anterior oblique position. The findings may be inconstant. Esophagoscopy is usually necessary for confirmation (see section on pseudotumors, Chapter 7). Dysphagia and vomiting are the usual complaints. Retrograde prolapse of esophageal mucosa into the stomach has also been reported (56).

Invagination

Transient invagination of the esophagus above or below the diaphragm may be observed occasionally (Fig. 129); it is more likely to occur in association with a hiatal insufficiency or hernia. A redundant esophagus characteristically presents with a "jack in the pulpit" appearance, at the distal end of the esophagus just above the level of the esophageal hiatus but demonstrated in the prone right anterior position (Figs. 130 and 131). This configuration must be differentiated from the "double ring" pattern of the paraesophageal hiatal hernia, which is usually unrelated (Fig. 132). Substernal discomfort may be a presenting symptom.

Volvulus

Occasionally, a mild degree of *physiologic volvulus* may be present, particularly in the presence of a sliding hiatal hernia (Figs. 133 and 134). Symptoms usually are absent.

Organic volvulus with actual obstruction of the esophagus is usually associated with a large paraesophageal hiatal hernia (see Chapter 8) or a markedly elongated and dilated esophagus.

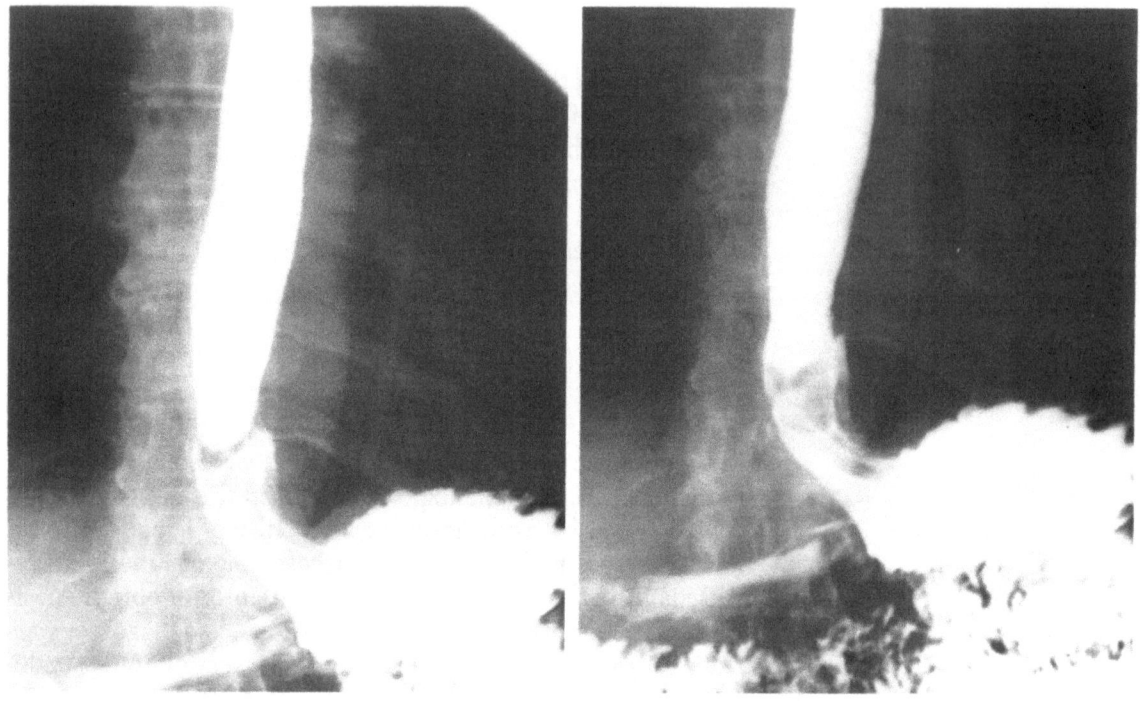

(A)

(B)

FIGURE 129.
(A and B) Esophageal
invagination.

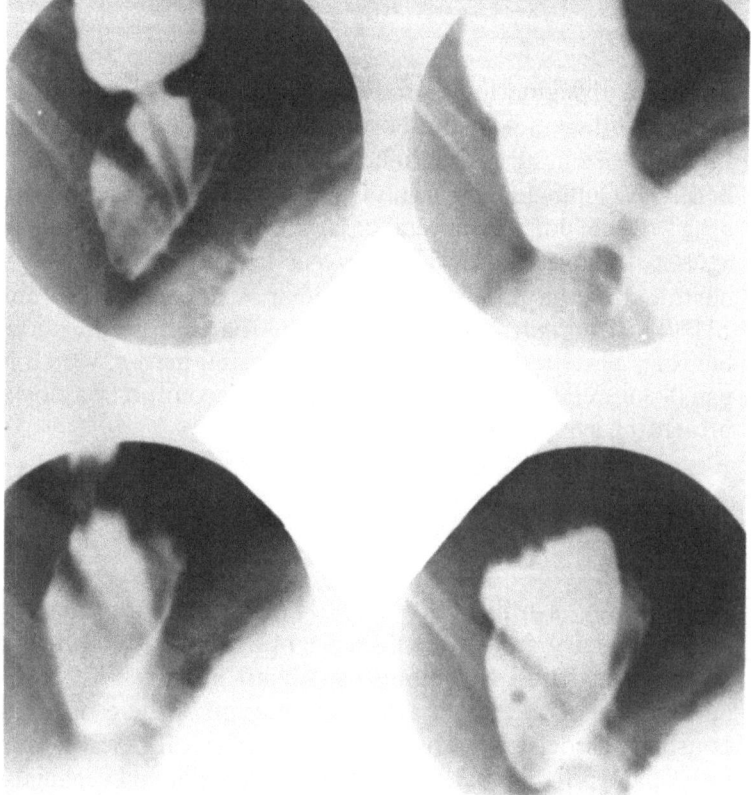

FIGURE 130.
Invagination in the presence of
a hiatal hernia (multiple spot
films).

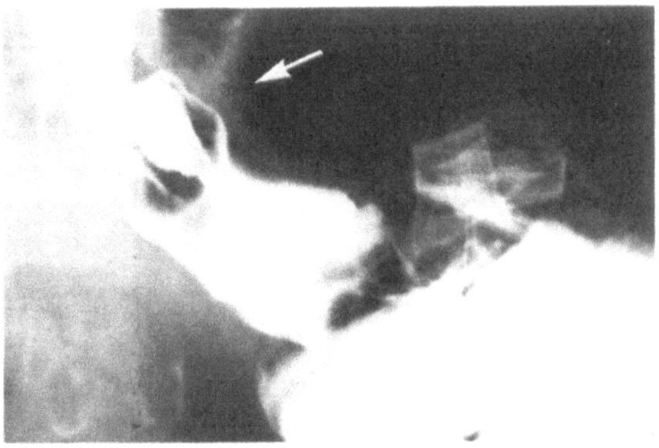

(A)

(B)

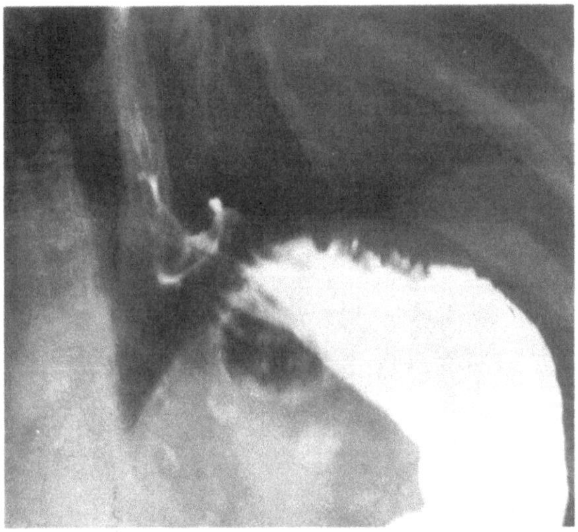

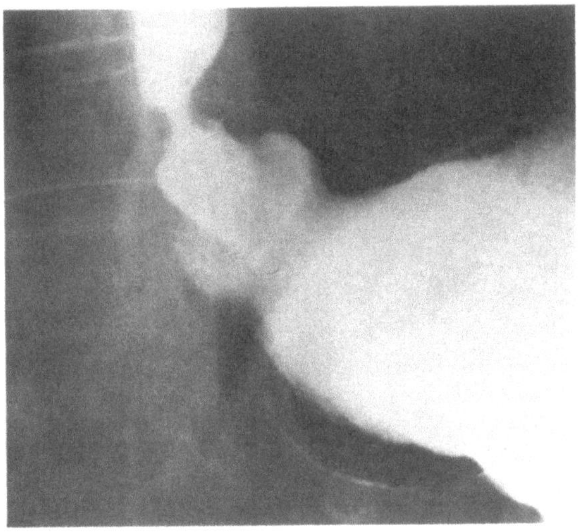

(C)

FIG. 132

FIGURE 131.
Invagination. In the presence
of: (A) hiatal hernia;
"Jack-in-the-pulpit" appearance
(at arrow). (B and C) Same
patient showing typical
esophageal invagination in the
presence of a hiatal hernia.

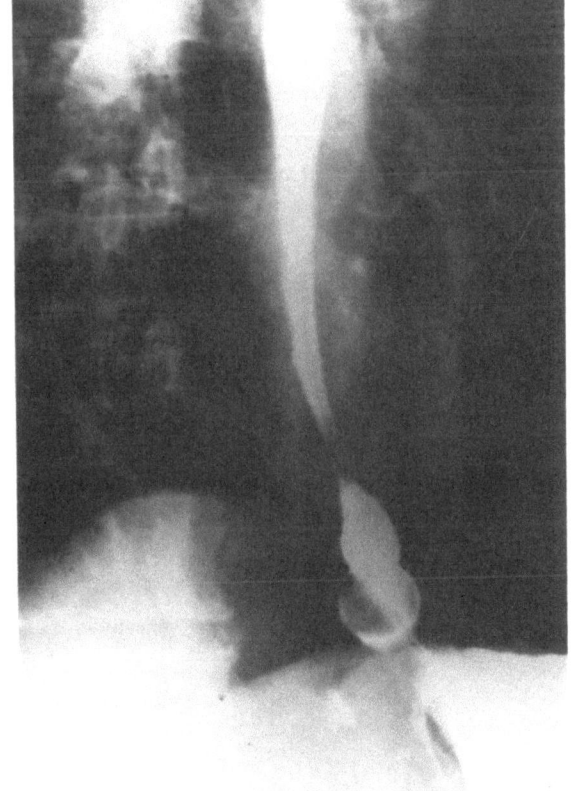

FIGURE 132.
Invagination resembling a ring shadow of a
paraesophageal hiatal hernia.

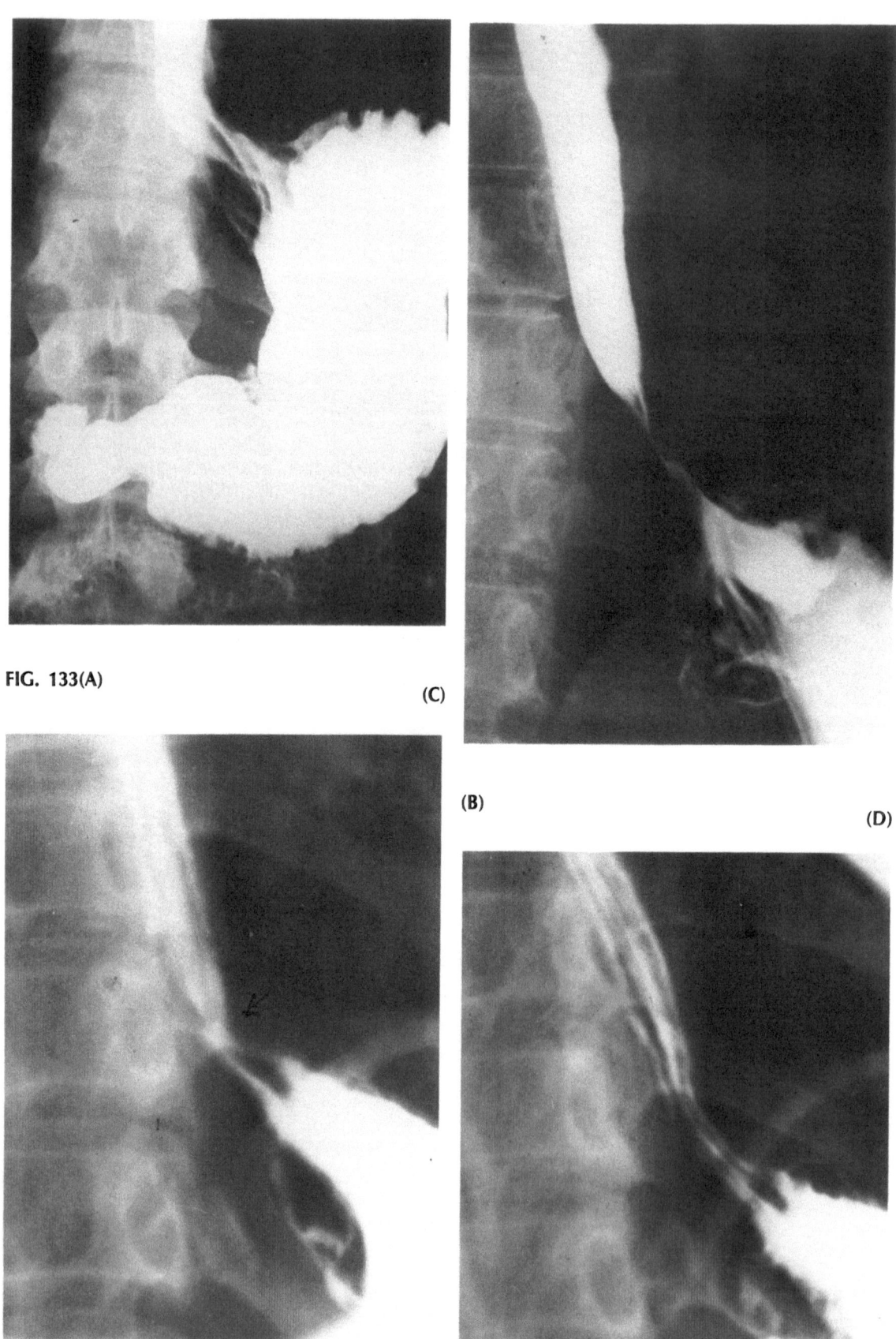

FIG. 133(A)

(B)

(C)

(D)

FIGURE 133.
Physiologic volvulus in normal esophagus. (A and B) Two different patients. (C and D) Films showing site of twist resembling an ulcer crater in (C) (another patient).

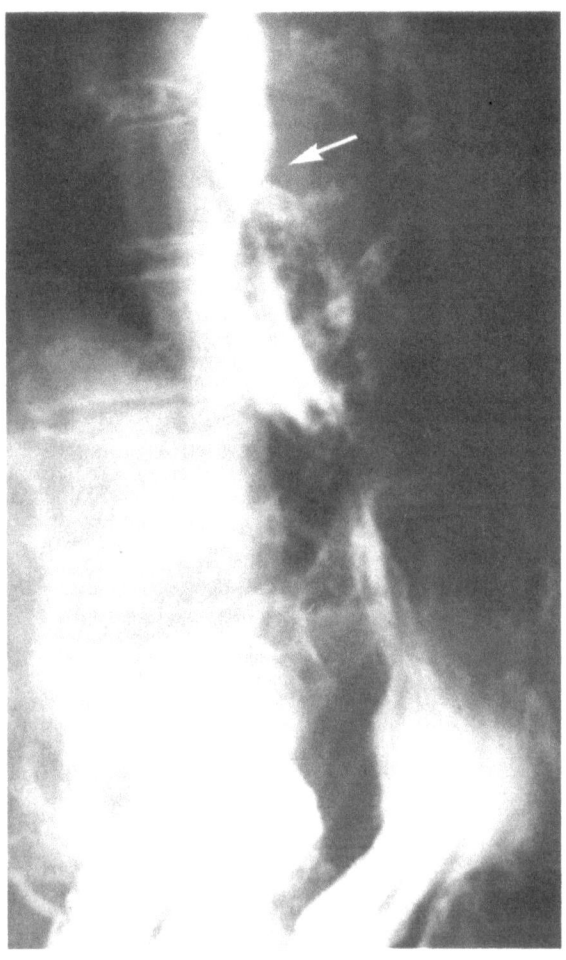

FIGURE 134.
Functional volvulus in the presence of hiatal hernia (at arrow).

Rumination (merycism)

Rumination refers to involuntary or voluntary regurgitation of gastric contents into the mouth. In involuntary rumination, remastication and reswallowing are accompanied usually by belching and aerophagia. Cineradiographic studies (91) in the erect position show normal swallowing to the level of the aortic arch. Distal to this point, the esophagus appears atonic, aperistaltic, and dilated, with the barium entering the stomach during expiration. Similar findings are noted in the supine position, with the addition of free regurgitation and pooling of barium in the lower end of the esophagus, which fills with air and barium to the level of the aortic arch. If this is followed by another expiratory effort with the glottis closed, the barium flows back into the patient's mouth.

Rumination is quite common in infants, in whom the normal neurogenic swallowing mechanism is not developed fully. Rumination may persist in older children with emotional problems and even into adulthood in individuals with emotional problems. The disorder resembles habitual vomiting, in which the patient voluntarily induces vomiting to obtain relief from epigastric discomfort. Curiously, only a small number of individuals who ruminate develop esophagitis. Mechanisms of voluntary rumination may be developed by special exercises and training. It is a process that reverses the normal swallowing pattern. No natural reversed peristalsis exists in the esophagus but, by training and practice, an increase in infraabdominal pressure with relaxation of the esophageal sphincters permits a reversed flow of gastric contents. The upward transit of food is aided by deep inspiratory efforts against a closed glottis (Muller's maneuver) accompanied by frequent belching and air swallowing, which relaxes or inhibits the sphincters. This series of events permits the Indian serpent eaters and sword swallowers to exercise their art. They train themselves to voluntarily counteract the effects of the autonomic system. Cineradiographic studies presented at the Eighth International Congress of Radiology in Tokyo illustrated the swallowing of live fish, frogs, snakes, and other objects that were then later regurgitated at will (41).

Belching

Belching or eructation of gas from the stomach is usually accompanied by some degree of regurgitation. This phenomenon occurs normally when the gas pressure in the stomach is greater than the tonus of the lower esophageal sphincter. Eructation occurs more easily and more often in the aged and in air swallowers. In this process, a sudden marked dilatation of the lower esophagus with disappearance of the cardiac incisura and shortening of the esophagus occurs. This shortening process is accomplished by marked contraction of the circular fibers of the mid-esophagus which may resemble a coiled spring (Fig. 135).

Belching becomes more frequent with advancing age because of relaxation of the sphincters and atonia of the esophageal musculature which facilitates air swallowing. The causes of aerophagia are many, including emotional, organic, local, or systemic factors. It may be self-induced in order to relieve epigastric discomfort or it may accompany excessive salivation.

DEGENERATIVE CHANGES

Degenerative changes are secondary to deterioration of body tissues as a result of localized or generalized wear and tear. Some of these changes involving the hypopharyngeal area have already been discussed, such as osteoarthritis and spondylosis of the cervical spine, fibrosclerotic changes of the prevertebral fascia, and vascular atheromatous changes of the aorta producing mechanical obstruction (see Chapter 4). However, degenerative changes also involve the neurogenic mechanism of the esophagus and sphincters, producing specific disorders.

Achalasia is included in this category here, although its etiology is still unknown. Achalasia signifies failure to relax; the term should be used specifically in describing a disorder involving the esophagus and lower sphincter, formerly referred to as cardiospasm.

Achalasia

Achalasia (71) is a neuromuscular disorder involving the entire esophagus, associated with degeneration of Auerbach's plexus. This degeneration presumably results in interruption of the normal parasympathetic innervation with loss of peristaltic action and failure of the lower sphincter to relax in response to the swallowing reflex. This purported pathogenesis constitutes the parasympathetic denervation theory and assumes that the disorder originates locally. Other investigators believe that the primary cause of the disorder is extraesophageal factors, probably cerebral or peripheral, particularly affecting the vagus nerve and acting on the ganglion cells, which then degenerate. Achalasia is a slowly progressive disorder characterized by fibrotic changes affecting the musculature, the sclerosis increasing with the progressive loss of the ganglion cells. Reduced enzymatic activity of the musculature and reduced levels of cholinesterase also are reported. Dilatation and thickening of the esophageal wall above the level of the contracted sphincter results. Progressive retention of food is part of the symptom complex.

Recently, impaired functional behavior of the lower esophageal sphincter has been linked to hypersensitivity to gastrin. Even hormonal effects have been suggested as the underlying cause of achalasia or other sphincteric motor abnormalities.

The radiologic changes vary with the state of the disorder. In its initial stages, minimal dilatation and only slight retention of barium above the contracted lower sphincter are observed. The primary peristaltic waves stop near the aortic arch or where the striated musculature ends. The contractions are replaced in the lower third of the esophagus by deranged, irregular waves resembling diffuse spasm. The lower sphincter remains contracted, resulting in some retention of barium. As the disorder progresses to its moderately advanced stage, dilatation of the esophagus increases in extent, with a conical narrowing at its distal end resulting in increased retention of barium (Figs. 136 and 137). The deranged motor activity of the lower third of the esophagus becomes less marked. Peristaltic contractions disappear and the esophagus begins to resemble a long sausage. In the advanced stage marked dilatation and uncoiling of the esophagus may be observed, resembling a dilated colon (Fig. 138). The sphincter remains contracted for long periods. Vomiting and spillage of foods into the trachea and lungs may occur, resulting in such severe complications as aspiration pneumonia, lung abscess, and bronchiectasis.

In the early stages, achalasia must be differentiated from dif-

FIGURE 135.
Belching showing "coil spring" effect. From Zaino, C., et al. *The Lower Esophageal Vestibular Complex*, 1963. Courtesy Charles C Thomas, Publisher, Springfield, Illinois.

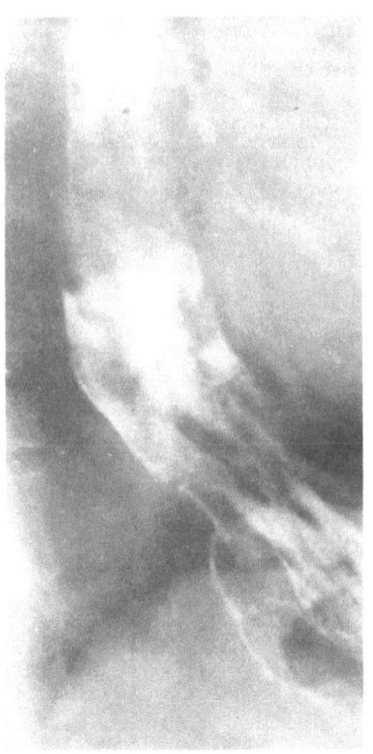

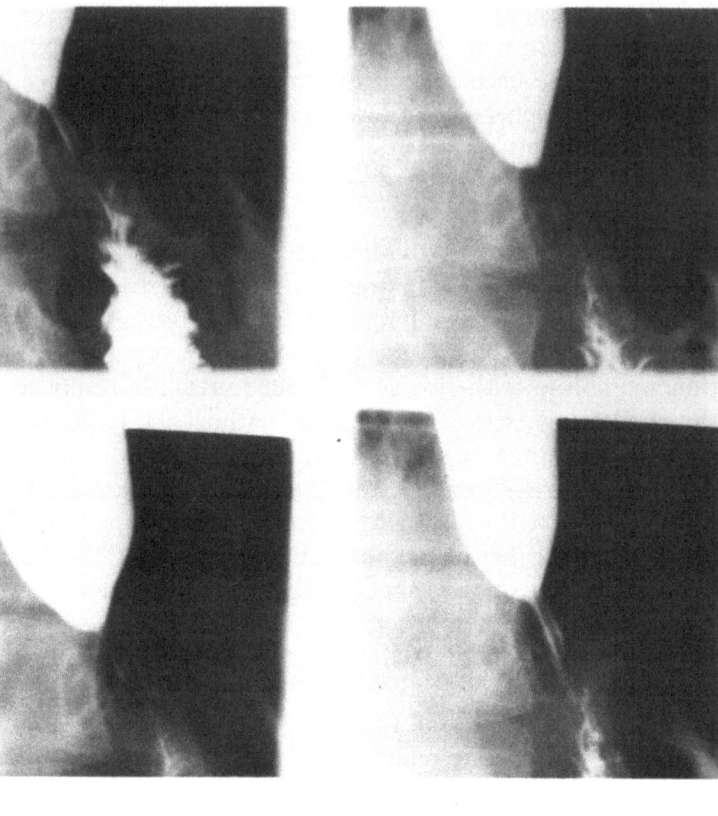

(A)

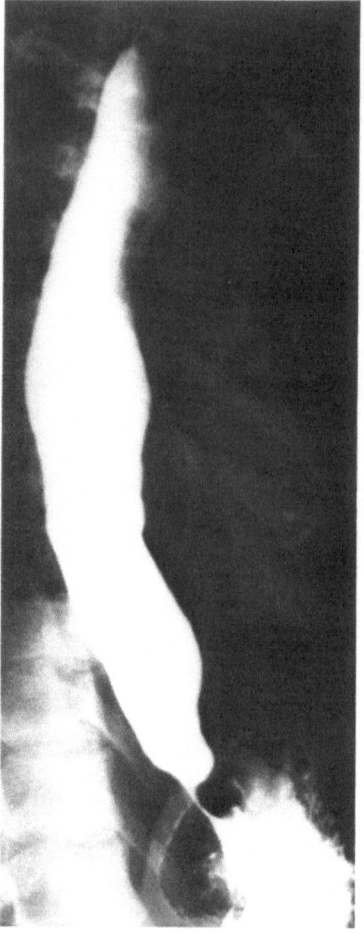

fuse spasm and/or vigorous achalasia. The lower sphincter zone in diffuse spasm is normal and there is no retention of barium. In vigorous achalasia, poor relaxation of the lower sphincter occurs, but no retention of barium takes place. In addition, spastic contractions are not repetitive. Esophageal manometric tracings may be essential for a true classification of the motor abnormality.

In the presence of a megaesophagus with obstruction, a number of other lesions may be considered. In South America, particularly in Brazil, Chagas' disease (a systemic parasitic disorder) is common and produces a radiologic pattern identical to achalasia. The underlying pathogenesis is similar to achalasia in the sense that destruction of Auerbach's plexuses is identified. The colon is affected similarly and myocardial involvement is also common, often associated with a fatal course (see Chapter 6)

Scleroderma, especially with esophagitis, will also produce a dilated and aperistaltic esophagus. This collagen disease is associated with mucoid and fibrinoid degeneration of collagen fibers, resulting in progressive thickening and rigidity of the submucosa and eventually complete loss of tone of the lower esophageal sphincter. This loss of tone permits free regurgitation and reflux of gastric contents into the esophagus (see section on esophageal reflex). Esophagitis with cicaterical changes

FIGURE 136. (B)
Achalasia in a moderately advance stage. (A) Spot films of sphincter zone; (B) showing the entire esophagus. Different patient from (A).

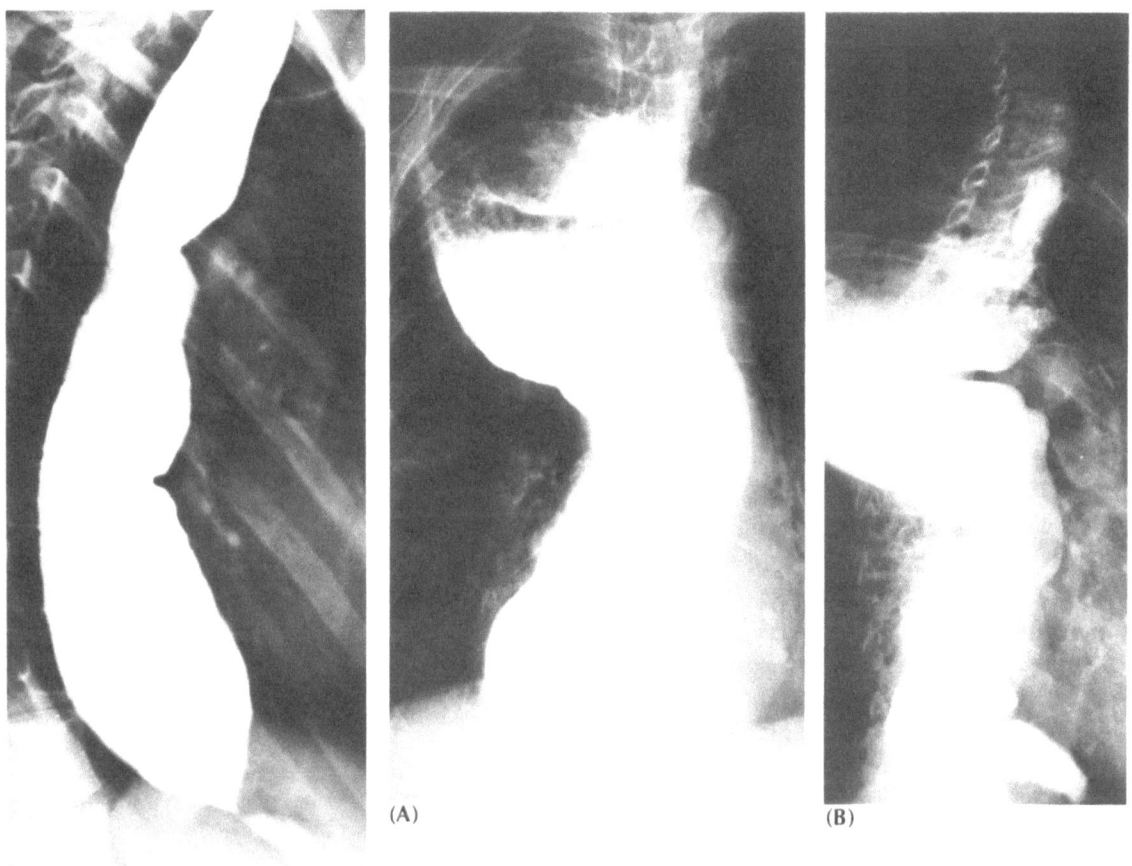

(A) (B)

FIGURE 137.
Achalasia, more advanced stage.

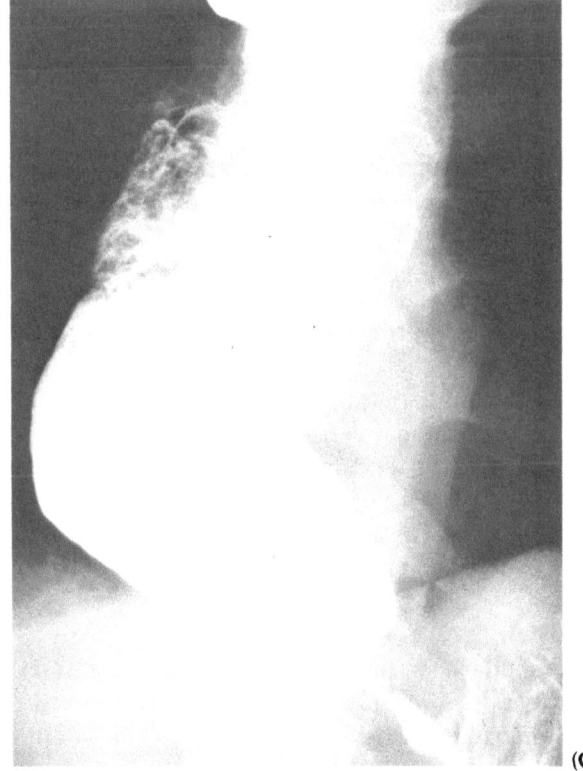

(C)

FIGURE 138.
Achalasia, advanced stages. (A and B) One patient, (C) different patient .

and dilatation of the esophagus ensues. In the early stage, in the upright position, barium flows into the stomach, in contrast to achalasia (see Chapter 6).

Carcinoma of the cardia and lower end of the esophagus at times produces a tapering effect, with dilatation of the esophagus above and retention of barium because of obstruction by the lesion. The area of lower esophageal narrowing is rigid, serrated, irregular, and eccentric. The motor pattern, however, is normal. Carcinoma of the esophagus can also develop in preexisting achalasia. The mid-esophagus is usually the common location. Such a neoplasm produces a filling defect that may be obscured by retained food in the esophagus associated with the achalasia.

The presence of hiatal hernia in achalasia is unusual. Occasionally, a web or ring is found in the lower esophagus. This is usually an incidental, unrelated finding and when present probably has preceded the onset of the achalasia.

Other conditions producing some occlusion of the sphincter zone include a hypertensive sphincter with dilatation of the esophagus, which may simulate achalasia. The history, a careful radiologic examination, and manometric studies usually indicate the correct diagnosis (121b).

In achalasia, the esophagus responds to cholinergic drugs, a feature that is useful in making a differential diagnosis between achalasia and carcinoma. Mecholyl usually produces vigorous contractions in the esophagus and some relaxation of the lower esophageal sphincter, permitting some degree of emptying of the esophagus. A positive mecholyl test generally is not observed in carcinoma. The technique of using Mecholyl radiologically is presented in Chapter 1.

Giant muscular hypertrophy

Giant muscular hypertrophy of the esophagus formerly has been thought a variant of achalasia but is probably the end result of severe segmental spasm (118). Dilatation of the esophagus also takes place but is not as pronounced as in achalasia. The lower sphincter is usually normal, although the dysfunction is chiefly located in the lower third of the esophagus. The chief cause appears to be vagal overactivity. On radiologic examination some dilatation of the lower end of the esophagus is noted, with irregular pseudo-diverticular formation. No definite obstruction is identified. The lower sphincter opens intermittently, allowing the passage of the barium. The thickening of the esophageal wall presents as a double contour density, associated with a narrowed and irregular lumen (Fig. 139).

"Curling"

"Curling" of the esophagus in the elderly is not an uncommon motor disturbance and is probably secondary to vagal overactivity and neuromuscular degenerative changes. In this condi-

FIGURE 139.
Giant muscular hypertrophy (at arrows). From Johnstone, A. S., Diffuse spasm and diffuse muscular hypertrophy of the lower esophagus Br. J. Radiol., *33*:726, 1960. The British Institute of Radiology, London.

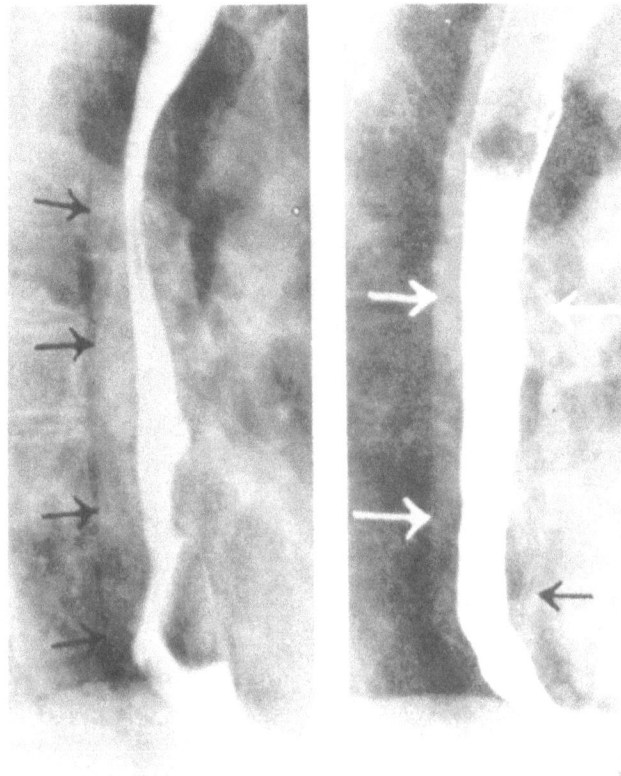

tion, the lower third of the esophagus becomes segmented, producing a beaded or corkscrew appearance (Fig. 140). This phenomenon has also been referred to as tertiary esophageal contractions. Secondary contractions are normal peristaltic waves initiated locally to clear residual food not transported into the stomach by the primary peristaltic wave. Teriary contractions are disorganized contraction waves resulting from the simultaneous contraction of the circular and longitudinal muscle fibers of the entire segment of involved esophagus. These contractions are not immediately relieved except by an additional swallow and a new sweeping primary peristaltic wave effaces them. Tertiary contractions are usually asymptomatic and occur more commonly in a relatively short esophagus. They appear and disappear spontaneously. The lower sphincter is normal and no obstruction to the passage of a barium bolus is observed. "Curling" is noted frequently with a sliding hiatal hernia and a relatively short esophagus. Occasionally a sudden impulse of vagal overactivity allows the longitudinal fibers of the lower half of the esophagus to contract, pulling the stomach up into the thorax. When the contraction

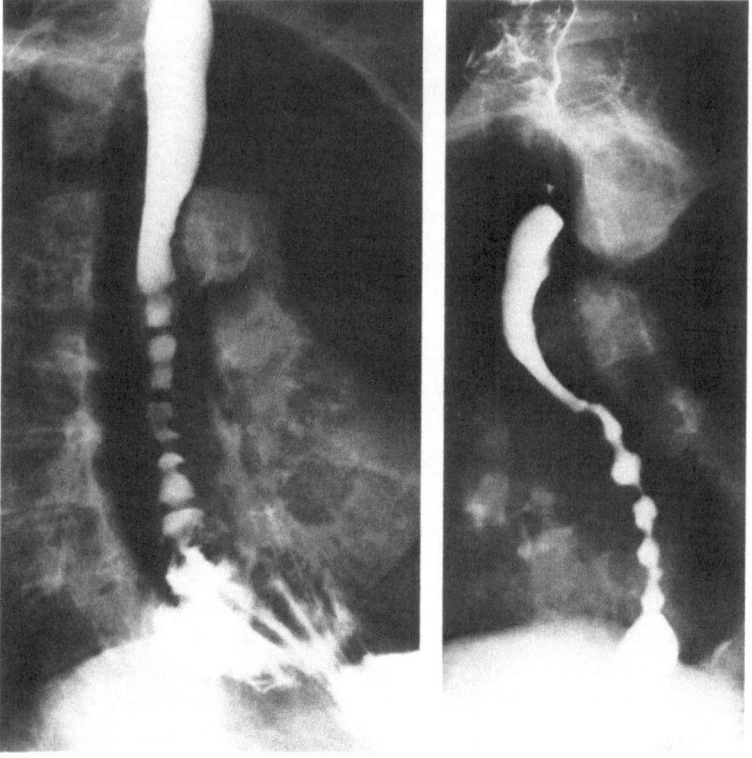

FIGURE 140.
"Curling" of the esophagus. (A and B) Two separate patients with hiatal hernias.

(A)   (B)

subsides, the herniated stomach can slide back into the abdominal cavity. "Curling" can be induced by the Valsalva maneuver and can be relieved by certain drugs, such as amyl nitrate, benzedrin, atropine, and tincture of belladonna (218).

Presbyesophagus

Presbyesophagus (273) is a more advanced motor dysfunction of the esophagus occurring in the aging and is caused by degenerative changes in motor nerves. Denervation of normal peristalsis with increased contractions in the lower third of the esophagus are observed in the presence of a hypertensive lower esophageal sphincter. On radiologic examination, dilatation of the esophagus is noted with intermittent tertiary contractions. Some degree of stasis of the barium bolus because of the irregular and uncoordinated contractions is noted fluoroscopically. In the upright position, a to and fro action may be reminiscent of an "elevator" esophagus. In the more severe forms of this condition, it is important to differentiate between early achalasia, diffuse spasm, scleroderma, and esophagitis. However, because presbyesophagus occurs chiefly in elderly, relatively asymptomatic individuals, the correct diagnosis generally is established easily.

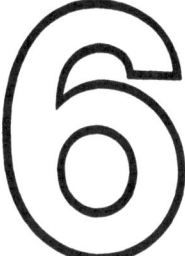
ORGANIC LESIONS (SYSTEMIC)

NEUROMUSCULAR DISORDERS

Multiple causes of neuromuscular disturbances involving the hypopharynx and esophagus exist. These disorders are manifested chiefly by impairment of the swallowing mechanism, with resultant dysphagia. This group of disorders usually is divided into lesions which interrupt the normal reflex arc controlling deglutition and local toxic myopathies or systemic diseases which affect the muscles involved in deglutition.

Lesions interrupting the reflex arc

A number of lesions interrupt the normal reflex pathway to the muscles of the orohypopharynx and esophagus. These may be grouped according to location as cerebral, intermediary, or peripheral. The ensuing disorders may be acute or chronic.

Acute cerebral lesions usually last longer and produce greater incoordination than acute peripheral lesions. Peripheral lesions tend to be shorter in duration and produce a lesser degree of dysfunction.

The radiologic features are generally nonspecific and multiple and indicate chiefly impaired function of the swallowing mechanism. Symptoms of dysphagia usually provide the first evidence of any serious disability, inevitably leading to additional studies. The age of the patient and the history are of paramount importance. Neuromuscular degenerative changes that occur in the elderly have to be differentiated from the more serious lesions of the nervous system. The radiologic findings are best noted during fluoroscopy or cineradiography (61) and involve a careful evaluation of the function of the oropharynx and hypopharynx. These areas are examined ordi-

177

narily with only cursory attention during an upper gastrointestinal tract investigation because of the rapid passage of the liquid bolus.

A careful search should be made for early difficulty in initiating the swallowing act, segmentation and asymmetrical passage of the bolus, patchy or irregular coating of the pharyngeal walls, nasal and or tracheal spillage, spasm of the pharyngoesophageal sphincter (Fig. 141), widening or overdistension of the hypopharynx, and failure of the epiglottis to fold over the larynx. Delay in the propulsion of the bolus because of sluggish or absent peristalsis and inability to swallow with force may also be present. Regurgitation of barium into the nasopharynx and trachea (pharyngeal incoordination) (Fig. 142)

FIGURE 141
Neurogenic dysfunction. Prolonged spasm of upper sphincter.
Retained barium 1 hour after ingestion of barium bolus.

FIGURE 142
Neurogenic dysfunction, pharyngeal incoordination in two patients.
(A) Regurgitated barium in the nasopharynx; (B) spillage of barium into the trachea.

FIG. 141   FIG. 142(A)   (B)

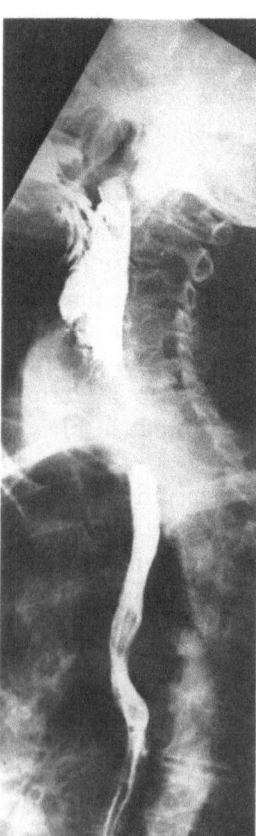
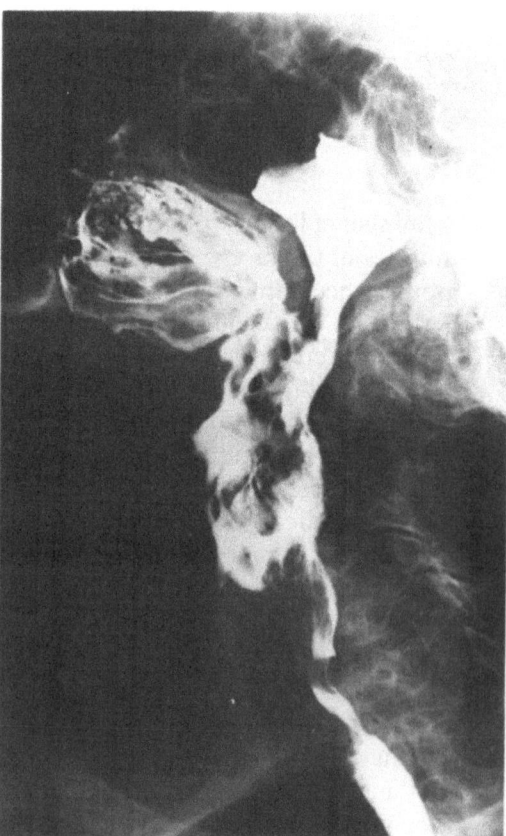
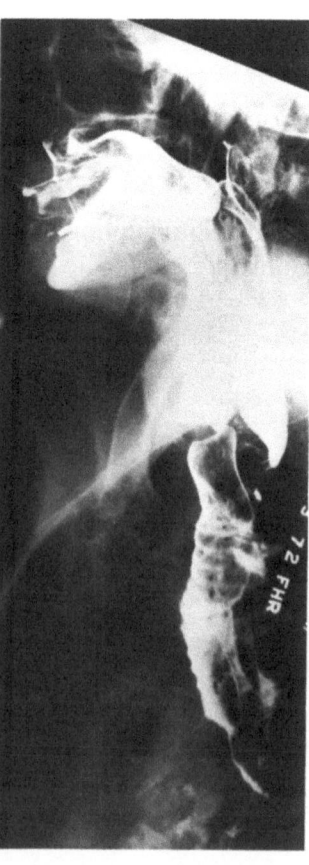

FIGURE 143
Neurogenic incoordination: the vallecular sign. Nasal tube passes through without obstruction but no barium can be swallowed in a patient with a cerebrovascular accident.

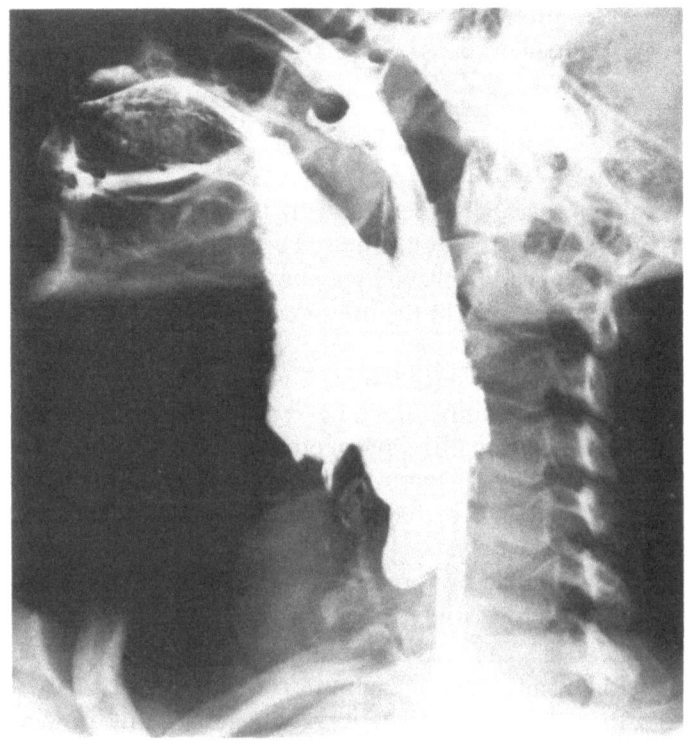

and the prolonged retention of barium in the valleculae (the vallecular sign) (Fig. 143) usually indicate a serious organic lesion. Although neuromuscular disorders affecting the swallowing mechanism have been grouped in relation to their locations, the causative lesion may exist at more than one site or even extend from one location to another.

Cerebral and intermediary lesions

Cerebrovascular accidents constitute the most dramatic cause of the sudden onset of dysphagia. The cerebral episode is usually secondary to vascular embolization, thrombosis, or hemorrhage, affecting the swallowing center or interrupting the reflex arc to the muscles controlling the swallowing mechanism. Although the degree of paralysis varies, in most instances, sudden involvement of the upper constrictors and sphincter produces failure of the propulsive mechanism in the oro- and hypopharynx. At fluoroscopy, the barium bolus progresses poorly beyond the hypopharynx. There, it collects and is retained for a considerable time, because of the failure of the upper sphincter to open. When additional barium is given, nasal regurgitation occurs and the barium spills into the larynx and trachea as the hypopharynx becomes flooded. This is indicative of a serious swallowing dysfunction. However, when the patient survives the initial cerebral insult, usually fairly rapid progressive improvement occurs and, at times, complete regression of symptoms takes place, depending on the underlying cerebral pathologic process.

Bulbar and pseudo-bulbar palsy

Bulbar palsy is a rare disorder resulting in difficulty of speech, deglutition, and mastication, chiefly because of atrophy of the muscles of the pharyngeal and hypopharyngeal area. Degenerative changes are present in the motor cells of the pons and medulla oblongata.

Pseudo-bulbar palsy results from a variety of other cerebral lesions affecting the bulbar nuclei and producing similar findings to bulbar poliomyelitis, syringomelia, epidemic encephalitis, parkinsonism, etc. Fluoroscopic examination will reveal a positive vallecular sign, spillage of barium into the trachea and atonia typical of paralysis of the muscles of mastication or deglutition controlled by cerebral centers.

In bulbar poliomyelitis paralysis of the inferior constrictor muscles as well as the muscular components of the sphincter zone develops. The paresis is asymmetrical, producing a partial paralysis that results in the barium bolus sluggishly flowing down one side of the lateral channels.

In parkinsonism the bulbar nuclei are involved, producing diminished peristalsis of the entire esophagus. In addition, difficulty in mastication because of muscular rigidity occurs. A specific sequence of changes has been reported on fluoroscopic examination with orally ingested barium, even before the onset of dysphagia (150). Initially, slowing of the swallowing time because of lingual impairment is observed. As the pharyngeal muscles become involved, dysphagia then occurs, with increased impairment of motility. The lower end of the esophagus eventually is affected with the appearance of tertiary contractions and esophageal reflux. Associated spasm of the pharyngoesophageal sphincter (180) is often present.

Brain tumors

Brain tumors or other cerebral mass lesions, such as a gumma, may also interrupt the nervous pathways controlling the muscles of mastication and swallowing. Tumors of the cerebellopontine angle and the glossopharyngeal nerve, lesions of the jugular foramen, trauma, and aneurysms can also similarly affect the swallowing mechanism. The radiologic findings depend on the extent and location of the lesion.

Avellis' syndrome

Avellis' syndrome (67) is an intramedullary lesion affecting the nucleus ambiguous or the vagal and spinal accessory

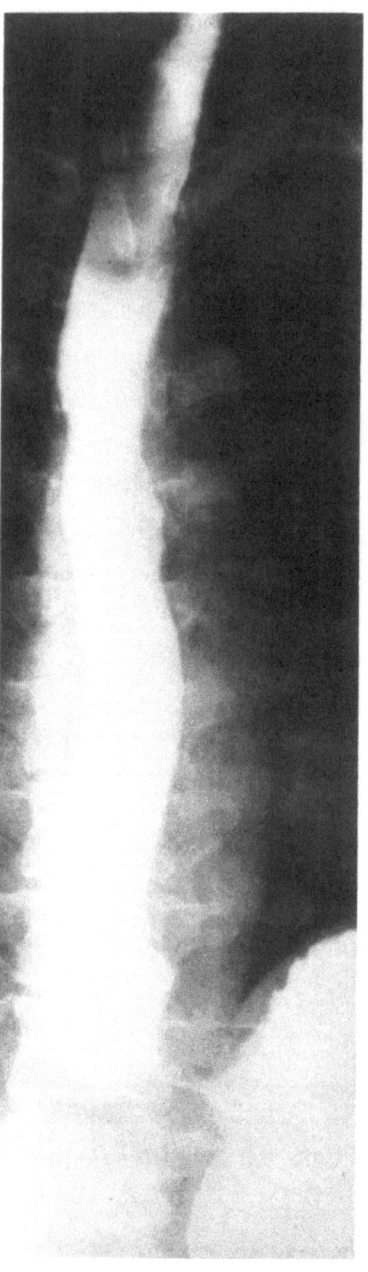

FIGURE 144
Multiple sclerosis, showing presence of an aperistaltic esophagus.

nerves supplying the soft palate and vocal cords. With more extensive involvement, a Horner's syndrome is also present. Avellis' syndrome may be caused by a number of disorders, including neoplasms, trauma, vascular accidents, inflammatory lesions, or even toxic agents.

On fluoroscopic examination, difficulty in swallowing is evident, with regurgitation through the nose. Unilateral transport of barium in the hypopharynx region take place and stasis of barium in the valleculae is observed. Tomographic studies of the larynx may be helpful in the detection of the unilateral paralysis of the vocal cords which is present commonly.

Amytrophic lateral sclerosis

In amytrophic lateral sclerosis degenerative changes affect the anterior horn cells of the spinal cord and pyramidal tract, producing diminished or absent peristalsis of the esophagus with involvement of both the upper and lower sphincters. At fluoroscopy, complete atonia or paralysis of the hypopharynx and esophagus may be apparent. Both sphincters become relaxed and patent and the esophagus itself is devoid of peristalsis. The caliber of the esophagus is markedly reduced and it appears uniform in size and unyielding. Following the ingestion of barium paste or liquid barium, the flow will be markedly reduced and only a thin, continuous, long strand of barium will be seen, extending from the oropharynx to the stomach, without the usual areas of sphincteric contractions. The esophagus will therefore resemble a long tube.

Multiple sclerosis

In multiple sclerosis disseminated degenerative changes of the motor pathways of the central nervous system takes place. If the motor pathways controlling the swallowing mechanism are involved, radiographic findings are similar to those in amytrophic lateral sclerosis (Fig. 144).

Peripheral lesions

Peripheral pathways affecting the swallowing mechanism can be affected by a number of lesions that may interrupt the reflex arc to the muscles involved in deglutition. The changes may be only partial and asymmetrical and are frequently unilateral. The vagus and recurrent laryngeal nerves may be involved by infective or inflammatory lesions and such neoplasms as carcinoma of the esophagus. Where toxic systemic effects and local factors are responsible, sensory as well as motor changes are present.

Diabetic peripheral neuropathy is produced by metabolic changes affecting the peripheral nerves. When the vagus nerve is involved, derangement of the swallowing mechanism occurs. Limited peristaltic activity of the esophagus is noted, producing delayed emptying (144). Tertiary contractions are also present. Such tertiary contractions, not unusual in the elderly where they are caused by degenerative changes, must suggest a diabetic neuropathy in a young individual.

A variety of disorders produces locally active and systemic toxins, which affect the muscles of mastication and produce dysphagia.

Toxic myopathies

Diphtheritic paralysis

Diphtheritic paralysis is secondary to the toxic effects of this infective disease. The muscles of the pharynx, the soft palate, and the larynx are usually involved, but the esophagus also may be involved. The autonomic innervation is implicated as well as the vagus nerve. Both motor and sensory activities are affected. The radiologic findings are those of a partial or even total paralysis, with sluggish to absent peristaltic action. This is especially apparent when the patient swallows thick barium paste. The transit time is markedly prolonged and the vallecular sign is usually present.

Botulism

Botulism can also produce paralysis, particularly of the constrictors of the pharynx. The paralysis is secondary to the effects of the botulism toxin on the cerebral swallowing centers. The symptoms are insidious, with progressive dryness of the pharynx and eventual paralysis of the pharyngeal muscles, including the soft palate. Liquids are ingested with difficulty. On fluoroscopic examination, the findings characteristic of pharyngeal and esophageal paralysis are noted, with absent peristalsis and a positive vallecular sign.

Tetanus

Tetanus results in clonic spasm of the muscles of mastication, secondary to the toxin produced in this disorder. The nervous pathways controlling these muscles are affected, resulting in impairment of swallowing mechanism.

Rabies

Rabies affects the central nervous system. In the early stages, impairment of swallowing and respiration may be present. Reflex spasm develops, with interference of the drinking and breathing processes. Paralysis then occurs. The features of an acute bulbar paralysis and even tetanus may be simulated. The history and other clinical data are helpful. The early radiologic features are those of impaired function with spasm of the pharyngoesophageal sphincter followed by the findings associated with a complete paralysis.

Other muscular lesions

Myasthenia gravis

Myasthenia gravis is a disorder of endocrine or metabolic origin, affecting the skeletal muscles. It is characterized by muscle weakness and early fatigue. A thymic tumor may be the cause. No sensory disturbance or muscle atrophy is present. The myoneural junction or terminal nerve end plates are "blocked," preventing muscle contraction. An oral phase, initially present, progresses into pharyngeal muscular weakness. Sluggish movements of the tongue interfere with deglutition. Paresis of the muscles of the orohypopharynx follows, with resultant stasis and dilatation. The sphincters are apparently not involved.

On fluoroscopic examination, the larynx fails to ascend and the epiglottis cannot fold over. Consequently, a positive vallecular sign, with spillage of the barium into the larynx and trachea, develops.

Because the underlying dysfunction includes a chemical block of the neuromuscular junction, a positive response to cholinergic drugs may be anticipated. The administration of prostigmine intramuscularly results in a temporary disappearance of the dysphagia. The effects of prostigmine in this regard may therefore be used as a diagnostic test.

Muscular dystrophy

Myotonic dystrophy (Muscular dystrophy) (134) is a disorder of unknown origin characterized by atrophy and myotonia of the skeletal muscles. The upper sphincter of the esophagus is affected; atony of this sphincter occurs, with free regurgitation of food from the esophagus into the pharynx (chalasia).

An anteroposterior view of the barium-filled cervical esophagus in an individual with myotonic dystrophy shows the handle part of the normally racket-shaped image of the dilated sphincter (see Chapter 2) to be wider and more tubular in appearance than usual because of atony of the sphincter. Spillage of barium into the trachea with subsequent pneumonia is common. The diminished peristalsis with associated dilatation and poor emptying of the esophagus produces radiologic findings similar to achalasia, scleroderma, or paralytic lesions involving the sphincters. In the presence of a dilated esophagus (and colon) without any evident explanation, myotonic dystrophy should be considered.

In this disorder, in addition to the changes just described, the skull may be enlarged with prominent frontal sinuses and a small sella turcica. An increase in the serum lysozyme has also been reported (227).

Stiffman's syndrome

Stiffman's syndrome (236) is a rare disorder of unknown cause characterized by progressive muscular rigidity and spasm. The onset may be gradual or rapid, with varying degrees of muscle stiffness and pain. The neck muscles concerned with swallowing and deglutition are almost invariably affected. Abnormal esophageal motility is apparent on fluoroscopic examination although there are no specific findings.

Cushing ulcers

Cushing ulcers of the esophagus are secondary to lesions of the central nervous system that affect the vagus nerve and hypothalamus, especially the tuber cinereum. The causative lesions in the brain include traumatic and spontaneous hemorrhage, neoplasm, and acute encephalitis. Hypersecretion and hypermotility are considered to be responsible for the development of an esophageal ulcer. Localized ischemia may result.

The esophageal ulcers are usually acute and readily perforate. The stomach and duodenal bulb are also commonly involved. The esophageal ulcers in this entity are usually located in the distal third.

Cushing and curling ulcers of the esophagus

Curling ulcers

Curling ulcers, secondary to extensive skin burns, may also occur in the esophagus, stomach, and duodenal bulb. These ulcers are usually acute and may remain "silent" until they perforate.

The radiologic findings for Cushing and curling ulcers include disturbed motility, spasm, and the identification of a niche or crater. The criteria for the diagnosis of ulcers are presented in Chapter 7.

Acute pharyngitis, tonsillitis, adenoiditis, and epiglottitis are responsible for respiratory as well as swallowing difficulties in children and adults. Of these, epiglottitis can be severe and, at times, even fatal.

INFLAMMATORY LESIONS
Oropharynx

FIGURE 145
Acute tonsillitis. Enlarged tonsil at arrows. From Forrest, J. V., and Lester, P. D. Roentgenographic evaluation in lingual tonsillitis. Reprinted from Arch. Otolaryngol. 97:482, 1968, American Medical Association.

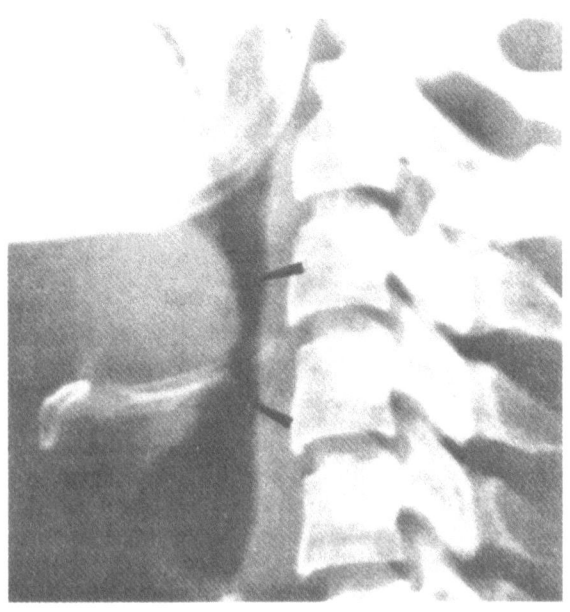

Acute pharyngitis

Simple acute pharyngitis may, on occasion, produce such severe edema and surrounding inflammatory reactions that interference with swallowing and normal relaxation of the pharyngoesophageal sphincter result.

Acute tonsilitis

In acute tonsilitis a lateral film of the neck may be valuable in detecting an area of soft tissue swelling, involving the area of the base of the tongue and valleculae, with downward displacement of the epiglottis (Fig. 145). Such swelling must be differentiated from abscess, lingular thyroid tissue, a thyroglossal duct cyst, and a neoplasm (82). The history of acute onset and the clinical findings on direct inspection of the throat usually suffice to establish the diagnosis. A barium swallow, in addition to a lateral film of the cervical region, is helpful in the differential diagnosis as well as in determining the extent of the inflammatory process.

Acute adenoiditis

Acute adenoiditis may also produce swallowing difficulties. The adenoids, which usually appear after the sixth month of life, are located in the middle of the roof of the nasopharynx and can be visualized on lateral plain films of the cervical region (39). A smoothly contoured soft tissue mass, rounded anteriorly and straightened posteriorly, may be observed. In the presence of infection or inflammation the adenoids are particularly prominent. Posterior irregularity of the contour of the adenoidal mass, especially in relatively asymptomatic adults, suggests a malignant neoplasm.

Acute epiglottitis

Acute epiglottitis is reflected in the rapid onset of swelling of the epiglottis, often causing complete obstruction of the airway and the hypopharynx. These features are demonstrated readily on a lateral film of the neck. The distension of the hypopharynx with air and a swollen epiglottis are diagnostic.

Distension of the hypopharynx with air may be secondary to the airway obstruction as well as involvement of the epiglottis or aryepiglottic folds, which produces dysphagia and inspiratory distress in the presence of a normal cry. Acute disorders affecting the larynx, such as laryngitis, croup, foreign body, or paralysis of the vocal cords secondary to congenital defects, will produce respiratory distress associated with a "hoarse cry." In acute epiglottitis the dysphagia is caused by edema interferring with the normal swallowing mechanism (122).

Chronic ulcerative pharyngitis

Chronic ulcerative pharyngitis is an infrequently encountered disorder usually associated with aphthous stomatitis (23). The cricopharyngeus muscle is affected by cicatrizing changes that may interfere with swallowing. On radiologic examination, a prominent cricopharyngeal impression is noted, apparently associated with spasm of the pharyngoesophageal sphincter and an ulcerating pharyngeal wall (Fig. 146).

Esophagus (esophagitis)

Inflammatory changes of the esophagus result from local causes or are secondary to systemic disorders. Esophagitis is frequently discovered at autopsy, especially in patients who have been elderly, debilitated, or chronically or seriously ill. Esophagitis is acute or chronic and of the catarrhal, follicular, fibrotic, phlegmonous, or corrosive type. Usually, however, it is exudative or desquamative. In exudative esophagitis, diffuse cellular infiltration that may also be associated with superficial erosions is present. In the desquamative type, partial separation of the epithelial lining of the esophagus from the underlying esophageal wall occurs.

The systemic factors responsible for esophagitis are associated with bacterial, fungal, and parasitic agents. Several skin disorders can affect the mucosa of the hypopharynx and esoph-

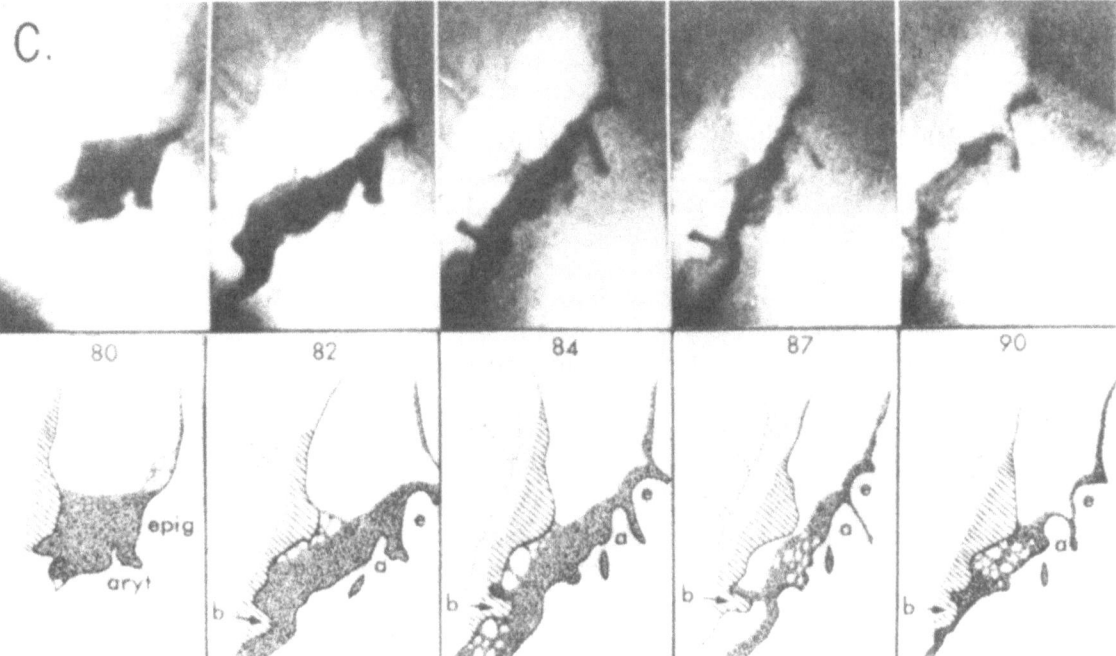

FIGURE 146
Chronic ulcerative pharyngitis (cine strip). (Note spasm of pharyngoesophageal sphincter at 80th frame). From Bosma, J. F. et al "Chronic ulcerative pharyngitis." Reprinted from Arch. Otolaryngol. *87*:86, 1968. Copyright 1968, American Medical Association.

agus, producing inflammatory changes. These are discussed in section on skin conditions. Acute esophagitis may completely resolve or progress to a chronic form, depending on the degree of damage to the underlying tissues and the extent of the subsequent reparative fibrotic process.

In general, the radiologic findings in acute esophagitis are not specific. The earliest changes to the esophageal mucosa are those of edema, with localized thickening of the mucosal folds. In the presence of superficial erosions, the mucosal surface becomes irregular with serrated edges. These findings can regress or disappear completely. Progressive changes are characterized by the persistence of spasm, irregularity, and narrowing of the involved area, with complete loss of the mucosal pattern. Diminution in peristaltic activity, secondary to the cicatricial changes, then ensues. Eventually stenosis results (see Chapter 7).

Acute catarrhal esophagitis

Acute catarrhal esophagitis is caused by direct extension of a number of inflammatory conditions, such as an upper respiratory infection—tonsillitis, pharyngitis, laryngitis, or even bronchitis and pneumonia. Radiologic findings are usually minimal and transient, consisting chiefly of irritability, hypermotility, and spasm. Typhoid fever and exanthemata, such as

measles and scarlet fever, also may be responsible for acute catarrhal esophagitis. Diptheria has been discussed in the section
on toxic myopathies. Hematogenous sources of infection, associated with septicemia, also may cause acute and even chronic
esophagitis. The radiologic findings are not specific.

Chronic bacterial esophagitis

Chronic bacterial esophagitis may be caused by a number of
systemic as well as local factors. It may exist in a number
of forms—follicular, ulcerative, cystic, granulomatous, or
fibrotic.

Chronic follicular esophagitis, usually related to pharyngeal
inflammation, is associated with systemic lymphoid hyperplasia, principally in children and young adults. This form also
may be present in megaesophagus. The chronic ulcerative type
of esophagitis usually clears, following removal or treatment of
the underlying cause. Chronic cystic esophagitis is characterized by occlusion if the mucosal glands of the esophagus with
resultant formation of retention cysts. These cysts may rupture spontaneously, leading to full recovery. A granulomatous
esophagitis may be primary or secondary to Crohn's disease
(see section on Crohn's disease later). Chronic fibrotic esophagitis is discussed in Chapter 7.

Ulcerative esophagitis

Acute or chronic ulcerative esophagitis associated with
chronic ulcerative colitis and chronic hepatitis has been reported (131). Although this type of esophagitis is not uncommon in debilitated and chronically ill patients, especially
those receiving treatment with corticosteroids, a more specific
correlation with chronic ulcerative colitis appears to be a
factor. Necropsy studies on patients with chronic ulcerative
colitis show a fairly high incidence of associated esophagitis
(45). In patients with idiopathic ulcerative esophagitis, therefore, an unsuspected chronic ulcerative colitis should be considered.

The radiologic findings are similar to those usually found in
moniliasis or other chronic ulcerative lesions of the esophagus.
An ulcerating and/or pseydopolypoid mucosal pattern with loss
of motility is observed. Subsequent perforation, stenosis, and
obstruction can take place.

Renal transplantation

Diffuse esophagitis can be a gastrointestinal complication of
renal transplantation (120). On radiologic examination diffuse

esophageal mucosal thickening caused by edema, without ulcerations, or a "cobblestone" appearance of the mucosal pattern is noted. Moniliasis infection may also be present. Pneumatosis cystoides intestinalis also may be associated (see section on pneumatosis cystoides of the esophagus).

Fungus infections

Thrush

Oral thrush is commonly observed in infants with congenital hypogammaglobulinemia and those who have no lymphoid tissue in the oropharynx. Superficial erosions are noted and an actual pseudo-membrane may develop with extension into the esophagus. In severe cases, complete esophageal obstruction can develop. The radiologic findings are generally confined to the hypopharynx and upper esophagus and are typical of esophagitis and its complications.

Moniliasis

Moniliasis, caused by Candida albicans, is usually associated with oral thrush especially in dehydrated infants or following severe burns. The germinating fungi produce extensive and varied pathologic lesions and associated radiologic changes when the esophagus is affected (30). Moniliasis often occurs in patients whose body defenses against infection are impaired. Prolonged antibiotic or steroid therapy, immunosuppressive drugs, and chemotherapeutic agents for malignant neoplasms are important contributory causes. (220). Moniliasis, however, has been reported in young people without any evident underlying disease (100). The entire esophagus may be involved but the changes especially affect the middle third.

The radiologic findings show rapid changes as the disease progresses (Fig. 147). In the acute phase, thickening of the mucosal folds caused by edema is followed by a "cobblestone" appearance of the mucosal pattern (97). An irregular, shaggy, or ragged esophageal outline develops as the mucosal surface becomes ulcerated. As the esophageal wall is further involved, some loss of motility and aperistalsis occurs, causing the lumen to narrow and occasionally obstruct. This phase is enhanced by the continued growth of monilia and collection of debris. Changes in motility follow the pattern of progressive involvement. Initially, slight impairment of peristaltic action of the involved segment is detected, followed by progressively slower transit, which advances to complete aperistalsis in the advanced cases. The esophagus, at first, is somewhat dilated in the affected segment and barium coating this area can be observed for a considerable time (as long as 1 hour) following the ingestion of a barium bolus. As the diseases advances, if un-

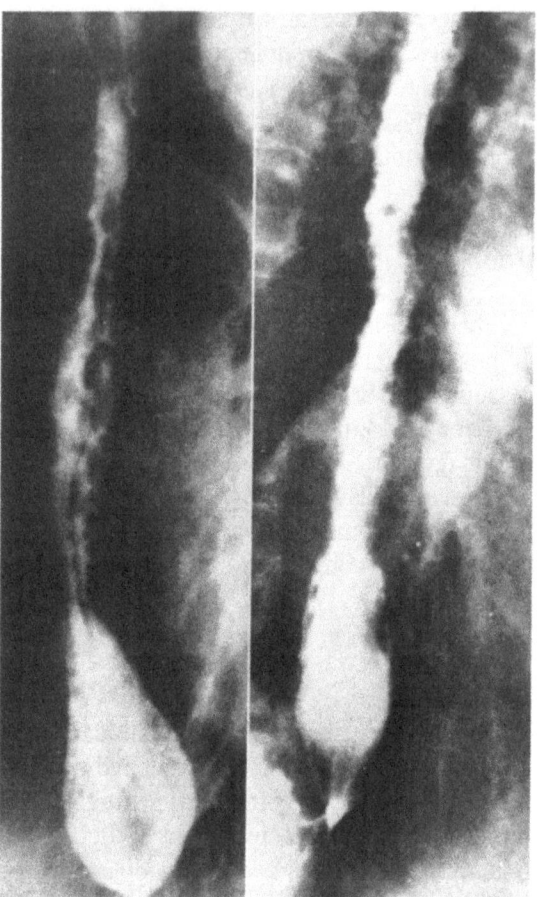

(A)   **(B)**

FIGURE 147
Moniliasis. (A) Edematous mucosa, (B) cobblestoning of mucosal pattern. Reprinted from Sheft, D. J., and Shrago, G. Esophageal moniliasis. J.A.M.A. *213*:1859, 1970. Copyright 1970, American Medical Association.

treated, narrowing of the involved esophagus occurs secondary to cicatricial changes and accumulated debris. Occasionally, the esophageal mucosal pattern resembles that of "esophageal diverticulosis" caused by dilated mucosal glands (247) (see Chapter 7). All abnormal findings disappear after successful treatment with fungicides.

Chagas' disease

Chagas' disease is the most common parasitic infection involving the esophagus. It is caused by the *Trypanosoma cruzi* organism and is endemic in Central and South America. The parasite invades the host cells of the reticuloendothelial system and eventually discharges into the circulatory system, reaching various body tissues. In the gut, escaping leishmania forms of *T. cruzi* are thought to release a neurotoxin, which destroys the submucosal, myenteric plexus (132). Years later, megaesophagus, indistinguishable from achalasia, can be demonstrated radiologically.

Parasitic infestations

The earliest radiologic findings are observed in the chronic stage of this disease, being related to esophageal motor dysfunction. Initially, excessive contractility and irritability are noted. As the slow process of denervation progresses, a gradual loss of peristalsis and progressive dilatation of the esophagus occurs. Failure of relaxation of the lower esophageal sphincter follows. Eventually, a megaesophagus develops; this viscus attains an enormous size, with complete aperistalsis and stasis of esophageal contents (Fig. 148). The colon may be affected similarly. Other organs also may be involved (197), helping to differentiate Chagas' disease from achalasia.

Schistosomiasis

FIGURE 148
Chagas' disease. Megaesophagus resembling achalasia. (A) Frontal view, (B) oblique view.

Schistosomiasis is a parasitic disease caused by a trematode or "blood fluke." The intermediary host is a snail. The disease is contracted by drinking or bathing in infected water. The larvae of the worms mature in the intrahepatic portal veins, producing chronic hepatitis and portal hypertension, resulting in

(A)   **(B)**

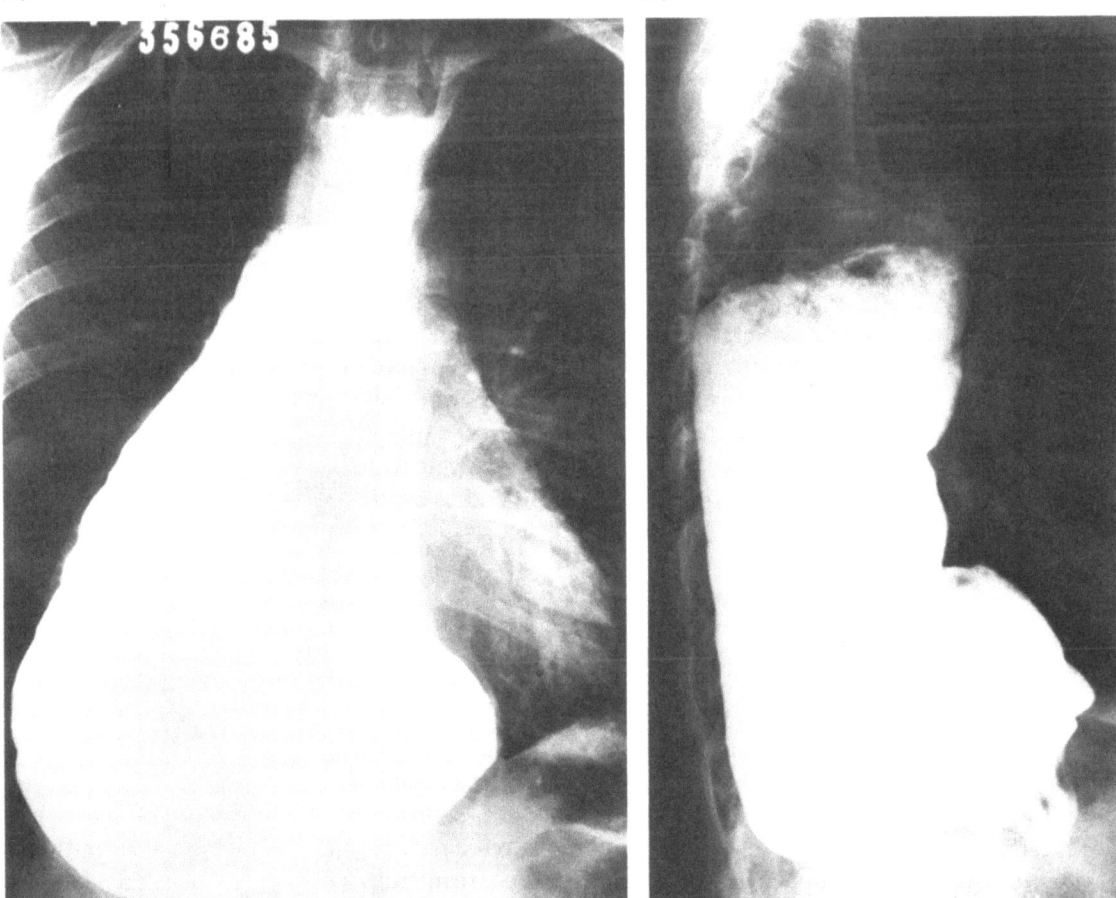

the formation of esophageal varices. *Schistosoma mansoni* and *Schistosoma japonicum* are the more commonly encountered organisms causing gastrointestinal disease with varices. This disease is a common cause of acquired esophageal varices in children (Fig. 149) in these areas of the world. *Schistosoma haemotobium* more often affects the genitourinary tract.

Pemphigus vulgaris

Pemphigus vulgaris affects the mucous membranes as well as the skin and may extend to the esophagus with accompanying dysphagia. Repeated exacerbations of the skin and mucosal lesions are common. With each attack, esophageal erosions may be present, producing gradual stenosis and eventually stricture formation. Abnormal radiologic findings are usually absent initially. However, with repeated attacks, areas of stricturing or webs may be noted. Therefore, this condition may be responsible for esophageal webs of apparent "unknown" etiology. Benign pemphigoid lesions and the rare bullous pemphigus variety occasionally also affect the esophagus, resulting in similar weblike strictures.

Herpes simplex

Herpes simplex can affect the esophagus of both infants and adults. Neonatal herpes may spread to the esophagus in infants afflicted with herpes simplex stomatitis, resulting in weblike strictures (135). Thus, periodic radiologic examination of the esophagus in the presence of this condition is warranted. An acute disseminated form, which may be fatal in newborn, also exists. In adults, following surgery or radiation therapy for esophageal carcinoma, herpetic esophagitis may be a complication. The radiologic findings are indistinguishable from a moniliasis esophagitis. The diagnosis is established histologically by the demonstration of cellular nuclear inclusion bodies typical of this disease in the involved esophageal mucosa.

Epidermolysis bullosa

Epidermolysis bullosa (212) is a rare inherited skin disorder appearing during infancy or at birth. Following minimal trauma, multiple bullous lesions develop in the skin and the esophageal mucosa. The esophageal lesions may be of a local stenotic or a diffuse ulcerating type, or both. When strictures develop, they are usually in the upper third of the esophagus, resulting in stasis with aspiration of food and pulmonary complications. When the distal third of the esophagus is involved, a stricture

Skin diseases affecting the esophagus

FIGURE 149
Schistosomiasis in a child, showing esophageal varices.

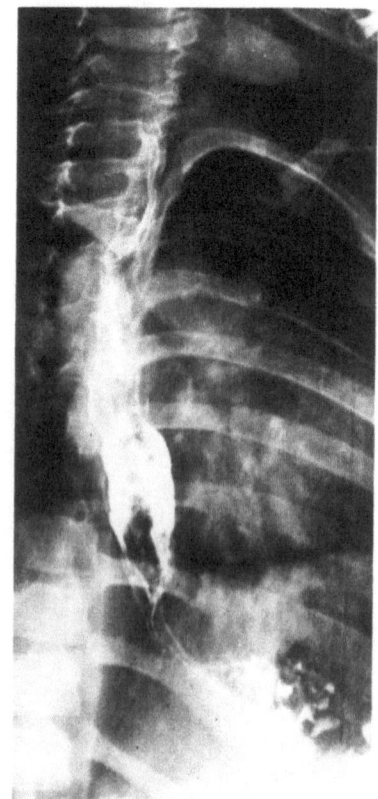

similar to peptic esophagitis develops. The region above the lower sphincter can become affected and produce findings similar to scleroderma or to the stricture of ingested caustics. Pseudo-diverticula also develop, secondary to the inflammatory changes.

The radiologic findings reflect the underlying pathologic changes. Obstructive symptoms are initially caused by edema and acute inflammatory changes, with progression later to stenosis and eventual stricture (Fig. 150). These findings begin in childhood and may persist to adult life. The radiologic features are not specific.

GRANULOMATOUS LESIONS

FIGURE 150
Epidermolysis bullosa. Stenotic changes in upper esophagus.

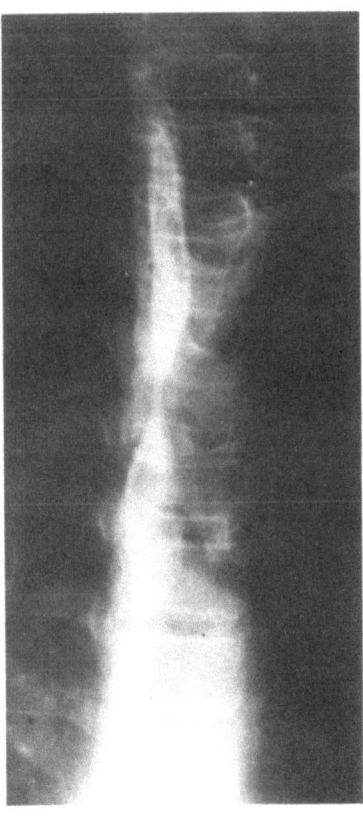

Tuberculosis

Tuberculosis intrinsic in the esophagus is rare. Esophageal tuberculosis may be part of disseminated miliary tuberculosis or follow esophageal trauma in a patient with active pulmonary tuberculosis who is ingesting bacteria-laden sputum. More often, the esophagus is involved secondarily by direct extension from surrounding tuberculous mediastinal lymph nodes or from a Pott's paraspinal abscess (203).

In intrinsic active disease of the esophagus, the pathologic changes in diffuse involvement are ulcerative or hypoplastic in type and the radiologic findings are those of a nonspecific chronic esophagitis (Fig. 151). With a localized disease, a narrowed esophageal segment is observed, usually in the middle third, with effacement of the mucosal pattern. Dilatation of the esophagus proximally takes place. A localized esophageal tuberculous granuloma is rare and may be impossible to differentiate from a neoplasm. External adhesions with compression, deviation, and occasional obstruction of the esophagus may occur. Enlarged tuberculous mediastinal lymph nodes may compress the esophagus, producing scalloped areas of compression and fixation of the esophageal wall. Fistulous tracts may develop following direct erosion of the esophageal wall.

Syphilis

Syphilis of the esophagus is a rare entity. It may occur as a result of a direct extension from syphilitic disease in the pharynx, larynx, or hypopharynx. Other types of involvement include a localized gumma and diffuse esophagitis. The upper end of the esophagus is involved principally in cases caused by direct extension. Ulcerating lesions occur initially; scarring and ultimately stenosis develop in the absence of treatment. A gumma may present as a mass lesion.

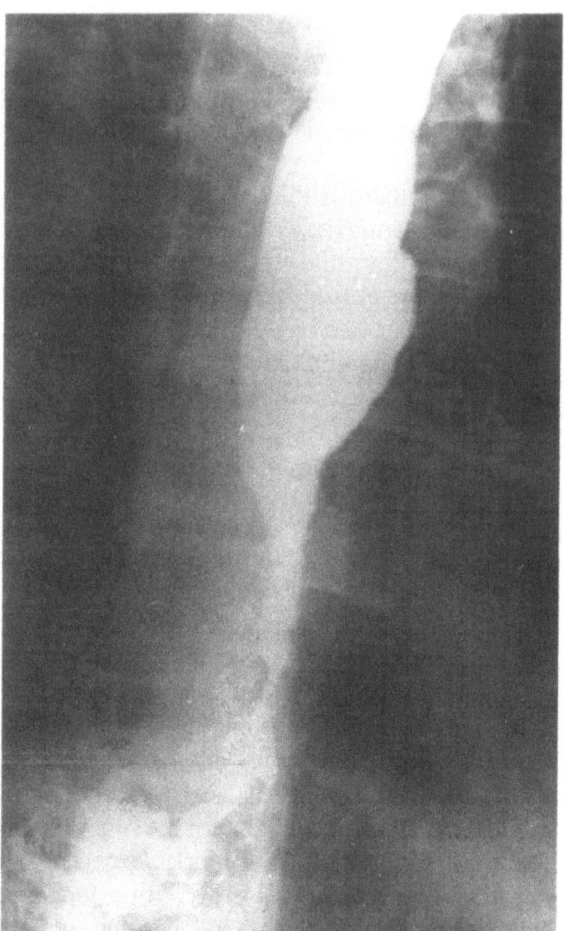

FIGURE 151
Tuberculosis. Esophagitis with stenosis of lower esophagus.

Radiologic findings are those of a nonspecific localized or diffuse esophagitis or in instances of a gumma or a mass lesion with irregularity and rigidity of the wall of the involved esophagus, simulating a malignant neoplasm. All these manifestations disappear following adequate antisyphilitic therapy.

Tabetic neuropathy produces degenerative changes of the posterior horn cells of the spinal cord and the posterior ganglia, which may affect the action of the upper and lower sphincters of the esophagus. Abnormal peristaltic waves can be observed in the esophagus.

Actinomycosis, blastomycosis and histoplasmosis

These entities rarely affect the esophagus, either in a primary form or as secondary extensions. The radiologic findings include multiple, small esophageal wall abscesses, which may perforate and produce sinus tracts and fistulae. Strictures may

FIGURE 152
Blastomycosis, stenotic changes. Courtesy of Drs. S. Glasser and P. L. Clemetson of Sunnyvale, California.

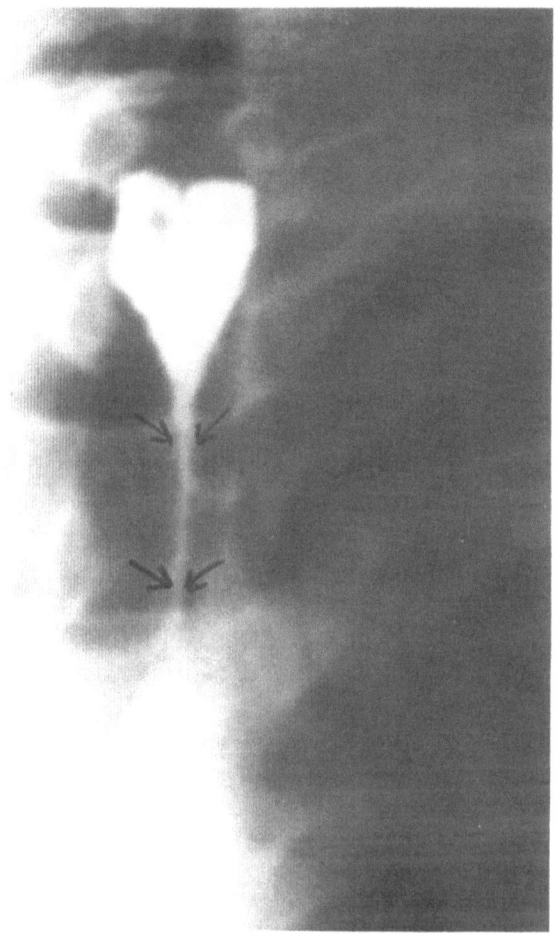

follow the healing process. The radiologic findings are not specific (Fig. 152).

Crohn's disease

Crohn's disease of the esophagus has been recently reported as an isolated lesion, unassociated with reflux esophagitis (157). The pathologic findings consist of a thickened esophageal segment which is markedly adherent to the underlying mediastinal structures and to adjacent affected lymph nodes. Extensive submucosal fibrosis with involvement of the muscularis and destruction of the mucosa is reported, similar to Crohn's disease of the small intestine (138). Usually, shortening of the esophagus may contribute to the development of an hiatal hernia.

The radiologic features consist of a cobblestone mucosal pattern of the area of involvement. Irregularity of contour of the esophageal wall, rigidity, and fixation because of the surrounding mediastinal inflammatory changes and adenopathy may suggest a malignant lesion. Fistulous tracts may be present. An individual with Crohn's disease of the small bowel (or colon) who complains of dysphagia should be studied for esophageal involvement.

Sarcoidosis

Sarcoidosis of the esophagus is extremely rare. A positive Kveim test has been used to differentiate this granulomatous disorder of unknown cause from other granulomatous processes. However, this test appears to be less than specific, being occasionally positive in Crohn's disease or in individuals with persistent adenopathy of other causes (259).

The esophagus in sarcoidosis is rarely intrinsically involved. Most commonly, the esophagus is compressed by enlarged hilar and mediastinal nodes. When the esophagus is directly invaded, marked thickening of the wall of the affected area is observed.

The radiologic findings in the very rare intrinsic form are nonspecific. Only minimal mucosal changes are observed, particularly early. A benign stricture, however, may represent the primary manifestation. Crohn's disease and other granulomatous disorder should be excluded. A therapeutic test with steroids may be attempted; steroids often produce improvement or even healing of sarcoid lesions, with regression and disappearance of the roentgenologic findings.

COLLAGEN DISEASES
Diffuse systemic sclerosis (Scleroderma)

Scleroderma is one of a number of collagen disorders that affect the esophagus. This apparently autoimmune disease is more frequent in women than in men, usually occurring between the ages of 30 and 50 years. A progressive systemic form may affect the esophagus before the appearance of any skin lesions. The most commonly encountered type is associated with acrosclerosis and atrophic types of skin lesions.

The underlying pathologic features of scleroderma, reflected in the esophagus, consist of fibrinoid degenerative changes of the collagen fibers. This process begins in the submucosal layer and extends eventually to the muscularis, producing atrophy of the muscularis and sclerosis of the submucosal layer. Eventually, both layers are replaced by fibrous connective tissue. Interference with the intrinsic innervation results. In addition, the muscularis involvement disturbs the contractility of the esophageal wall, producing atonia. The skin changes, which often precede esophageal motor disturbances,

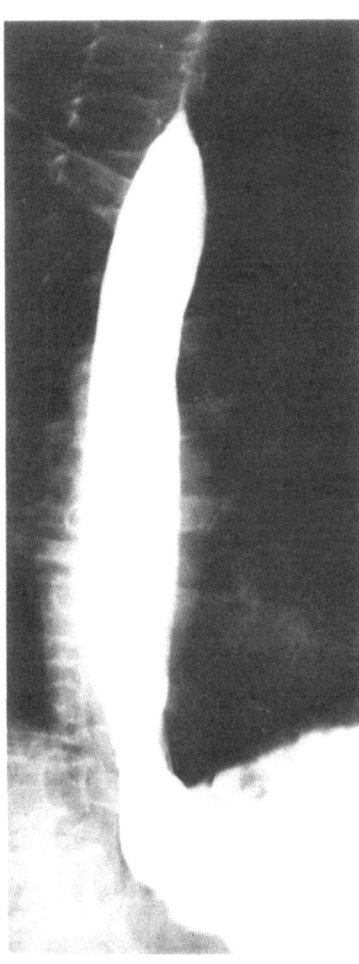

FIGURE 153
Scleroderma, showing patent lower esophageal sphincter and aperistalsis.

are characterized by subcutaneous edema followed by induration and eventual atrophy. The skin of the face and fingers becomes particularly involved and may be accompanied by the clinical manifestation of Raynaud's disease. These changes are primarily caused by vasospasm of the peripheral vessels of the fingers, resulting in diminished blood flow and in the development of cutaneous sclerosis and atrophy of the ungual tufts of the phalanges. Subcutaneous deposits of calcium are commonly encountered, although this finding is not specific and is also observed in dermatomyositis (see section on dermatomyosis). In systemic scleroderma other organs besides the esophagus are affected. The small bowel, colon, lungs, and heart may all exhibit abnormalities of collagen.

Motor dysfunction of the esophagus occasionally predates the appearance of any other detectable abnormality so that the radiologic examination is of great importance. The radiologic findings mirror the underlying pathologic changes. The earliest mucosal abnormality in the esophagus is submucosal edema, followed by sclerotic changes. This affects the motility of the esophagus and produces, initially, diminished peristalsis followed eventually by complete absence of normal contractability. As the mucosa thickens and the muscularis degenerates, the mucosal pattern suggests smooth atrophy. The lower esophageal sphincter becomes incompetent (Fig. 153). The lower segment of the esophagus resembles a rigid tube, which, in the prone horizontal or supine position, retains barium for hours. The esophagus empties readily in the upright position because of the effects of gravity—a feature that may be used to differentiate achalasia from scleroderma. Because of the failure of the lower esophageal sphincter to contract, gastric regurgitation into the esophagus is present (208). In addition, the dilated esophagus is easily filled with air, which can be demonstrated on plain films, particularly in the horizontal position.

Because of free gastric reflux into the esophagus, complications are common. Acute and then chronic esophagitis, with ulceration and stenosis, are commonly observed at different stages. Pseudo-diverticula and esophageal hiatal hernia secondary to the shortening of the esophagus are also noted in association with cicatrizing changes which produce upward traction of the stomach.

The colon in scleroderma may become significantly distended following a barium enema examination showing accentuated haustral pouches (pseudo-sacculations). The small bowel may also present with a malabsorption or "sprue" pattern not specific of scleroderma (also present in dermatomyositis and other collagen disorders).

Other significant radiologic changes are observed in the chest. Disseminated interstitial fibrosis in the lungs presents as a reticulonodular pattern, particularly in the basis. Cardiac enlargement is not uncommon.

Acrosclerosis

Acrosclerosis is a form of scleroderma associated with Raynaud's phenomenon. Esophageal changes occur late but are similar in character to the radiologic findings associated with classical scleroderma. Acrosclerosis is differentiated from scleroderma by virtue of the associated vasomotor disturbance involving the hands in the former.

Dermatomyositis

Dermatomyositis (polymyositis) is a collagen disease that, in contrast to scleroderma, affects chiefly the upper end of the esophagus. Edema and fibrotic degenerative changes of the muscles of deglutition, as well as of the muscularis of the upper end of the esophagus, develop.

Radiologic findings, on fluoroscopy, reveal delayed passage of the barium bolus because of muscular weakness and impaired esophageal motility, especially present in the upper third of the esophagus. Nasal regurgitation is frequent in dermatomyositis and is rare in scleroderma. Involvement of the lower end of the esophagus with pseudo-diverticula or sacculations may also be observed in scleroderma. Ulcerations and strictures are infrequently encountered and the lower esopha-

Other collagen disorders

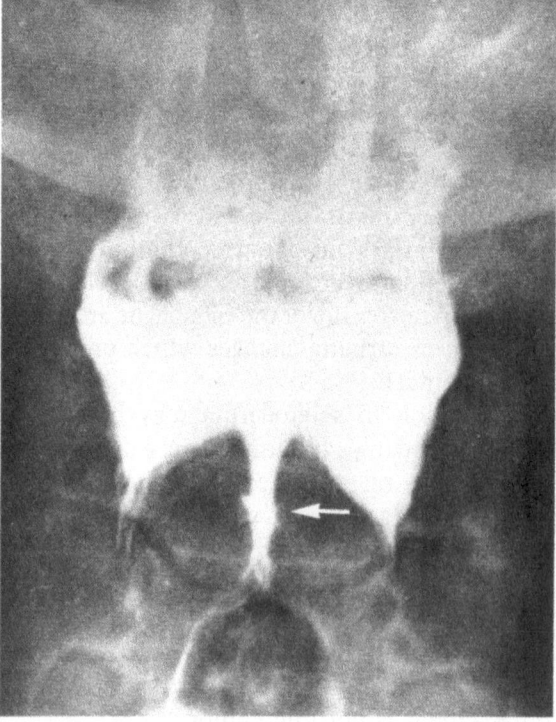

FIGURE 154

Dermatomyositis. Arrow at pharyngoesophageal junction. Note stenotic changes of the cricopharyngeus muscle above and the contracted sphincter below. Reproduced from Porubsky, E. S., et al. Cricopharyngeal achalasia in dermatomyositis. Arch. Otolaryngol. *98*:429, 1973. Copyright 1973, American Medical Association.

geal sphincter is not involved, in contrast to scleroderma. Other radiologic features noted in the esophagus are atonia, distension of the middle third, segmental contractions, weak peristaltic activity, delayed transit time, and atrophic mucosa (186). Impaired function of the upper and lower esophageal sphincters may also be present. Other gastrointestinal abnormalties may be present, particularly of the small bowel, in which a "sprue" pattern may be demonstrated.

Cricopharyngeal muscle involvement has also been reported in dermatomyositis (191). Stenotic changes of the cricopharyngeus muscle and contraction of the sphincter segment below the identifiable pharyngoesophageal junction can be demonstrated on radioloigc examination. Histologic studies of biopsy material from the cricopharyngeus muscle show the characteristic pathologic changes indigenous to this disorder. The associated symptoms can be relieved by a myotomy (Fig. 154).

Subcutaneous calcifications in the soft tissues of the extremities and periarticular areas, particularly the digits of the hands, are often present. Contractures of the digits in the later stages is not uncommon. Disseminated, interstial pulmonary fibrosis, although less common than in scleroderma, does occur.

Lupus erythematosis

Disseminated lupus erythematosis shows changes similar to dermatomyositis. (162) Muscle weakness may be present in the oropharynx, which may progress to dysphagia and even complete paralysis. Loss of contractile power and muscle tone of the esophagus with impaired motility often develops, resulting in abnormal or absent peristalsis, with a delay in emptying of the esophagus.

Rheumatoid arthritis

Rheumatoid arthritis, in its advanced stages, also may affect the esophagus, resulting in considerable loss of esophageal motility.

DEFICIENCY DISORDERS   Sideropenic anemia

Sideropenic anemia (Plummer–Vinson or Patterson–Brown–Kelly syndrome) (165) is a disorder of unknown cause related to iron deficiency. This entity is most frequent in middle-aged females, although it may also occur in males (33). It is most prevalent in Sweden. Some investigators believe the disease to be secondary to hormonal dysfunction, whereas others believe a deficiency of vitamin B is the major cause.

In the acute phase, a diffuse esophagitis is present in addition to inflammation of the tongue and mouth. The pharyngoesophageal sphincter becomes particularly involved, with atrophic changes in the submucosal layer. Later, the muscularis may also be affected and eventually fibrotic changes occur, producing mucosal atrophy and webs, with or without symptoms of obstruction. Narrowing of the sphincter zone may result (113), with an associated hypochromic microcytic anemia and achlorhydria. The fibrosis and webs may persist after the treatment of the anemia. An increased incidence of carcinoma of the hypopharynx is reported in this syndrome.

The webs in this disorder have a characteristic location and appearance (Fig. 155A). They are found chiefly anteriorly, at the pharyngoesophageal junction near the lower pole of the cricoid

FIGURE 155
Plummer-Vinson disease. (A) Typical web, (B) web and stenotic sphincter zone. (A) from McNab Jones, R. R. The Patterson-Brown Kelly syndrome Part II. J. Laryngol. Otol. 75:551, 1961. Headley Bros., Ltd., Invicta Press, Ashford, Kent, England.

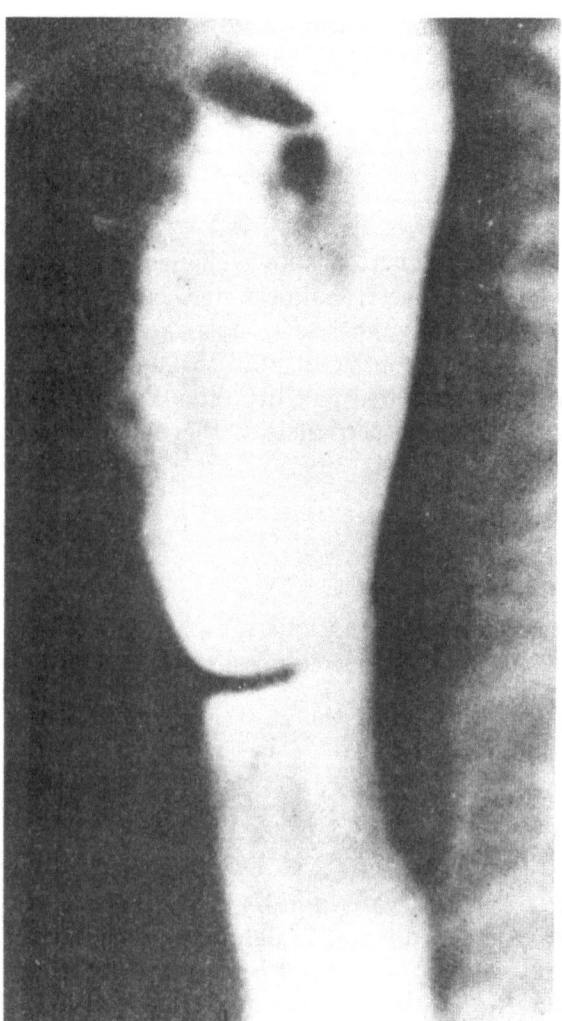

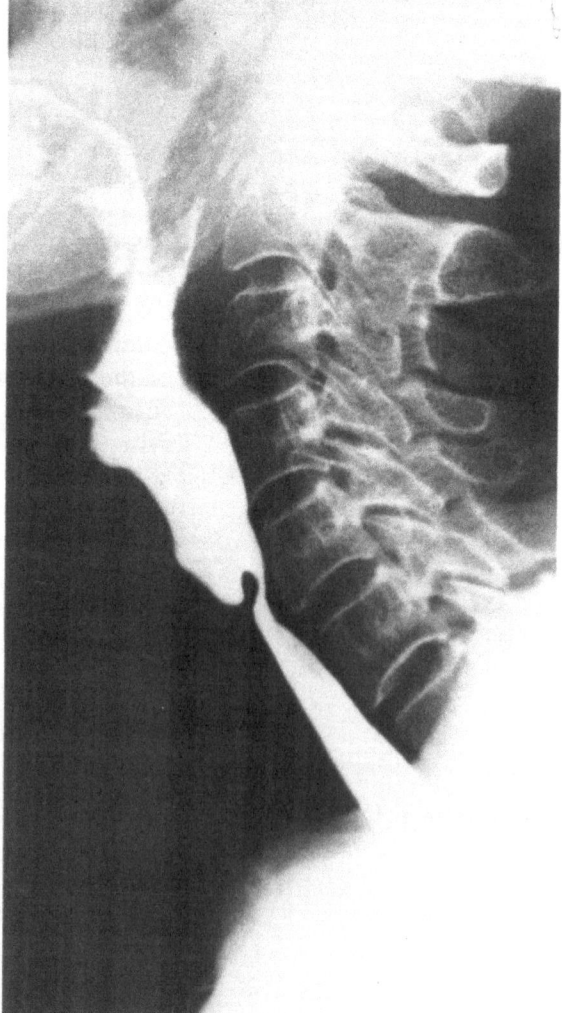

(A)

(B)

lamina. Frequently only an incomplete ring is observed, although occasionally a complete ring may be demonstrated. A cufflike constriction corresponding to the upper sphincter zone segment may also be present directly below the web (Fig. 155B). The narrowing and irregularity of this segment produces obstruction and dysphagia. An additional web at the distal end of the upper sphincter may on rare occasions also be present.

Radiologic examination requires special care in demonstrating the webs. Considerable distension of the upper sphincter zone with barium is essential in delineating the incisura characteristic of the web. Views of the cervical region in the lateral, oblique, and anteroposterior positions during swallowing should be outlined. In the presence of obstruction, stasis of the barium in the hypopharynx can be observed and a positive vallecular sign often is associated.

Esophageal webs are also related to local causes, which are discussed in Chapter 7. Mucosal atrophy secondary to avitaminosis, pernicious anemia, Sjogren's syndrome, and senility must all be considered in the differential diagnosis of esophageal webs. The radiologic features in these entities may be grossly similar to the Plummer–Vinson syndrome.

Avitaminosis

Severe avitaminosis alone may also affect esophageal motility, producing radiologic findings similar to achalasia.

LEUKEMIA AND LYMPHOMAS OF THE ESOPHAGUS

In children and adults with acute leukemia and widespread involvement, the esophagus may show gross or microscopic evidence of leukemic infiltration, reflected in coarsening of the mucosal folds of the esophagus radiologically. Necropsy studies have shown esophageal erosions, especially in terminal cases, and frequently associated moniliasis (96).

Because the lymphomas (40) usually involve the mediastinal lymph nodes, the esophagus often is secondarily involved by direct extension. Ulceration and obstruction may occur. Occasionally, as part of widespread involvement, the esophagus may show intrinsic lymphomatosis infiltrations producing dysphagia. Lymphomas in the cervical region may also occur (Fig. 156).

Hodgkin's disease rarely specifically produces intrinsic infiltration of the esophagus. The radiologic findings are those of narrowing of the esophageal lumen and ridigity of the esophageal wall resembling carcinoma (Fig. 157A). The esophageal mucosa may show ulcerating lesions.

Any of the lymphomas (and leukemia) generally respond well to radiation therapy with regression and eventual disappearance of abnormal radiologic changes (Fig. 157B). Recurrences, of course, are not unusual.

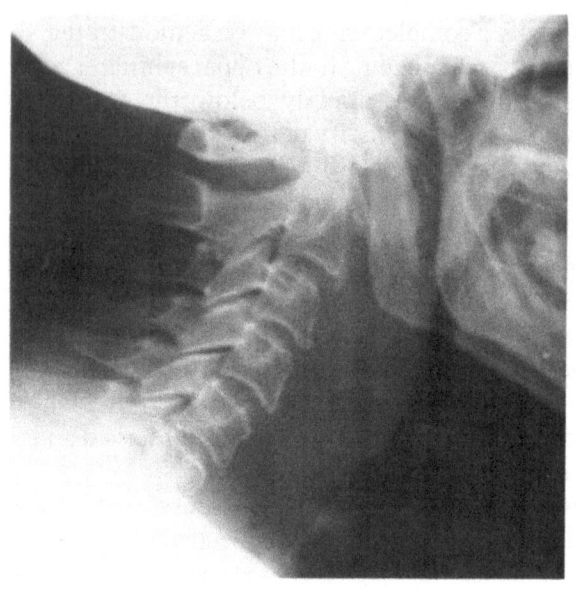
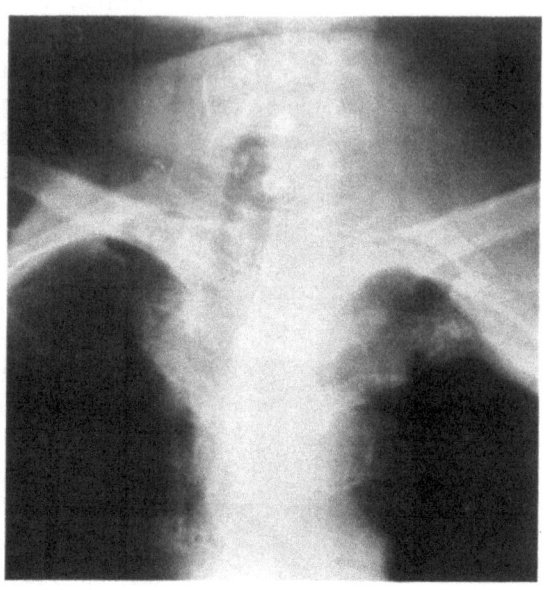

(A) (B)

FIGURE 156
Cervical lymphoma. (A) Retropharyngeal space mass. (B)
Anteroposterior view, showing symmetrical soft tissue mass in
lower neck region and deviated trachea.

FIGURE 157
Hodgkin's disease. (A) Lower esophageal changes, (B) normal
esophagus following radiation therapy.

(A) (B)

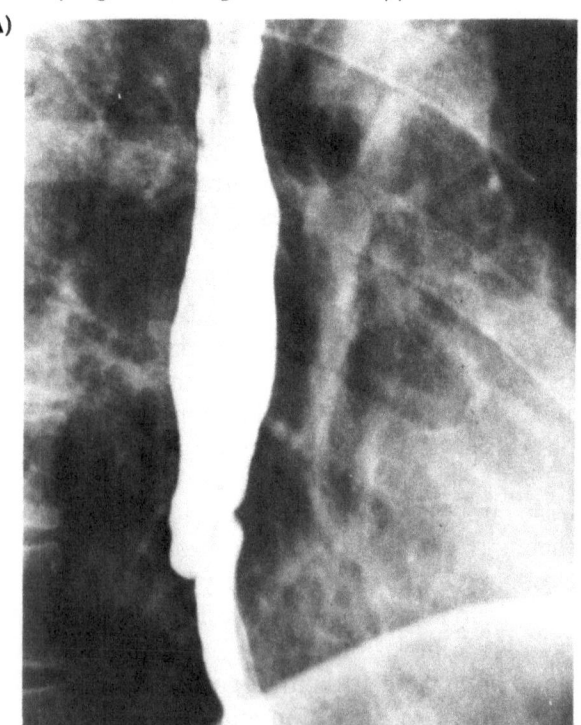
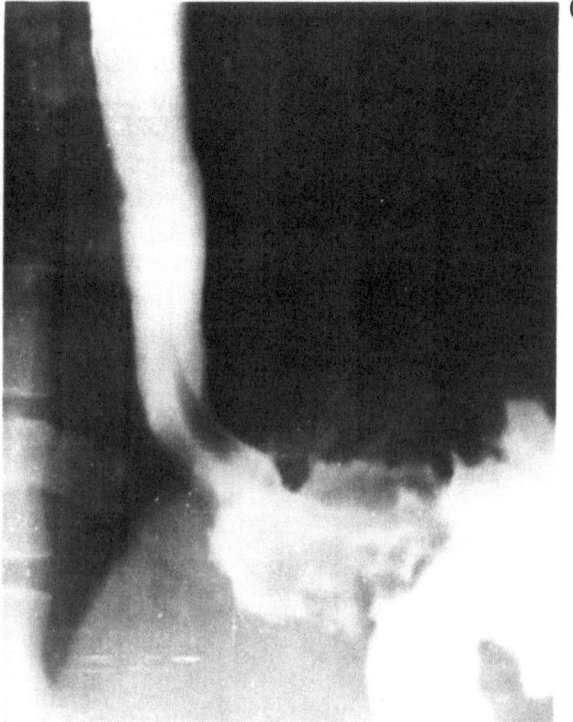

AMYLOIDOSIS

Amyloidosis is a disorder of unknown cause in which amyloid is deposited in various tissues, including smooth and striated muscles. It is considered to be related to the plasma cell dyscrasias. The primary form shows absence of other underlying disorders. The secondary and more common variety is associated with prolonged inflammatory lesions or infections, particularly chronic debilitating disorders (neoplasms), rheumatoid arthritis, and multiple myeloma. Currently the division into primary and secondary forms is no longer considered tenable.

Amyloidosis of the esophagus is a rare disorder. The esophagus is affected as part involvement of the entire gastrointestinal tract or the disease may be present primarily in the esophagus, without evidence of amyloidosis elsewhere (109). Amyloid is deposited, initially, in the submucosa of the esophagus around blood vessels, later involving the muscularis.

In amyloidosis of the esophagus, widening of the mucosal folds is a common finding on radiologic examination. The normal motor responses of the esophagus are affected, with resultant atonia and dilatation. On occasion a mass lesion caused by amyloid deposition may cause obstruction, simulating a neoplasm (Fig. 158).

ESOPHAGEAL VARICES

Abnormally dilated esophageal veins are observed in a variety of disorders in children and adults. Although varices are more

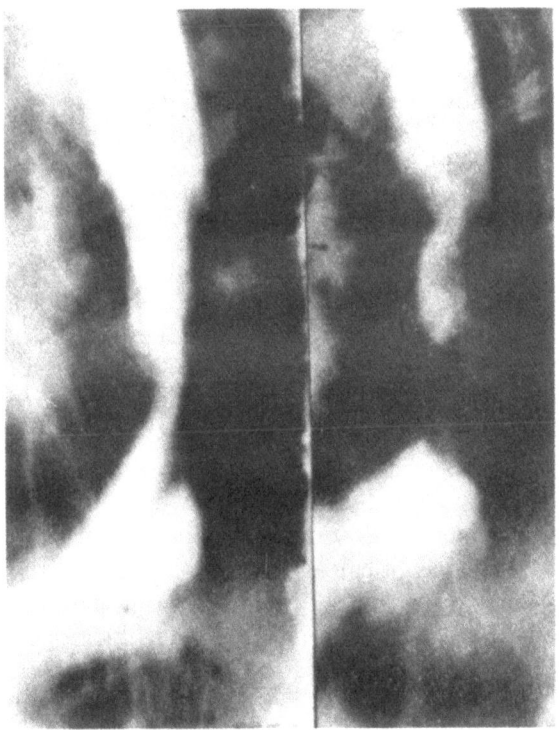

FIGURE 158
Primary amyloidosis of the esophagus. Reprinted from Heitzman, E. J., et al. Primary esophageal amyloidosis. Arch. Intern. Med. *100*:141, 1962. American Medical Association.

often present in the lower end of the esophagus, they may also be present in the upper end of the esophagus (downhill varices).

In children, varices may be secondary to congenital malformations, portal venous thrombosis, or extra- and intrahepatic portal hypertension. In adults, portal hypertension of extra- or intrahepatic origin is the major cause. "Downhill esophageal varices" are secondary to obstruction of the superior vena cava. Tumors extending into the mediastinum or fibrosing mediastinitis for any reason may produce superior vena cava obstruction and "downhill varices."

The radiologic examination of the esophagus for the detection of varices requires specialized techniques. The findings are chiefly dependent on (a) the dynamic changes of the esophagus during swallowing, (b) intrathoracic pressure (c) abdominal pressure, and (d) the stage of development of the varices. In Chapter 1, on technique, a number of special examinations have been listed. Because these examinations cannot be used in all circumstances, the choice of study must be patterned individually.

Cinefluoroscopy and/or cineradiography offer the simplest and best methods for the early detection of esophageal varices (2). Radiologic demonstration depends on the degree of engorgement of the varices during the examination. With cine studies, the esophagus can be examined in active inspiration and expiration and while the patient performs Valsalva and Müller maneuvers. In this way the changing pressures and dynamics permit the abnormally dilated veins to be more readily detected.

The earliest radiologic finding is localized thickening of the mucosal folds, with a wavy appearance of the borders of the esophagus and slight dilatation of this viscus (Fig. 159). The mucosal pattern therefore must be well visualized in order to detect very early changes. A thin barium mixture is preferable to a thick mixture. Double contrast studies often are helpful. Various methods to accomplish this have been advocated and described in Chapter 1.

As the varices enlarge, the diagnosis becomes easier. The key finding is the changing character of the mucosal pattern, with varying engorgement of the varices at different stages of the examination and even on successive films. This is helpful in differentiating the early mucosal changes associated with varices from an infiltrating carcinoma. As the size of the varices increases, the esophagus becomes more dilated and peristalsis decreases (Fig. 160). Spasm of the lower esophageal sphincter from the constant irritation of the engorged varices may occur, producing stasis of barium in the lower end of the esophagus. Varices may even appear and disappear in patients with advanced cirrhosis. Eventually rigid, finger-like ridges, representing the enlarged venous channels, may involve virtually the entire esophagus.

Downhill esophageal varices characteristically are delin-

FIGURE 159
Esophageal varices, early stage.

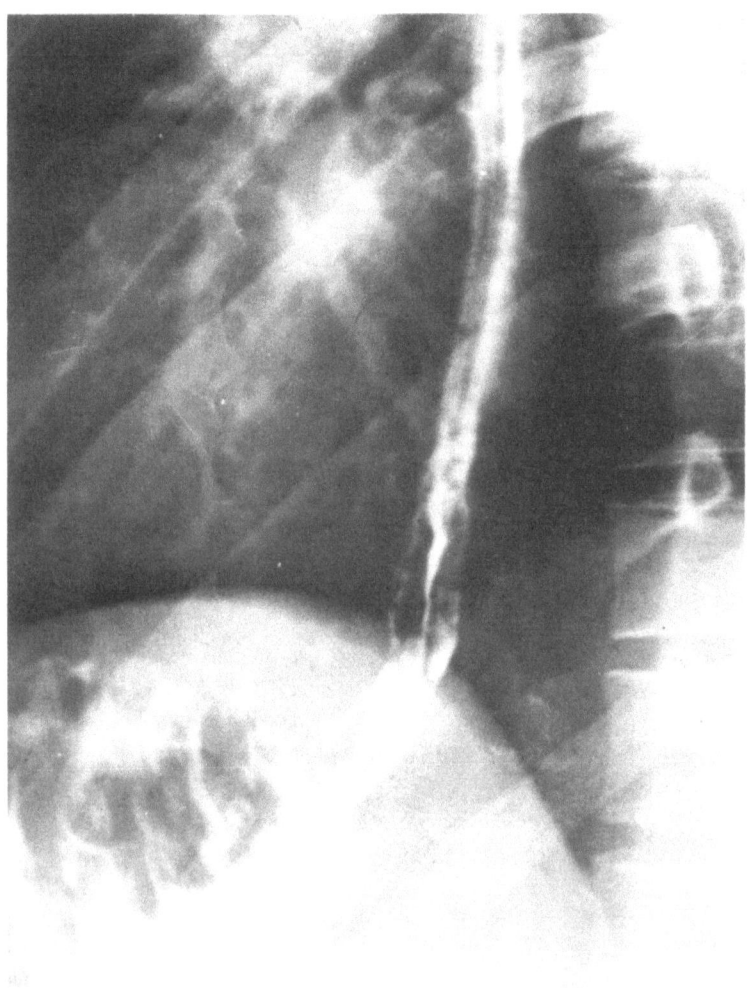

eated only in the upper end of the esophagus, associated with superior vena cava obstruction and mediastinal fibrosis. Congestive heart failure, aneurysms, or mediastinal tumors rarely may be responsible. Even less commonly, downhill varices may be demonstrated in the aged, without any evident cause. The roentgenologic techniques for their demonstration are similar to the methods used in delineating varices in the lower end of the esophagus.

Before a shunting operation is contemplated in the treatment of esophageal varices, splenoportography or other angiographic procedures are performed to delineate the collateral circulation (see Chapter 1). The findings following surgery are discussed in Chapter 8.

In the differential diagnosis, hiatal hernia, hernia with funneling of the lower end of the esophagus, carcinoma, lymphosarcoma, and polypoid esophagitis must be excluded. Infiltrating carcinoma in particular may produce polypoid mucosal changes that are difficult to differentiate from large varices,

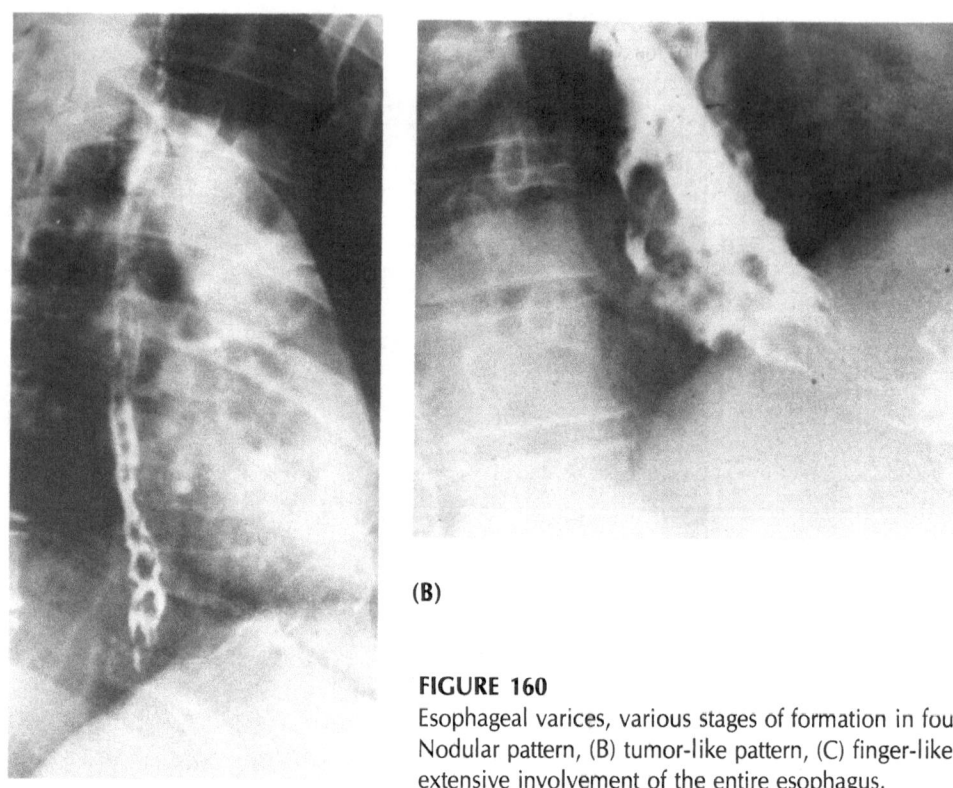

(B)

FIGURE 160

Esophageal varices, various stages of formation in four patients. (A) Nodular pattern, (B) tumor-like pattern, (C) finger-like pattern, (D) extensive involvement of the entire esophagus.

(A)

(C)

(D)

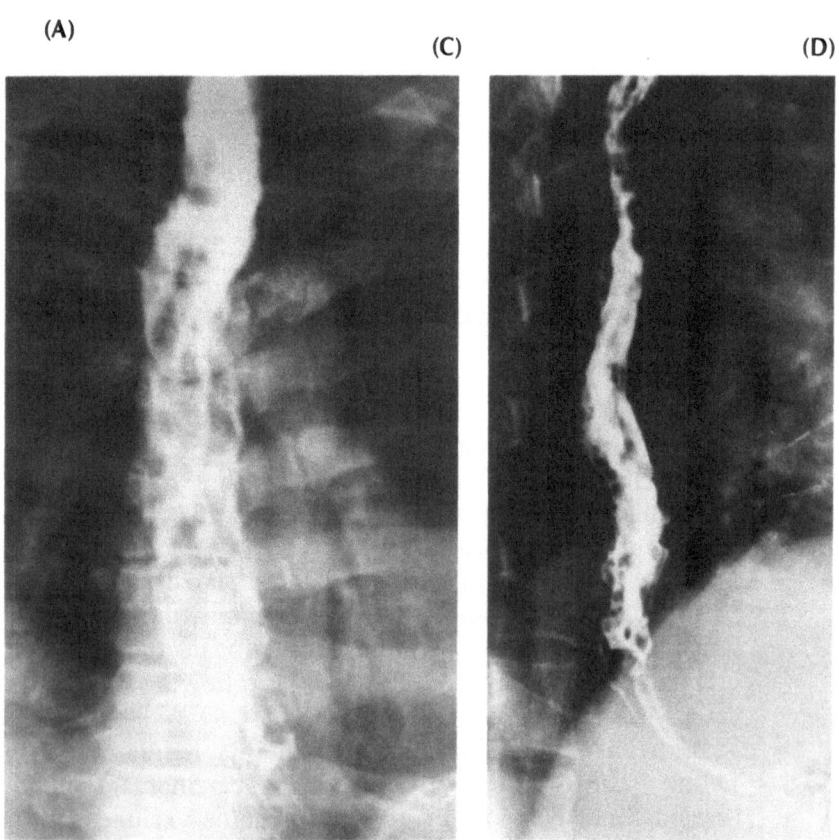

which may present in a static pattern. However, in varices, the esophageal wall is pliable and even though the esophagus may be dilated and peristaltic waves are sluggish, rigidity is absent. In polypoid esophagitis, there is irritability and spasm exceeding that associated with varices. In hiatal hernia, the demonstration of the contracted lower sphincter segment above the herniated portion of the stomach is diagnostic. Funneling of the distal end of the esophagus may present a difficulty because of the coarsened herniated gastric mucosal folds. However, tortuosity and irregularity of the mucosal folds are absent.

MISCELLANEOUS CONDITIONS

Allergic reactions

Allergic reactions secondary to drugs may result in acute angioneurotic edema with a form of multiple, giant urticaria affecting the esophagus. Total obstruction of the esophagus may occur in severe cases. Radiologic examination usually is not performed, except possibly in establishing the degree of esophageal obstruction.

Schizophrenia

Schizophrenia also may affect the swallowing mechanism. Cinefluoroscopic studies have been reported (26) showing occasional impairment of the swallowing mechanism secondary to motor disturbances.

Hypothyroidism

Hypothyroidism in infants may produce a thickening of the retropharyngeal soft tissues detectable on a lateral film of the cervical region. This area may be evaluated by the Arbran–Kemp method, i.e., by measuring the soft tissue thickness from the vertebra to the pharyngeal lumen. Normally, the anteroposterior diameter of the retropharyngeal soft tissues in a lateral film should be no more than three-fourths of the anteroposterior diameter of the body of the fourth cervical vertebra (102). This measurement is facilitated by using a thick barium bolus which coats the posterior pharyngeal wall after the barium has traversed this area.

Sydenham's chorea

Sydenham's chorea is probably an autoimmune disorder that is the result of a streptococcal infection, most commonly observed in childhood, characterized by muscular twitching and mental changes. Motor changes in the pharyngeal area result in hypermotility, which affects the swallowing mechanism and is detectable on fluoroscopic examination following a barium swallow.

Intramural hematomas

Spontaneous hematoma of the esophagus is a rare disorder, increasing in frequency because of the use of anticoagulant drugs. Hemorrhage can result from a number of systemic causes in addition to the use of anticoagulant drugs, including bleeding diatheses, liver disease, leukemia, and renal failure (42). Intramural dissection by the accumulated blood, similar to a dissecting aneurysm (115), occurs. Dysphagia usually is the presenting complaint. On radiologic examination the findings are similar to those of an intramural tumor, resulting in obstruction of the esophageal lumen. Rapid disappearance of the dysphagia and resolution of the tumor mass result after correction of the cause of the bleeding.

Intramural esophageal hematoma may also develop as a result of trauma, particularly of the esophagus.

Pneumatosis Cystoides of the Esophagus

This rare disorder, reported in an autopsied case (249), is characterized by multiple submucosal or subserosal air pockets or cysts. It is much more common in the colon and small intestine. It occurs chiefly in the presence of chronic, obstructive lesions of the gastrointestinal tract, particularly strictures. It is assumed that as a result of trauma to the mucosal surface above the level of obstruction, seepage of air into the submucosal layer takes place. In other instances a pulmonary cause is assumed, with air seeping into the wall of the involved segment of bowel (or esophagus) through the mediastinum, following rupture of pulmonary alveoli. This disorder in the bowel has been reported recently as one of the gastrointestinal complications or renal transplantation (98a.)

No radiologic demonstration of pneumatosis cystoides esophagi has been reported to our knowledge but the finding of air pockets along the affected esophageal wall, especially after the lumen is outlined by a barium swallow, can be anticipated.

CHAPTER
7

ORGANIC LESIONS (LOCAL)

Acute inflammatory involvement of the oropharynx and esophagus is relatively common. Many causes exist. An inflammatory process may go unrecognized both clinically and even radiologically. The radiologic findings concerning systematic causes are described in Chapter 6. Inflammatory changes due to local causes are now considered.

Most acute forms of esophagitis usually subside when the causative factors are removed and adequate treatment is given. Untreated esophagitis may result in permanent damage, characteristic of the chronic form. The sequence of the changes from acute to chronic esophagitis can best be followed radiologically.

Local causes of esophagitis have been divided into three main groups, consisting of mechanical, chemical, and thermal factors. Esophagitis, secondary to surgical procedures and radiotherapy, is considered in Chapter 8.

ESOPHAGITIS
Classification of local causes of esophagitis

I. Mechanical factors
  A. Posttraumatic
    1. Intubation
    2. Endoscopy
    3. Bouginage
    4. Foreign bodies
    5. Cardiac catheterization
  B. Chronic stasis
    1. Megaesophagus

    2. Internal or external obstruction from neoplasms or vascular mediastinal masses

  C. Ingestion of coarse (irritating) foods

II. Chemical factors

  A. Ingestion of caustics and drugs

    1. Alkalis

    2. Acids

    3. Other poisons and drugs

  B. Inhalation of chemical dusts and fumes, e.g., occupational

  C. Excessive use of alcohol and tobacco

  D. Regurgitated, highly acid gastric contents (peptic esophagitis)

III. Thermal factors

Posttraumatic

Mechanical factors

Posttraumatic causes are numerous. Any injury to the mucosal surface of the hypopharynx or esophagus may be responsible for inflammatory changes. At times, these changes are quite severe and may lead to the death of the patient. Initially, in the acute stage a localized cellulitis or abscess may develop. This is followed by intramural extension of the inflammatory process, with ulceration and erosions of the mucosal surface, leading to perforation.

The radiologic findings are similar to those described in part under the systemic causes of esophagitis. In addition, specific types of trauma may result in specific changes. A localized abscess produces the appearance of a mucosal or intramural lesion. Marked irritability, localized spasm, and rapid alteration in appearance on subsequent examinations help to distinguish an inflammatory process from a neoplasm. Persistent narrowing, unrelieved by antispasmodic medication, will suggest an early stenosis or stricture.

INTUBATION In prolonged intubation, because of the artificially created patency of the lower sphincter zone and a free reflux of gastric contents into the lower end of the esophagus, localized esophagitis can develop. Marginal ulcerations at the gastroesophageal junction may then ensue.

ENDOSCOPY Endoscopy can cause abrasions or tears of the mucosal wall, with resultant infection. This is more frequently encountered with the use of the rigid endoscope.

BOUGINAGE Bouginage, with frequent dilatations, commonly produces mucosal trauma. This procedure, although mechanically helpful in enlarging the lumen of the esophagus, contributes to exacerbation of the inflammatory changes.

FOREIGN BODIES Inflammation and perforation secondary to trauma from foreign bodies is a significant clinical challenge (see Chapter 4). Unrecognized nonopaque foreign bodies may lead to foreign body granulomas, which can mimic mucosal tumors.

CARDIAC CATHETERIZATION Retropharyngeal and mediastinal hemorrhage may be a complication of cardiac catheterization, producing compression of the esophagus and/or enlargement of the retropharyngeal space with dysphagia and respiratory distress. On radiologic examination considerable widening of the retropharyngeal space may be observed, with anterior displacement of the larynx.

Chronic stasis

MEGAESOPHAGUS Disorders resulting in direct or indirect esophageal obstruction usually also produce acute esophagitis. Megaesophagus, regardless of the cause, is frequently associated with esophagitis because of the mechanical trauma for retained coarse foods, bacterial contamination, and vascular congestive changes. However, the inflammatory changes may be difficult to detect radiologically because they often are obscured by the retained food. Esophageal lavage may be necessary preceeding a barium study of the mucosa, especially in the presence of underlying neoplasms.

INTERNAL AND EXTERNAL FACTORS Obstruction from internal and external factors also may be responsible for esophagitis. In the presence of a primary neoplasm, secondary inflammatory changes are common, often obscuring the neoplasm. Spasm and irritability on radiologic examination can mask a malignancy, especially when an infiltrating neoplasm with localized ulcerations is present. Inflammatory changes tend to obscure the extent of an underlying lesion. An obstructing intrinsic esophageal or extrinsic neoplasm also may result in stasis of ingested food with secondary esophagitis.

Ingestion of coarse foods

Ingestion of coarse and spicy foods can traumatize the esophageal mucosa, producing acute esophagitis that may become chronic. Radiologic features of a cicatrizing process may result. Individuals who habitually ingest spicy and coarse foods are particularly prone to such a development.

Intramural rupture of the esophagus may occur, secondary to hurried or overzealous ingestion of coarse foods. Radiologic examination with a barium swallow may reveal a small intramural collection of contrast medium. This is usually detected in the distal third of the esophagus and is associated with reduced or absent peristalsis in the involved area. Healing usually occurs spontaneously within several weeks (160).

Caustic agents

The ingestion of caustic agents dramatically produces progressive inflammatory changes in the esophagus with associated radiologic findings (86). Accidental ingestion of caustics, chiefly in children, and ingestion for suicidal purposes in adults are the chief causes. The most common caustic agent ingested is lye, but other strong alkali-containing agents produce oral, hypopharyngeal, esophageal, and gastric burns. The effects are dependent on the concentration and amount of the ingested material.

ALKALIS Alkalis produce precipitation of proteins, with deeply penetrating burns. The immediate spasm resulting from alkali ingestion stimulates vomiting of the chemical, which tends to minimize the severity of damage. In children, extensive mouth and subglottic burns usually develop. Edema of the larynx with respiratory obstruction requires prompt tracheotomy. Perforations, mediastinitis, and death may follow.

ACIDS Acids, as a rule, produce superficial coagulation necrosis and only minor esophageal burns. The stomach is usually more extensively involved. Esophageal damage develops chiefly in the areas of normal esophageal constrictions where some delay in the transit of the chemical occurs.

The radiologic findings with barium have been well described by Martel (161). In the immediate acute phase (several hours after the ingestion of a caustic agent), a diffuse blurring of the esophageal mucosa occurs, secondary to edema. Slow transit of the barium column is followed by changes in the mucosal pattern, with linear streaks and placquelike collection of barium in deep crevices or ulcers. Gaseous dilatation of the esophagus can also be observed on occasion on plain films. This dilatation is caused by the atony resulting from muscular necrosis, which occurs within 4 to 5 days of the acute episode. If the patient survives the acute period, the esophagus becomes denuded and a soft, granulomatous, occasionally ulcerating surface develops. The esophageal wall then shows serrated edges in the area of involvement. During this period, secondary infection may produce a diffuse, severe esophagitis, requiring several weeks to heal. A fibrotic process ensues, which continues for months. In this interval, in the absence of effective therapeutic measures, progressive narrowing of the involved area and stricture formation are observed.

Chemical factors

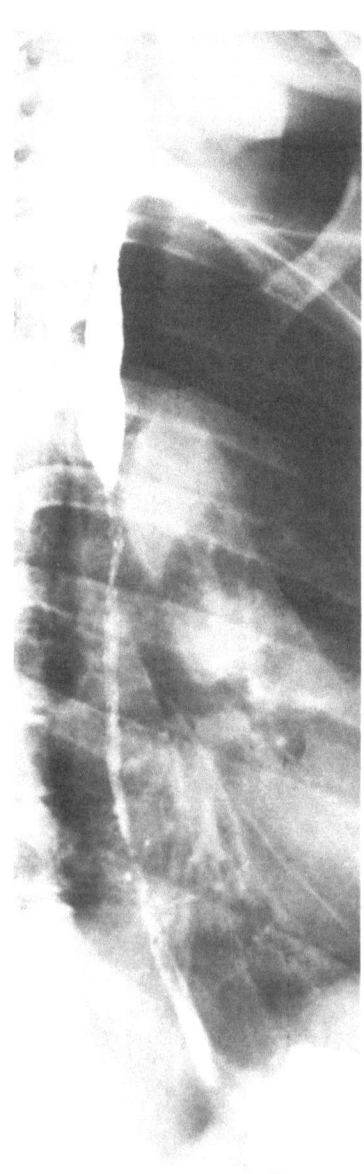

FIGURE 161
Lye esophagitis. Typical chronic, beaded, stenotic changes.

Eventually, complete stenosis with obstruction and an aperistaltic channel develop.

The course and extent of esophageal involvement depends on the degree of damage and the response to prompt and effective therapeutic measures. With the onset of stenosis, funneling of the barium above the site of narrowing and hyperperistalsis proximal to the stricture develops. More than one stricture may exist. The residual stenosis is usually beaded in radiologic appearance (Fig. 161).

Inhalation of toxic dusts and fumes

In certain occupations, workers inhale fine chemicals in the form of dust and fumes. In addition to the lung changes the esophagus may become involved, with the development of a chronic superficial esophagitis. Histologically, this form of esophagitis is characterized by irregular shallow ulcerations, cellular infiltration, and fibrotic changes of the submucosa. The radiologic findings reflect the underlying pathologic changes.

Excessive alcohol and tobacco

Excessive use of alcohol and tobacco may also be responsible for esophagitis. In chronic alcoholics the findings result from the chemical irritation locally or secondary to cirrhosis of the liver in the systemic process. Esophageal varices with periphlebitis is often present. In addition, peripheral neuropathy of the vagus nerve can occur secondary to the toxic effects of the alcohol. This results in sluggish peristalsis and delayed emptying of the lower esophagus, with some dilatation. The lower sphincter is usually not involved (262).

In heavy smokers and in individuals who chew tobacco, cancer *in situ* has been reported in addition to chronic superficial esophagitis. Gastroesophageal reflux appears to be much more common in smokers than in nonsmokers (229). This phenomenon has been traced to a fall in the resting pressure of the lower esophageal sphincter, resulting from the relaxing effects of nicotine on the sphincter, facilitating reflux and hence esophagitis. Symptoms probably depend on the acid contents of the stomach and the degree of reflux.

Peptic esophagitis

Peptic esophagitis actually represents a chemical esophagitis secondary to gastroesophageal acid reflux (209). Patients with excessive acid are more prone to develop symptoms. The hyperchlorhydria is secondary to a number of systemic causes but very often is associated with a chronic duodenal ulcer. However, peptic esophagitis can be present without hyperchlorhydria and reflux can occur without the development of esophagitis.

The most important accompanyment of peptic esophagitis is persistent vomiting of acid gastric contents. The resultant esophagitis is at first acute, but with prolonged or recurrent attacks a chronic form develops. In addition to the hydrochloric acid, increased pepsin, regurgitated bile salts, and peptic juices, particularly during persistent and prolonged bouts of vomiting, may also be responsible for the esophagitis. The degree of damage produced probably varies with the mucosal resistance, which may be weak initially or may weaken progressively with prolonged and repeated attacks. At first only the surface epithelium is involved, but later erosion into the submucosal surface and muscularis mucosa occurs.

The earliest radiologic findings of peptic esophagitis consist of alteration in the mucosal pattern of the lower esophagus with irritability and spasm and ulceration (Fig. 162), followed by some degree of funneling as cicatrizing changes set in (Fig. 163A).

(A)   **(B)**

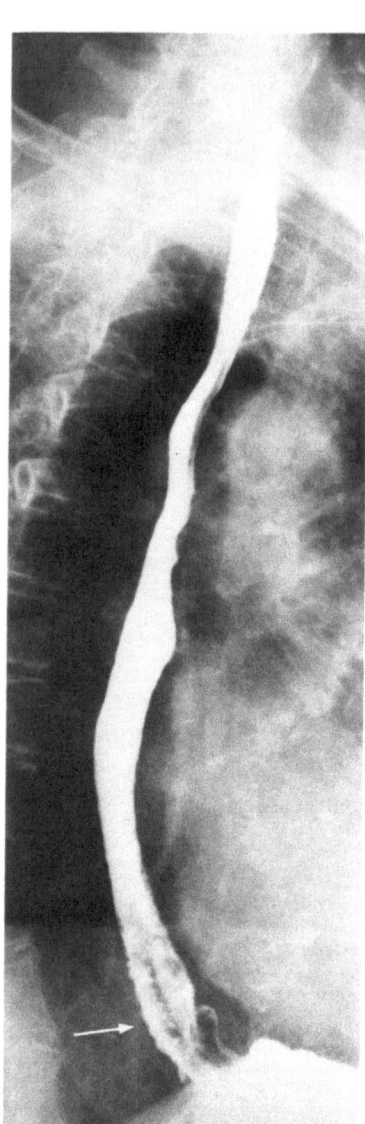

FIGURE 162
Localized early peptic esophagitis (at arrows).

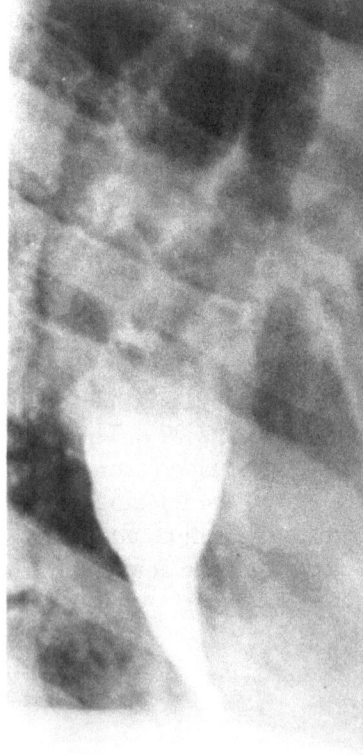
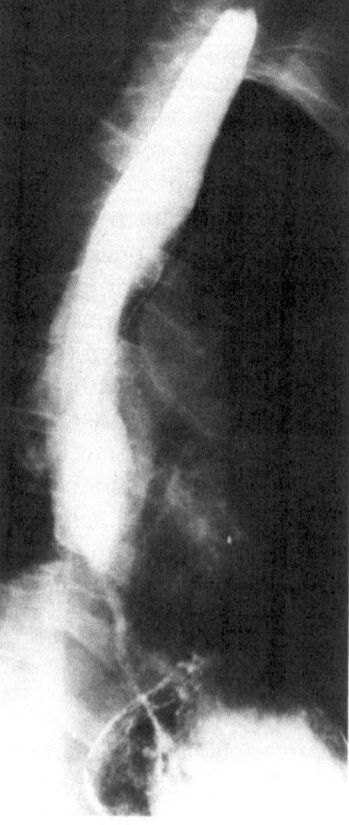

FIGURE 163
More advanced states of peptic esophagitis. Two different patients.

Damage to the esophageal mucosa by gastric reflux is determined in a number of ways. The burning substernal sensation is probably the most common symptom. Confirmation of peptic esophagitis can be obtained by the diluted hydrochloric acid perfusion test, motility studies, electrical potential determination (EPD) data, and finally by direct endoscopic examination with biopsy. The acid barium test (see Chapter 1 for technique) is performed by having the patient ingest acidified barium. In patients with esophagitis, increased, disordered peristaltic action is noted as the patient swallows the acid barium mixture. In patients with a normal esophagus no significant change in peristalsis is noted. The perfusion test is based on the assumption that dilute hydrochloric acid produces no symptoms in contact with a normal esophagus, whereas in an individual with esophagitis typical burning substernal sensation is experienced. In esophagitis, motility studies show evidence of hypermotility similar to that of diffuse spasm. The EPD test depends on the status of the epilithelial layer of the esophageal mucosa, which transmits a normal electrical polarity curve, whereas a damaged epithelium records an abnormal curve.

Peptic esophagitis secondary to chronic hyperacidity eventually produces a long tubular type of stenosis, without obvious ulcerations (264) (Fig. 163B).

Upward pull is created, secondary to the shortening of the esophagus by the stricture, often resulting in a sliding type of hiatal hernia.

The presence of an hiatal hernia formerly was presumed to be a *de facto* cause for peptic esophagitis. The high incidence of hiatal hernia now encountered without any symptomatic manifestations or gastric reflux, especially in the elderly, has altered present day concepts of this disorder. The normal acid production of the stomach decreases with age, so that hyperacidity is less frequently a factor. In a preexisting hiatal hernia and associated peptic esophagitis, an incompetent lower esophageal sphincter is usually present. The portion of the esophagus involved appears to be much shorter, with the sphincter segment affected chiefly. This type of esophagitis is more likely to show localized marginal ulcerations, without aberrant epithelium. The earliest radiologic manifestations of peptic esophagitis with an hiatal hernia are irregularities of the mucocal pattern or a serrated appearance of the sphincter zone segment (Fig. 164). Subsequently, a short localized area of stenosis with or without ulcerations develops (Fig. 165). If untreated, a stricture results, giving the appearance of congenitally short esophagus with peptic esophagitis (Fig. 166), the history and age of the patient being helpful in establishing the distinction.

In neonates, infants, and children, an incompetent lower esophageal sphincter results eventually in peptic esophagitis

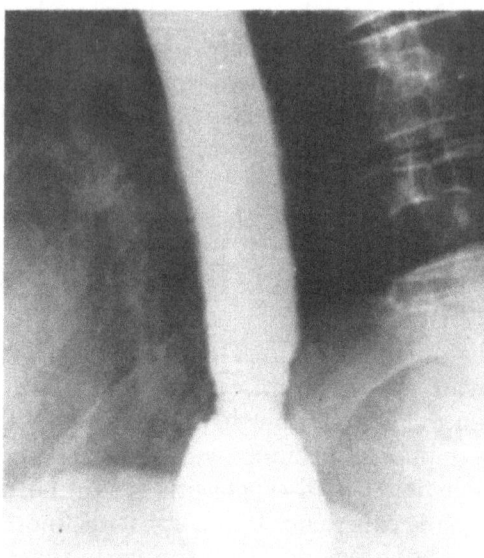

FIGURE 164
Early peptic esophagitis in the presence of a hiatal hernia.

FIGURE 165
Peptic esophagitis with ulceration in the presence of a hiatal hernia.

FIGURE 166
Esophageal stricture in the presence of a hiatal hernia.

FIG. 165   **FIG. 166**

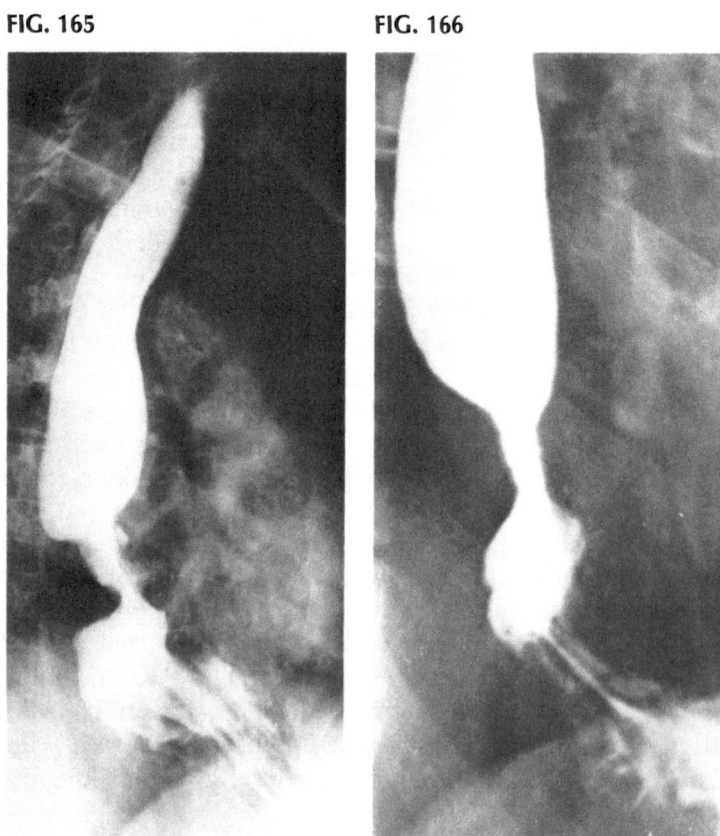

followed by a sliding type of hiatal hernia. This may also be confused with a congenitally short esophagus.

Thermal factors

Ingestion of very hot or cold foods may produce an acute edematous esophagitis, secondary to the thermal trauma to the mucosal lining of the esophagus. Perforation of the esophagus may even occur as a later sequela. The radiologic findings reflect the underlying pathologic changes.

ESOPHAGEAL ULCERS

Ulcers of the esophagus have systemic as well as local causes. The ulcers are usually single but may occasionally be multiple. Ulcers most commonly occur as a result of acute or chronic esophagitis (Fig. 167).

A distinction should be made between esophageal erosions and minute ulcerations. Erosions are usually localized, irregular areas of denuded mucosa, whereas minute ulcerations are multiple, small, symmetrical, superficial excavations, producing radiologically a serrated appearance of the esophageal lumen.

(A)

(B)

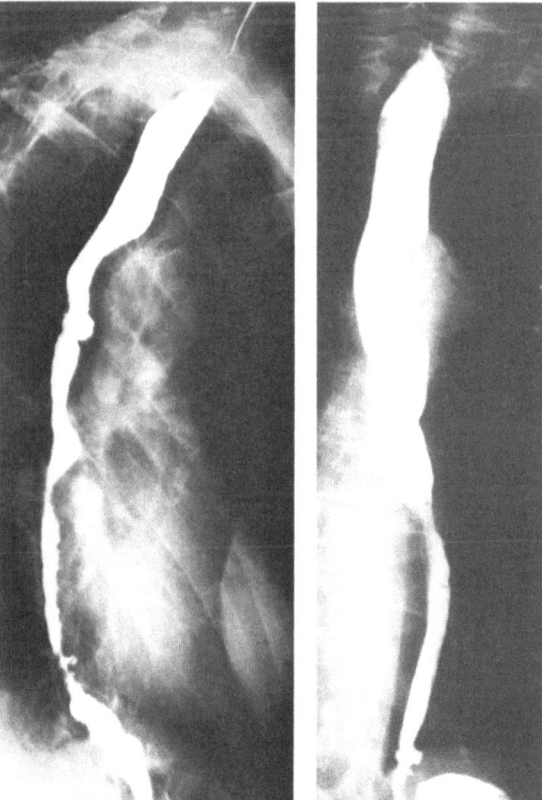

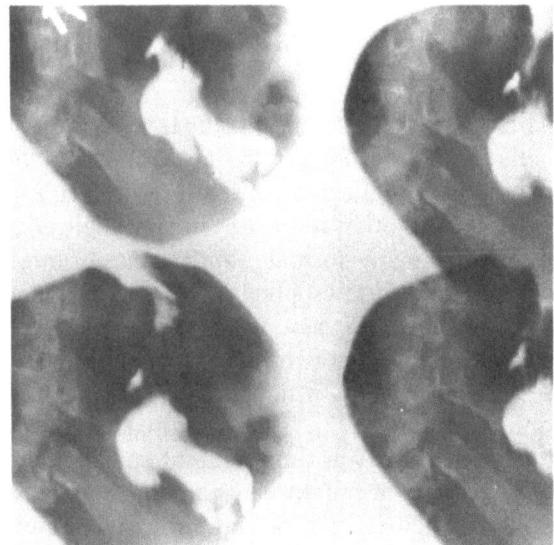

FIGURE 167
Esophageal ulcerations. (A) In the presence of acute peptic esophagitis; (B) in the presence of chronic esophagitis secondary to the ingestion of lye; (C) in the presence of acute esophagitis following surgery of the lower end of esophagus (spot films).

(C)

Esophageal ulcers are referred to as "peptic" ulcerations, similar to those observed in the stomach and duodenal bulb. The distinction between an acute or chronic ulcer depends on the degree of irritability, depth of ulceration, and rapidity of change on subsequent examinations, as well as the response to medical treatment. Ulcers may be benign or malignant. The latter are discussed in the section on esophageal malignancies.

The radiologic criteria for the diagnosis of an esophageal ulcer are the same as for any other peptic ulcer. An ulcer is an excavation of the mucosal surface which may be superficial or may extend deep into the muscular coat and may even perforate. The demonstration of an ulcer niche or crater radiologically with barium is the critical diagnostic feature. The niche is a barium opacity extending beyond the outline of the opacified lumen, projecting as a small collection of barium within the excavation in the tangential plane. The density of this collection is less than that of the lumen because it contains only a small amount of barium. When the ulcer is seen "en face," it is called a crater. The crater appears as a small localized area of increased density identified through a partly coated (with barium) esophagus. The crater may be overlooked or obliterated by a densely opacified esophagus. The location, shape, size, contour, and depth of the ulcer, as well as the relationship to the surrounding wall and the degree of disturbed motor function at the ulcer site, help in differentiating a benign from a malignant process.

A small esophageal diverticulum must always be excluded. The latter outpocketing is usually smooth and even inconstantly present. A neck generally is present, leading to the diverticulum. A small ulcer may occasionally appear separated from the main lumen. An ulcer is usually more irregular, retaining the barium longer; its shape is more constant throughout the examination.

The Barrett esophagus

This type (265) is an esophagus lined with columnar epithelial cells in place of the normal squamous cells (also see Chapter 3). In its uncomplicated state, the Barrett esophagus appears normal in all other respects. On radiologic examination, no difference from any normal esophagus is observed, in contrast to a congenitally short esophagus where the apparent lower portion of the esophagus is actually herniated stomach. The columnar epithelium lining of the Barrett esophagus is heterotopic and resembles cardiac, fundal, ciliated, or intestinal epithelium microscopically (37). The columnar lining may be mixed in type, particularly at the proximal end of the esophagus, where interspersing of squamous and columnar cells occurs. In addition, isolated islands of ectopic gastric mucosa may coexist

Peptic ulcerations

**The Barrett esophagus
and ulcer**

with squamous epithelium in other areas of the esophagus, particularly in the upper and middle segments. No cases of Barrett esophagus involving the entire esophagus have been reported.

Columnar epithelium in the lower end of the esophagus may also be acquired secondary to an inflammatory process. This may produce a columnar epithelial surface, originating from underlying ectopic gastric glands in the lamina propia. These glands are the remnants of faulty descent during embryologic development (182). Acquired heterotopia is found in elderly individuals, usually in association with a sliding type of hiatal hernia and chronic esophagitis.

Ectopic epithelium in the esophagus is more susceptible to the effects of regurgitated gastric juices than the normal esophageal epithelium. Inflammatory changes with ulcerations occur more frequently, therefore, and specifically, the Barrett esophagus is more susceptible to chronic ulceration than a normal esophagus (226). Also, whereas ulcerations occur in an esophagus lined with squamous epithelium, such ulcers tend to be more superficial, resulting in localized, generally short stricture. Ulcers associated with ectopic gastric mucosa are deeper, more chronic, and less prone to result in cicatrization and stenosis.

Columnar epithelial cells are also found high in the thoracic esophagus with or without ulceration. Therefore, an inflammatory process in this area can also produce a stricture that may mimic a malignant neoplasm.

A recent study of a stricture in a Barrett esophagus (108) including manometric, histologic, and acid determinations, suggests a congenital rather than an acquired origin. The diagnosis of a Barrett esophagus can be established occasionally by scanning with Tc 99 mm pertechnetate, which is selectively concentrated by the gastric type of mucosa found in this disorder (21).

Barrett ulcer

The Barrett ulcer (peptic ulcer of the esophagus) is usually a single, large ulcer, in the region of the middle third of the esophagus in an area of ectopic gastric epithelium. On radiologic examination, the ulcer persists as a deep, elongated, sharply defined, large niche (Fig. 168). Cicatrizing stenosis is usually absent, with only a minimal degree of functional disturbance apparent, consisting of slight spasm or abnormal motility. No fixation or mass at the site of the ulcer and no displacement or abnormal angulation of the esophagus are apparent. Although such ulcers often are resistant to medical treatment, they eventually heal. Perforation is an occasional complication. The Barrett ulcer must be differentiated from a

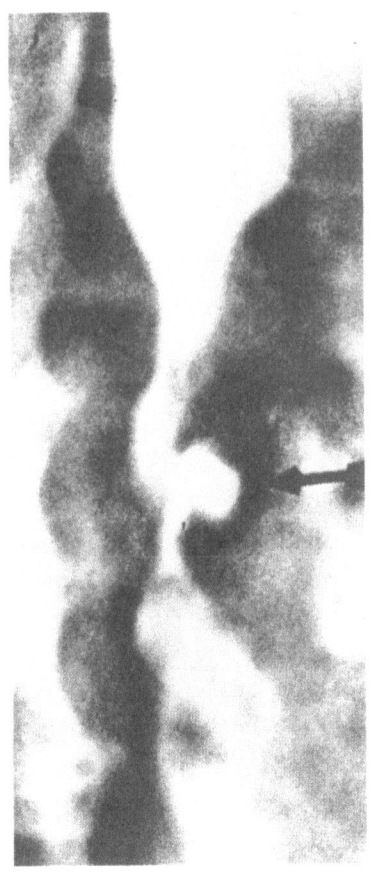

FIGURE 168
The Barret ulcer (at arrow). Reprinted from Som, M., and Wolf, B. S. Peptic ulcer of the esophagus and esophagitis in gastric-lined esophagus. J.A.M.A. *162:7*, 641, 1956. Copyright 1956, American Medical Association.

diverticulum. Ectopic and heterotopic gastric epithelium of the esophagus predisposes to malignancy so that a neoplasm must also be included in the differential diagnosis.

A marginal ulcer occurs at the gastroesophageal junction, secondary to a preexisting esophagitis (Fig. 169). An often associated hiatal hernia may or may not be identified. This type of ulcer tends to be acute and subsides after appropriate medical treatment. Such ulcers occur with or without heterotopic gastric epithelium. A marginal ulcer may also be present at the base of a short stenotic segment, secondary to inflammatory changes affecting the sphincter zone. In such instances, a hiatal hernia which either preceded or resulted from the inflammatory disease, usually is present. A congenitally short esophagus with ulceration and esophagitis shows similar changes but occurs in younger patients. Figure 170 shows the development of a stricture in the presence of an untreated esophagitis and hiatal hernia.

Marginal ulcer

FIGURE 169
Marginal ulcer (at arrow) in the presence of a sliding hiatal hernia.

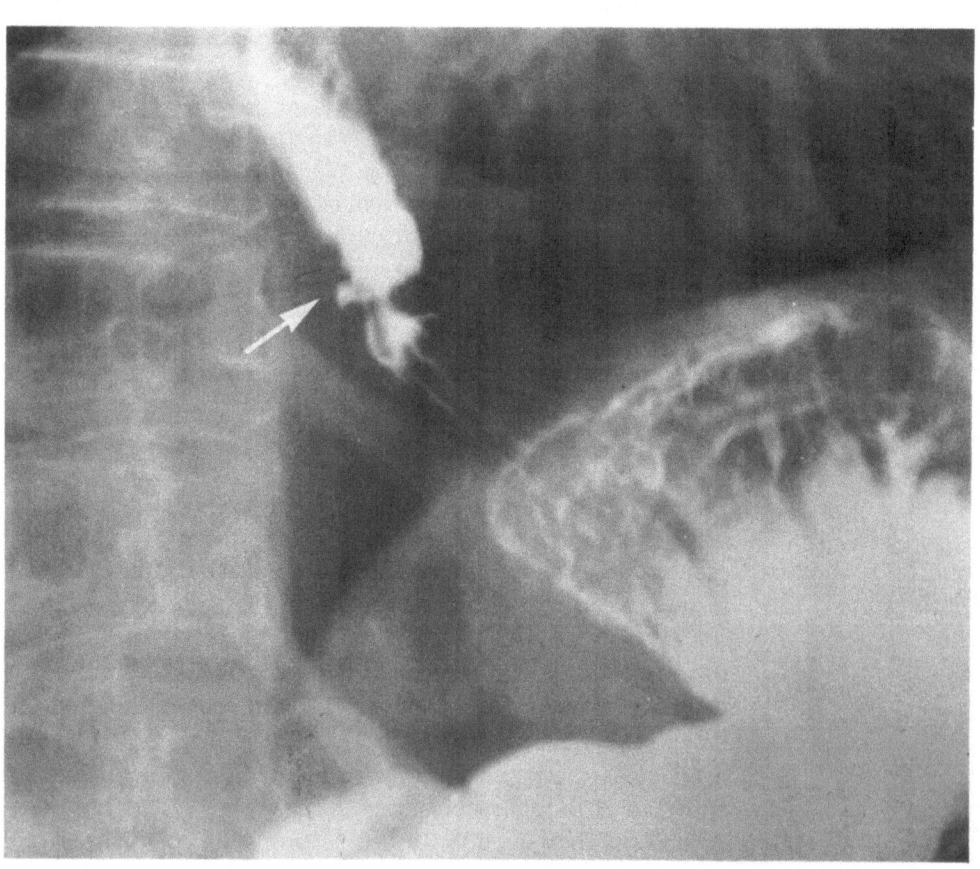

FIGURE 170
The development of a stricture in the presence of untreated esophagitis and hiatal hernia. (A) Initial examination; (B) one year later, same patient, showing a stricture with obstruction.

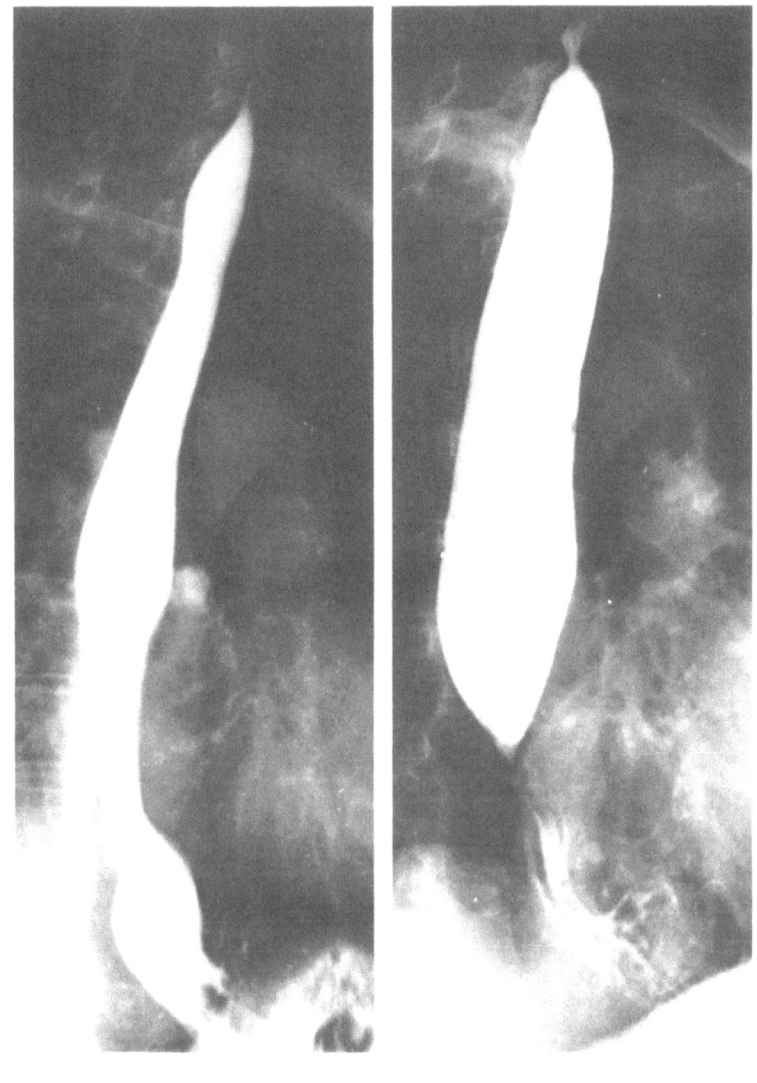

(A)   (B)

Iatrogenic ulcers

Iatrogenic ulcers are not unusual after prolonged esophageal or gastric intubation. These ulcers are usually located at the gastroesophageal junction (marginal). Esophageal as well as gastric ulcers may occur, following prolonged treatment with corticosteroids. Such ulcers are usually acute and clear rapidly after medical treatment. Iatrogenic ulcers also may follow any form of induced trauma from endoscopy or the ingestion of a foreign body.

"Kissing ulcers"

"Kissing ulcers" are rare, pressure-contact ulcers that usually are located in the hypopharynx (postcricoid region) and observed in elderly individuals with generalized cachexia. A large, heavily calcified cricoid cartilage that produces ischemic pressure changes and subsequent ulceration in the anterior and posterior walls of the hypopharynx may be responsible. These "kissing ulcers" also may follow intubation or use of tracheotomy tubes or may be caused by vascular changes secondary to prolonged lodgment of foreign bodies. Marked spasm is usually present because of the severe inflammation. On radiologic examination during the ingestion of a barium swallow, such ulcers may be demonstrated, although infrequently. These "kissing ulcers" are often only discovered at necropsy (244).

BENIGN STRICTURES

Strictures are principally the end result of some form of esophagitis. They are located anywhere in the esophagus and vary from thin annular rings to a cordlike constriction of the esophagus. Strictures may be the result of systemic as well as local disease processes. The location, appearance, and association of the stricture with a hiatal hernia helps in determining the cause.

A general classification of strictures follows.

Residual damage from systemic causes
1. Acute and chronic infections
2. Various granulomatous disorders
3. Crohn's disease
4. Ulcerative colitis
5. Chronic duodenal ulcer
6. Pemphigus, epidermolysis bullosa, herpes
7. Mediastinitis
8. Scleroderma
9. Dermatomyositis

Local causes
1. Ingestion of corrosive agents
2. Reflux esophagitis
3. Ulcer of esophagus
4. Trauma (especially secondary to foreign bodies)
5. Hiatal hernia
6. Ectopic and heterotopic gastric epithelized esophagus
7. Congenital disorders

Benign strictures must be differentiated from malignant strictures, acquired or congenital webs and rings, localized areas of muscular hypertrophy, and physiologic areas of spasm. The systemic causes of strictures are discussed in Chapter 6.

Radiologic considerations in examining strictures

The location of a stricture is an important first observation. The length, shape, character, and degree of obstruction then must be evaluated next.

In the cervical region, chronic esophageal trauma as a result of prominent cervical vertebral osteophytes may produce a small annular stricture located at or below the level of the upper sphincter.

A localized area of stenosis in the region of the aortic arch must be studied carefully to exclude a neoplastic process. Smooth, centrally located funneling of the stricture favors a benign lesion. Eccentric, irregular funneling above the stricture favors a neoplasm. Rigidity of the stenotic segment with a localized aperistaltic area also favors a malignant process, whereas some distensibility of the involved segment with normal or hyperactive peristalsis supports a benign disorder.

At the level of the mid-esophagus, the evaluation of strictures secondary to surrounding mediastinal disease provides important challenges. It is necessary to evaluate enlargement of mediastinal lymph nodes, fixation of any stenotic segment, abnormal angulation, and thickening of the esophageal wall and diverticula. A smooth, residual, stenotic, short segment slightly below the bronchial bifurcation may be the result of a healed Barrett ulcer. Here, the esophagus above and below this segment appears normal with normal mobility.

Strictures in the lower third of the esophagus are most common, being associated usually with an hiatal hernia (Fig. 170). It is necessary to determine whether the hernia has preceded or has been the result of the stricture involving the sphincter. A large hernia associated with a stricture usually signifies reflux esophagitis, secondary to the hernia. A long, stenotic, funneled segment above a hiatal hernia may be secondary to heterotopic gastric epithelium. A stricture may involve the sphincter zone alone (Fig. 171). Strictures may also result from healed, traumatic perforations (Fig. 172).

Chronic strictures, secondary to the ingestion of caustic agents, usually are long and produce a residual beading of the stenotic segment as well as rigidity. Following persistent bouginage, a benign stricture may resemble a malignant lesion because of the destruction of its mucosal surface.

A benign stricture eventually may undergo malignant transformation and the transition can be sufficiently slow in development and subtle diagnostically to pass undetected. Periodic radiologic examinations are essential and doubtful lesions should be biopsied. Cine studies are also very helpful. Benign strictures, to some degree, are more pliable than malignant lesions and demonstrate a degree of mobility. Benign strictures often change position during inspiration and expiration and are influenced by cardiac pulsations. In a malignant lesion, the wall is immobile or rigid; the lumen can be forced open by a passing bolus but only to a minimal degree. The bolus remains for a longer period above the stenotic area, which is not as readily affected by respiratory action or cardiac pulsations. Small annular strictures must be differentiated from webs, rings, and localized areas of muscular hypertrophy.

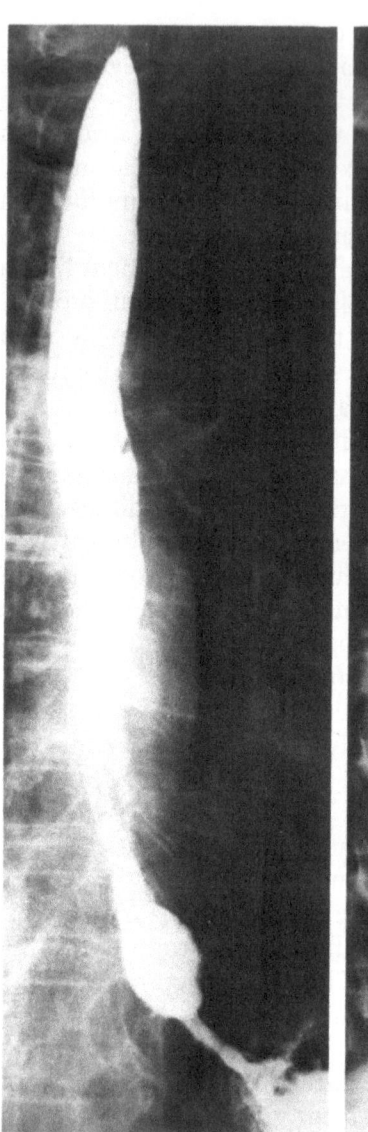
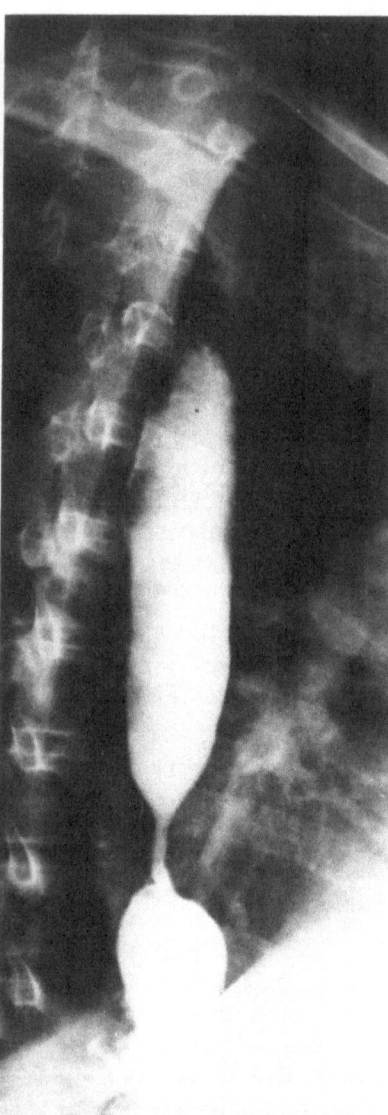

FIGURE 171
Stricture of the sphincter zone.

FIGURE 172
Stricture of the lower end of the esophagus, secondary to an old healed perforation following endoscopic examination.

FIG. 171   FIG. 172

Webs

Webs are thin membranes that partly or completely encircle the lumen of the esophagus (215). They are congenital in origin or acquired through systemic as well as local factors. Congenital webs are described in Chapter 3. Plummer–Vinson syndrome is the most common systemic cause for esophageal webs and is described in Chapter 6. Webs should not be confused with normal inconstant notchings chiefly observed at the pharyngoesophageal junction (Chapter 2). Cervical webs also may occur secondary to lye strictures (Fig. 173). Idiopathic web-like lesions in the area of the upper sphincter zone may also be a cause for dysphagia (Fig. 174).

The clinical significance of hypopharyngeal and cervical webs has been questioned recently (177). Asymptomatic webs

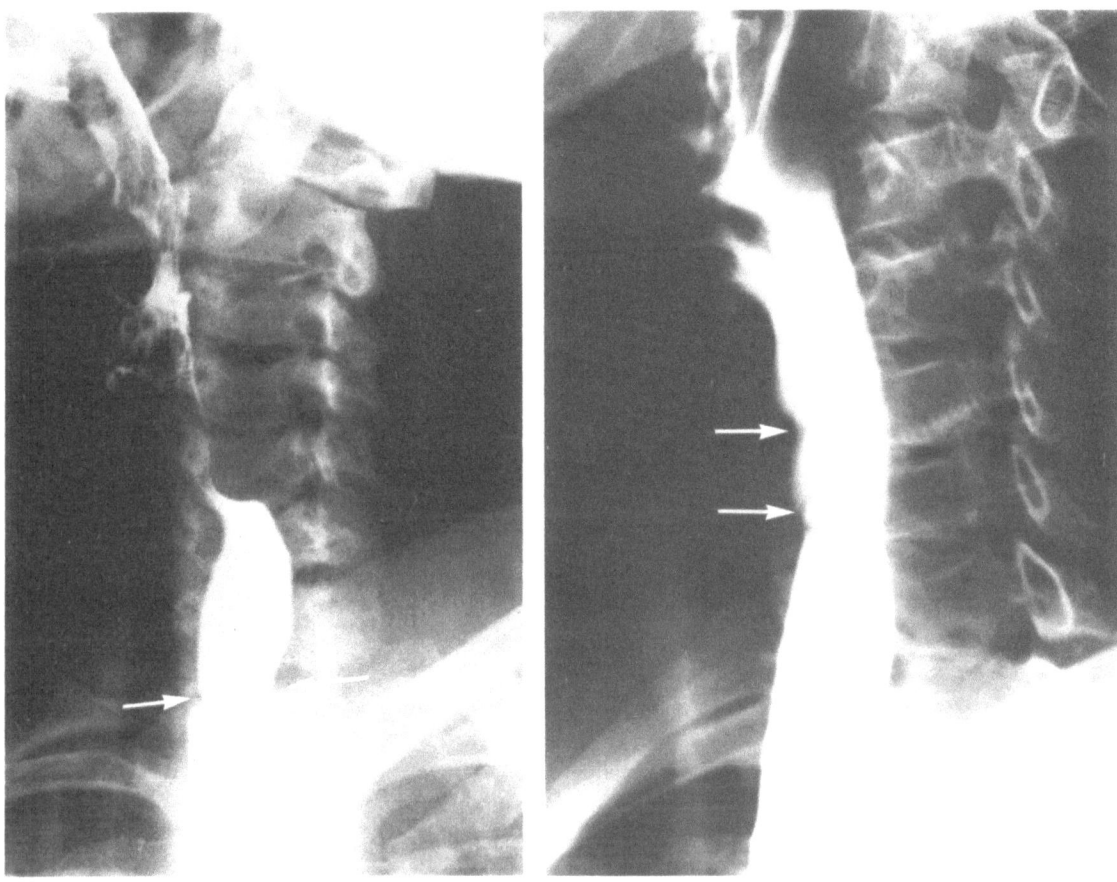

FIG. 173   FIG. 174

FIGURE 173
Web of cervical esophagus
secondary to a lye stricture (at
arrow).

FIGURE 174
Idiopathic web sectioning off the
upper sphincter zone (arrow),
associated with dysphagia of
many years duration.

Rings

in this region are not uncommon and may be of no clinical importance unless they produce an element responsible for dysphagia.

On radiologic examination, webs are best identified in a distended hypopharynx or esophagus (Fig. 175). The maximum narrowing produced by the web (as well as rings and strictures) is best noted just prior to the stripping action of an advancing peristaltic wave. Webs appear as thin notchings or incisura at the periphery of the barium column and are usually asymmetrical.

Ringlike strictures are usually more rigid and wider than webs and may also be asymmetrical; they are congenital or acquired. In the lower end of the esophagus, a demonstration of one or more rings is not unusual. These must not be confused with inconstant notchings outlining the upper and lower attachments of the phrenoesophageal membrane. These notches are frequently associated with hiatal insufficiency and hernia, as described in Chapter 5. On radiologic examination, these

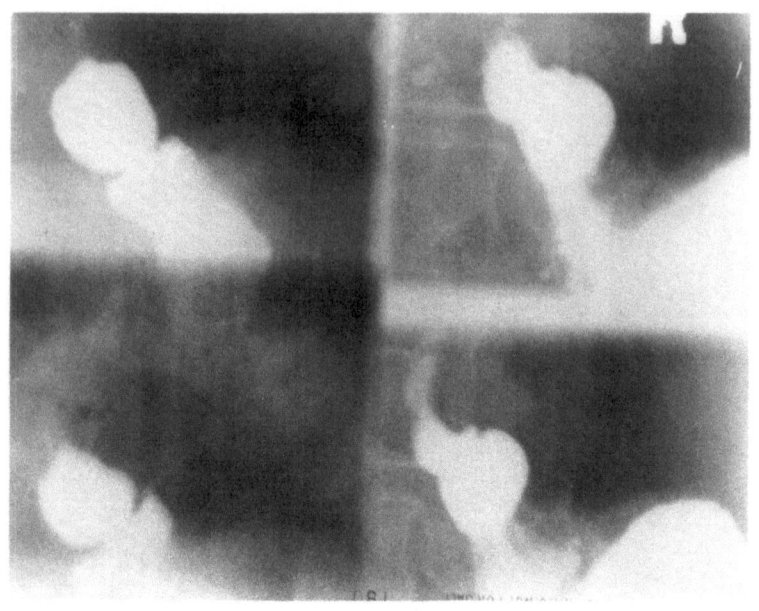

FIGURE 175
Annular inflammatory stricture, lower esophagus (spot films). From Zaino, C., et al. *The Lower Esophageal Vestibular Complex,* 1963. Courtesy Charles C Thomas, Publisher, Springfield Illinois.

FIGURE 176
(A) Schatski's ring. (B) Compare with ordinary notches demarcating the gastroesophageal junction (at arrow). From Zaino, C., et al. *The Lower Esophageal Vestibular Complex,* 1963. Courtesy Charles C Thomas, Publisher, Springfield, Illinois.

Fig. 176 (A)   **(B)**

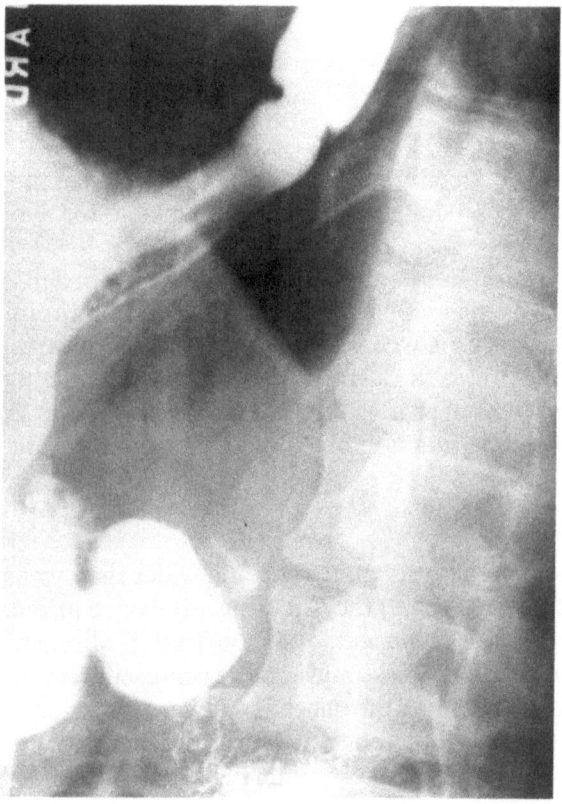 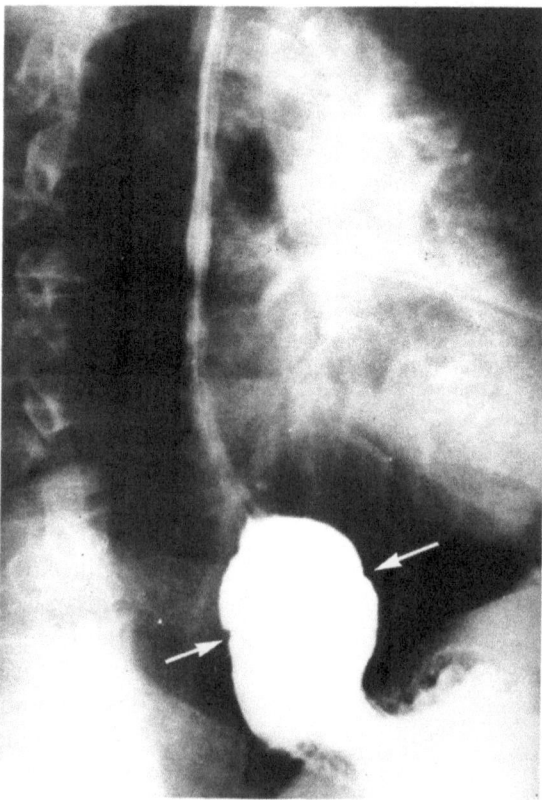

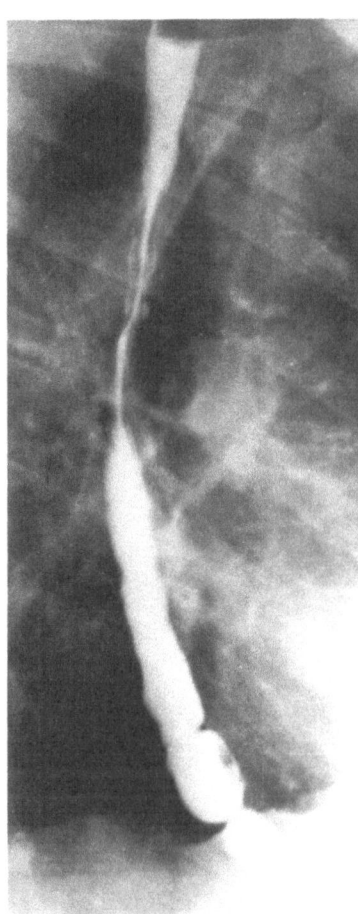

FIGURE 177
Double esophageal rings in the presence of an hiatal hernia.

Muscular hypotrophy

notches are small, inconstant, triangular, incisure-like defects that are unilateral or bilateral. A true ring is wider and usually encircles the entire esophagus.

Schatski's ring

Schatski's ring (101, 211) is located at the gastroesophageal junction and is associated with a sliding esophageal hiatal hernia. On radiologic examination the notches are square, thin, smooth, and symmetrical, being optimally demonstrated in a fully dilated esophagus (Fig. 176). No obstruction occurs, but the size of the esophageal lumen at the site of the ring varies according to the extent of the ring which is demonstrated. The Schatski ring is more frequent in males than females and may be responsible for intermittent attacks of dysphagia in both sexes. The ring is probably associated with the results of localized acid pepsin regurgitation because it is more frequent in individuals with reflux esophagitis secondary to chronic duodenal ulcer (68). The Schatski ring must be differentiated from rings produced by strictures secondary to healed marginal ulcers at the gastroesophageal junction. This type of ring is usually asymmetrical and more rigid.

Double ring

Several cases of a double ring have been observed in the association with hiatal hernia (Fig. 177). The lower ring is located at the gastroesophageal junction and the upper ring appears to be located at the level of the upper attachment of the phrenoesophageal membrane. In addition to a mucosal fold, these rings, especially at the level of the upper attachment of the membrane, may be caused by a localized band of muscular hypertrophy (see next section).

Annular idiopathic muscular hypertrophy of the circular muscular layer of the lower esophagus has been described. A smooth, localized, pliable area of annular narrowing is observed on radiologic examination. Zaino et al. (271) have reported similar findings in a number of gross esophageal specimens at the level of the upper attachment of the phrenoesophageal membrane. Hypertrophy or achalasia of the cricopharyngeal sphincter has been described by several authors who believe that the cricopharyngeal muscle is the upper sphincter. This has been related radiologically to a prominent cricopharyngeal impression, with associated symptoms of dysphagia. However, this radiologic observation also may occur in asymptomatic individuals. Cricopharyngeal hypertrophy is a

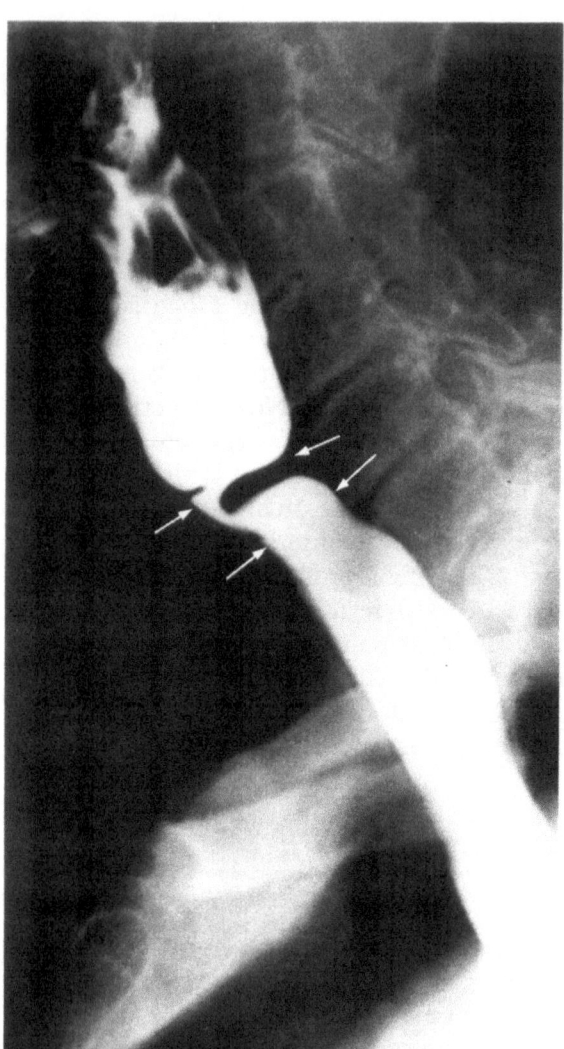

(A)

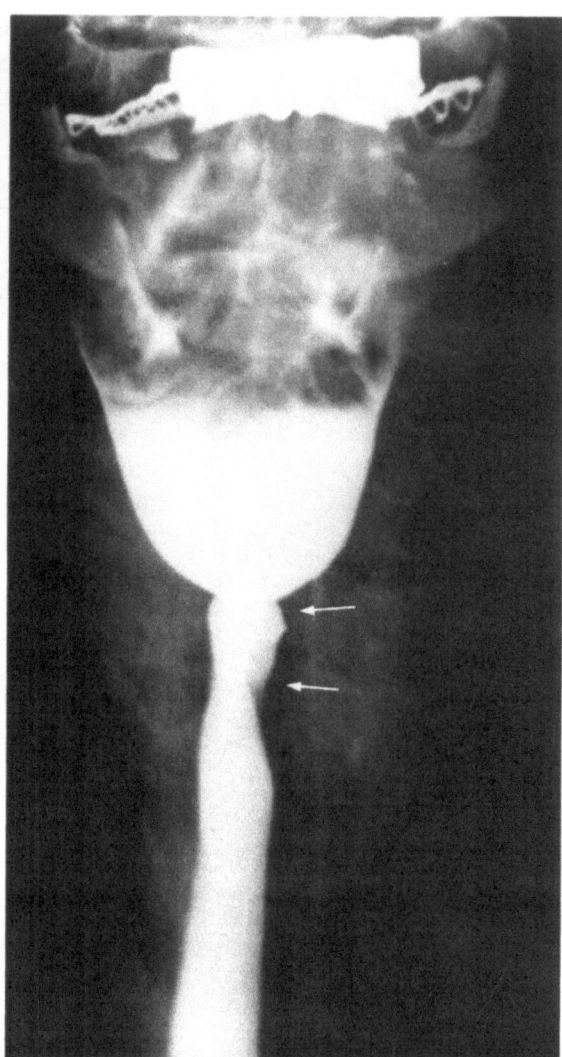

(B)

FIGURE 178
Cricopharyngeal hypertrophy
(unconfirmed). Sphincter zone
between arrows. (A) Lateral
view, (B) anteroposterior view.

compensatory phenomenon, usually secondary to hypertonic-
ity of the pharyngoesophageal sphincter, located directly inferior to the cricopharyngeus muscle. In asymptomatic individuals, the prominent cricopharyngeal muscular impression
represents a greater muscular contribution of its fibers to the
normal sphincter. In patients with dysphagia, this is an acquired muscular hypertrophy and is amenable to a myotomy
for symptomatic relief. The radiologic appearance is that of a
more sharply localized indentation than normal (Fig. 178).

A form of ulcerative esophagitis has been described (23) associated with an apthous stomatitis that produces cicatrizing
changes and hypertrophy of the cricopharyngeus muscle. In
such instances, a persistent cricopharyngeal impression may
be noted on radiologic examination and is probably the result
of pharyngoesophageal spasm.

Hypertrophy of the pharyngeal sphincter probably occurs but is very rare. Watson and Bancroft (251) have reported a case that appears to represent this entity. The authors are unaware of any case reports of hypertrophy of the lower sphincter.

DIVERTICULA

Diverticula are abnormal outpocketings of the gastrointestinal tract, which occasionally are noted in the hypopharynx and esophagus. A true diverticulum contains all the layers of the wall in which it is located. A false diverticulum consists primarily of the mucosal layer, protruding through a tear or defect of the muscular wall. The etiology of false diverticula varies. Diverticula are most frequently associated with other disorders of the esophagus (50).

Diverticula can be classified into congenital or acquired types. Acquired diverticula in turn can be subdivided into pulsion, traction, pulsion–traction, pseudo-, inconsistent, resilient, or intramural diverticula. They can also be grouped according to location—hypopharyngeal, cervical, thoracic, or epiphrenic.

Congenital diverticula are rare and usually represent residual buds from the embryonal development of the upper digestive tract (see Chapter 3).

Acquired diverticula are more common and generally more readily recognized.

Pulsion diverticula are thought to be the result of increased intraluminal pressure that permits a protrusion of the mucosal lining through a structurally weak, damaged, or diseased area of the hypopharynx and/or esophagus. This often is associated with deranged or abnormal neuromuscular function, all of which contributes to the development of a pulsion diverticulum.

Traction diverticula are secondary to an external pull from adhesions or fixation of surrounding structures. All layers of the esophageal wall are affected, producing a true diverticulum.

Pulsion–traction diverticula are produced by the combined factors of external traction and internal pulsion.

Pseudo-diverticula are functional outpocketings resembling diverticula on a single film. Actually these pseudo-diverticula represent segmentation of the esophageal lumen by abnormal contractions.

Inconsistent diverticula are caused by minimal wedging of the mucosal sac within the wall of the esophagus.

Hypopharyngeal and cervical diverticula

Hypopharyngeal diverticula are located most commonly between the oblique fibers and the "pars fundiformis" of the

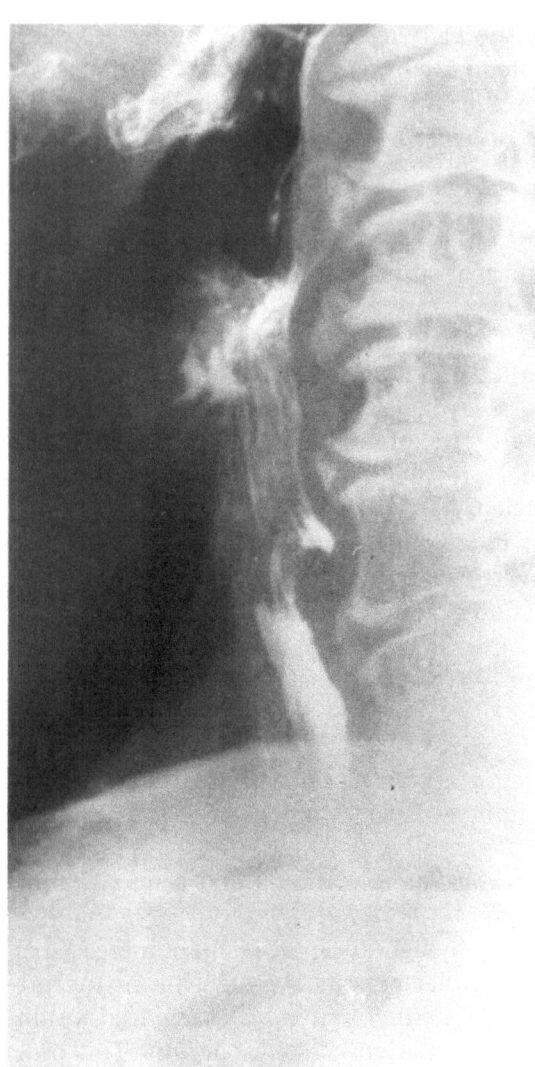

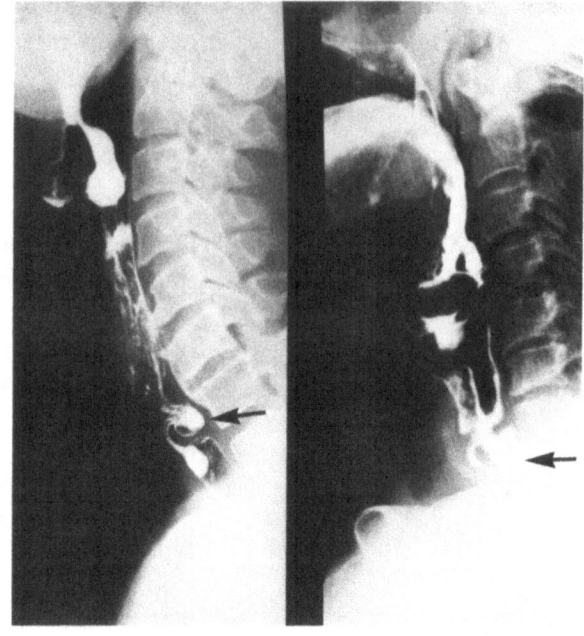

FIG. 180(A)   (B)

FIGURE 179
Zenker diverticulum, early stage.

FIGURE 180
Zenker diverticulum (at arrow). (A and B) Two different patients. From Zaino, et al. The Pharyngoesophageal Sphincter, 1970. Courtesy of Charles C Thomas, Publisher, Springfield, Illinois.

FIG. 179

cricopharyngeus muscle, just posterior and slightly to the left side, above the level of the pharyngoesophageal sphincter (Fig. 179). These are usually called "Zenker's diverticula" (Figs. 180 and 181). Rarely, two Zenker diverticula may be present, or a single Zenker diverticulum may be lobulated. A less frequent site of diverticulum formation is the Killian–Jamison area, which is a laterally placed opening separating the cricopharyngeus muscle and the proximal longitudinal fibers of the esophagus attached to the lower pole of the cricoid lamina. The recurrent laryngeal nerve and accompanying vessels reach the larynx through this area. These laterally located diverticula occur to the right or left side of the pharyngoesophageal junction, above the level of the sphincter zone (34, 35). Posterior, midline diverticula can also occur in any weakened or structurally defective midline location.

The majority of hypopharyngeal diverticula are of the pulsion type. They occur most frequently in middle-aged or elderly individuals in whom some degree of neurogenic incoordination or muscular atrophy exists. Because these diverticula are located above the level of the pharyngoesophageal sphincter, the sphincter itself probably causes the increased hypopharyngeal pressure in this area when sphincteric dysfunction produces delayed opening or increased pressure. Rarely, traction diverticula may occur in the hypopharyngeal area secondary to adhesions from chronic inflammatory changes, fibrositis, trauma, or an infiltrating malignancy.

Zenker's diverticula are more common in men than women, possibly because of the added pressure from a larger larynx. Their growth and appearance in various stages have been well described by Brombart (29). Careful examination of the dynamic changes in the pharyngoesophageal area with cine and fluoroscopy often visualizes very small Zenker's diverticula.

Stasis of barium at the pharyngoesophageal junction, above

FIGURE 181

Large-sized Zenker diverticulum. (A) Frontal view, (B) oblique view.

(A)

(B)

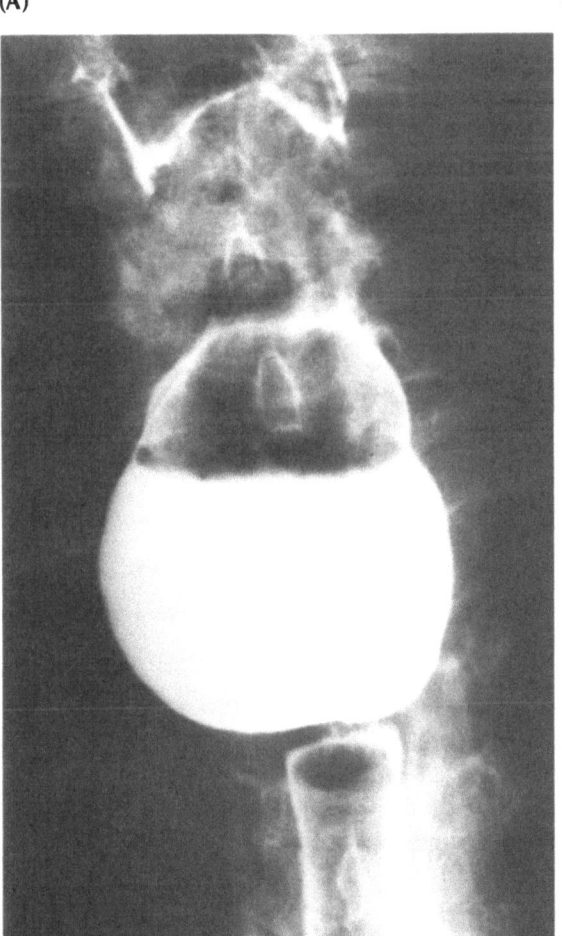
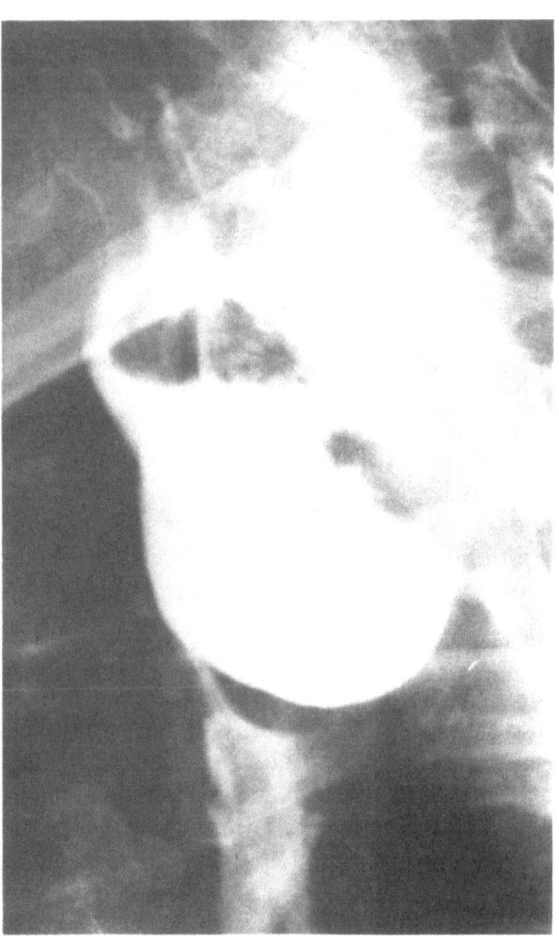

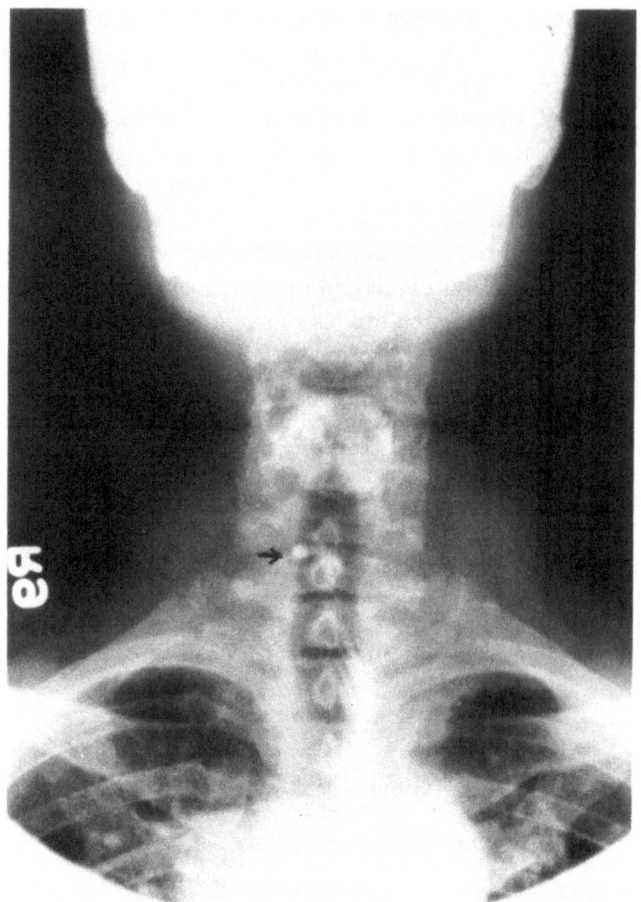

FIGURE 182
Small lateral hypopharyngeal
diverticulum (at arrow).

the level of the contracted sphincter, is not unusual and should
not be mistaken for a diverticulum. This stasis occurs more
commonly in the elderly, because of the relative loss of muscular tone of the hypopharyngeal muscles and the sluggish action of the sphincter. Such pseudo-diverticula are inconstant
and rapidly change shape and size. However, the demonstration of a small authentic diverticulum can also be inconstant. In its initial stage such a true diverticulum may be identified as a thornlike projection from the opacified lumen,
which may disappear during the actual swallowing act as the
mucosal pocket becomes inverted. At rest, however, the thornlike projection reappears, with a virtually identical pattern,
form, and size. As the diverticulum progressively enlarges, it
loses its elasticity and develops a pedicle. The sac of the diverticulum then progresses through stages in which it becomes
oval and pear shaped before becoming pendant.

Diverticula may become large enough to compress and displace the cervical esophagus. In all instances, however, the
contracted sphincter zone is identified in the resting stage as a

contracted segment several centimeters long, below the level of the pharyngoesophageal junction. In the larger diverticula, considerable retention of barium occurs because of the absent muscular layer which prevents contraction and emptying. In the upright position, a fluid level can be observed. In this connection, on a plain film of the cervical region a retained pocket of air may be noted, requiring consideration of abscess, pharyngocele, and laryngocele.

The modified Valsalva maneuver is helpful in the early detection of Zenker's diverticula. The degree of mobility, their location, and the direction in which they point may be determined. This maneuver also is helpful in distinguishing a traction- from a pulsion-type diverticulum. Traction diverticula are usually fixed in location by surrounding adhesions. In the anteroposterior view small diverticula may be identified as midline or lateral oval specks or retained barium. The anteroposterior view is particularly helpful in detecting lateral diverticula (Figs. 182 and 183) as well as upper lateral pharyngeal pouches or pharyngoceles. Diverticula in the sphincter zone have not been reported.

FIGURE 183

Lateral acquired diverticulum (at arrows). (A) Anteroposterior view, (B) lateral view. Reprinted from Buckstein, J., and Reich, S. Lateral pharyngeal diverticula as a cause of dysphagia. J.A.M.A. *144*:14, 1950. Copyright 1950, American Medical Association.

(A)

(B)

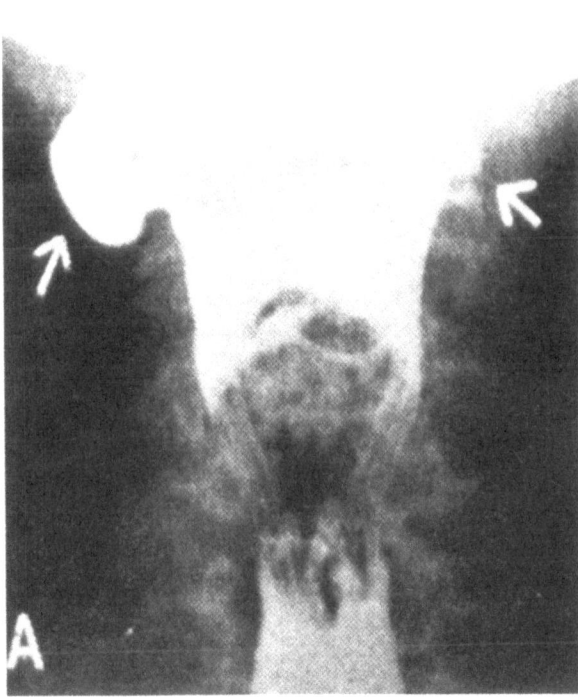
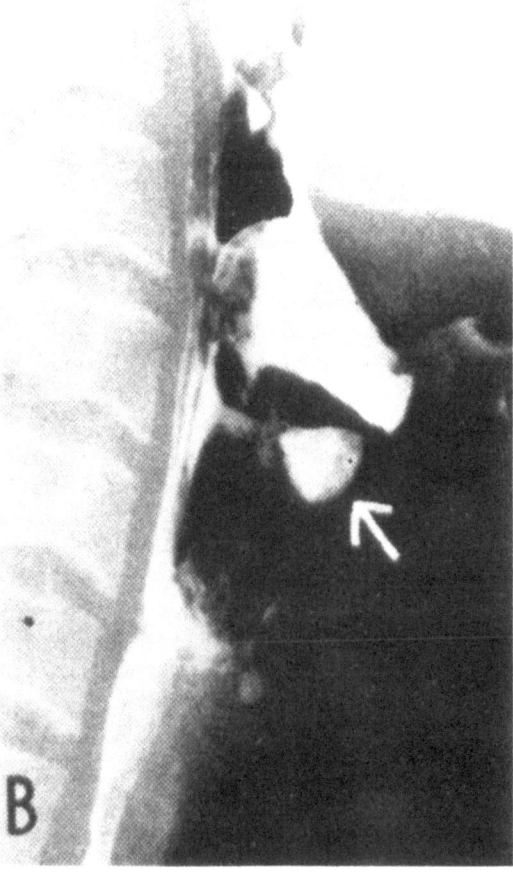

Lateral pharyngeal pouches

Lateral pharyngeal pouches can be true congenital diverticula or acquired pharyngoceles (261). Congenital diverticula are usually located in the tonsillar fossa and have long pedicles. Acquired pharyngoceles are superior or inferior to the level of the hyoid bone, usually occurring through a bulge or tear in the thyrohyoid ligament. The pouch extends into the pyriform fossa below or the tonsillar fossa above (Fig. 184). Lateral pharyngeal pouches are most common in glass blowers or musicians who use wind instruments. They may also occur in the elderly with weakened or relaxed ligaments. These pharyngeal pouches are pulsion diverticula and can easily be demonstrated with a barium swallow.

Laryngoceles

Laryngoceles are rare (83, 155). They are either acquired or congenital, saccular or cystic dilatations of the ventricular appendage of the larynx. Laryngoceles occur internal to the larynx but may herniate through the thyrohyoid ligament into the soft

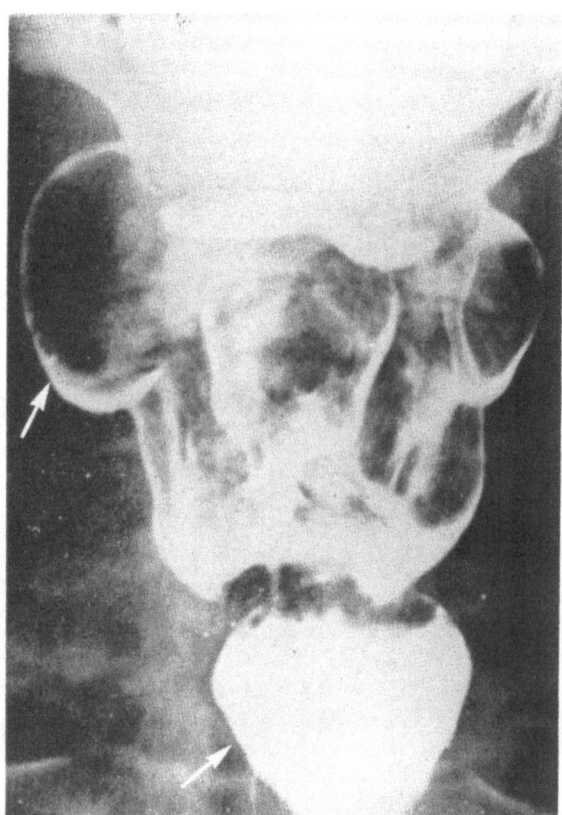

FIGURE 184
Pharyngocele (upper arrow) in the presence of a Zenker diverticulum (lower arrow). From Wilson, C. P. Diverticula of the pharynx. J. Roy. Coll. Surg. Edinburgh 4:11, 1959. Royal College of Surgeons, Edinburgh.

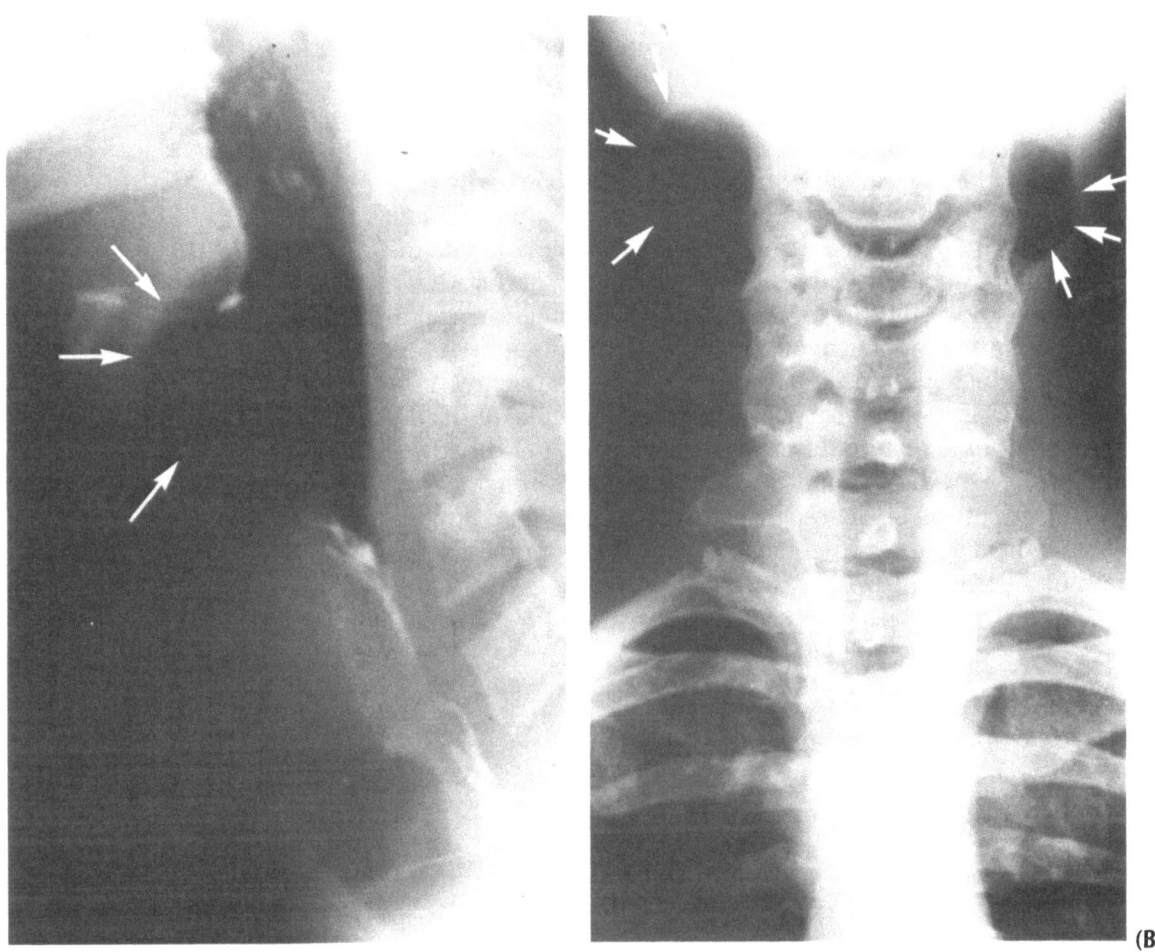

(A)

(B)

FIGURE 185
Laryngocele (at arrows). (A)
Lateral view, (B) frontal view.

tissue of the neck where they can be confused with pharyngoceles. Laryngoceles, however, are not opacified during a barium swallow because they are located in the larynx (Fig. 185).

Acquired laryngoceles occur most frequently in professional horn musicians because of the prolonged intermittent increase in intraglottic pressure needed to perform with these instruments.

Diverticula of the thoracic esophagus

Pseudo-, traction, or pulsion–traction diverticula of the uppermost segment of the thoracic esophagus are observed in individuals with chronic inflammatory disease of the apical lung segments, resulting in deviation and displacement of the esophagus. Pulsion diverticula in this area also occur, although less frequently. Diverticula at the aortobronchial triangle are inconstant and are chiefly of the resilient type (Fig. 186). In the elderly, air is frequently trapped in this area of the esophagus, causing bulging of this segment. Occasionally, the longitudinal muscles in this region of the thoracic esophagus separate and an inconstant bulge through this opening of the muscular layer produces a fanlike dilatation of this segment of the esophagus or a resilient diverticulum. Eventually, a fixed diverticular pocket results.

The most common site of esophageal diverticula formation is at the carina. The diverticula in these regions are of the traction type (Fig. 187a) or a combination of both the pulsion and traction varieties. At the carina, chronic inflammation of the peribronchial nodes usually will affect the esophagus. Calcified lymph nodes in this location are common, indicating previous inflammatory changes that are chiefly caused by tuberculosis or histoplasmosis. Rarely, a congenital attachment of the esophagus to the tracheobronchial tree accounts for the development of a diverticulum. In addition, spasm of the lower end of the esophagus, coupled with hyperactive peristalsis of the upper portion of the esophagus, may produce a high pressure gradient in the mid-esophagus, which aids in the formation of diverticula.

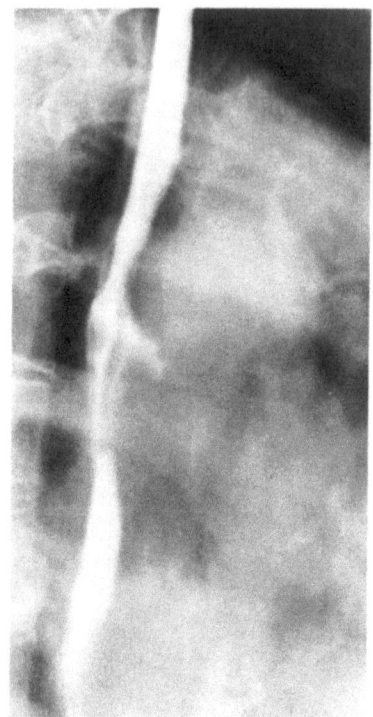

FIGURE 186
Resilient diverticulum at aortic-bronchial triangle.

(A)

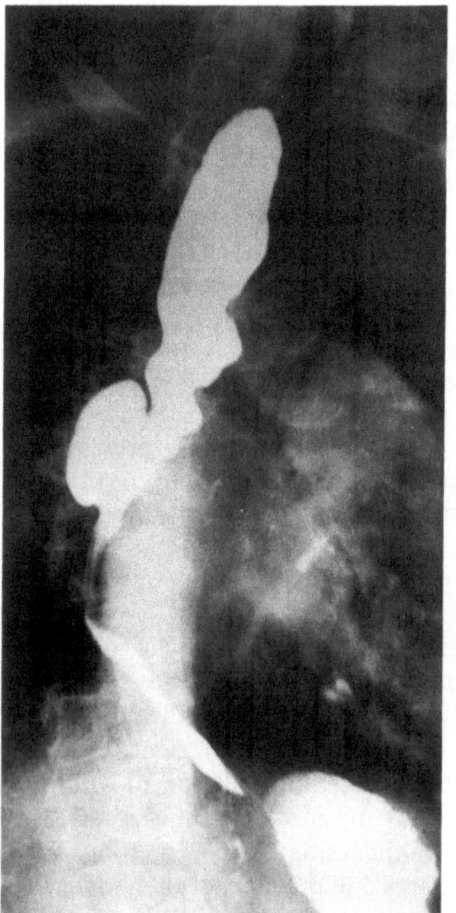

(B)

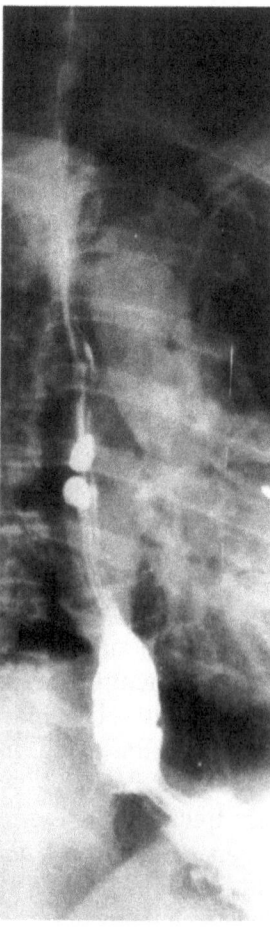

FIGURE 187
(A) *Traction diverticulum,* mid-esophagus. (B) *Pulsion diverticula,* mid-esophagus, in the presence of a hiatal hernia.

Traction diverticula (single or multiple) are readily missed. They are most often located in the right anterior wall of the middle third of the esophagus. In the anteroposterior view, such a diverticulum may be obscured by superimposition of the barium-filled esophagus. Hence, rotational and lateral views are necessary. Fluoroscopic and cine examinations are important. When a peristaltic wave sweeps over the site of a diverticulum, it becomes more readily visible. Traction diverticula may not be identified in an esophagus at rest. In addition, diverticula may change their shape on repeated examination, depending upon the degree of filling and distension. A broad necked diverticulum may empty rapidly contributing to the difficulty. Diverticula inferior to the tracheal bifurcation are located anteriorly; they usually are small, conical, or oval pouches with irregular walls. They must be differentiated from ulcer niches.

Pulsion diverticula are infrequently encountered in the mid-esophageal region. They are usually small, have distinct narrow necks, tend to move freely with the esophagus, and usually retain barium. Such diverticula also require differentiation from esophageal ulcers (Fig. 187B).

Pulsion–traction diverticula show the characteristics of both types, the traction and the pulsion, but are generally fixed in location by surrounding adhesions or other disease processes. A distinct neck usually is present.

Functional or pseudo-diverticula occur mainly in the lower two-thirds of the esophagus. They are most often identified on contraction of the esophageal musculature. They are usually multiple and disappear during the relaxation phase of the esophageal motility patterns. Although their shape and number tend to vary initially, chronic spasm ultimately may produce fixed pulsion-type diverticula at the site of pseudodiverticula as bulging occurs through areas of weakened or torn muscular fibers. Such diverticula are observed in instances of disturbed innervation without associated muscular hypertrophy.

Epiphrenic diverticula

Epiphrenic diverticula (121a) are located in the lower esophageal segment, just above the level of the diaphragm. They may be associated with hiatal hernia, achalasia, or any other disorder producing spasm or a hypertensive lower esophageal sphincter (32). Epiphrenic diverticula primarily are of the pulsion type and are usually demonstrated anteriorly and to the right or left side of the cardia of the stomach (Fig. 188). Their shapes depend on the size, location, and degree of filling of the sacs. They may displace the esophagus as they enlarge and, when flattened by the spine or mediastinal structures, may result in a "collar button" appearance (Fig. 189).

When epiphrenic diverticula are small, they are easily

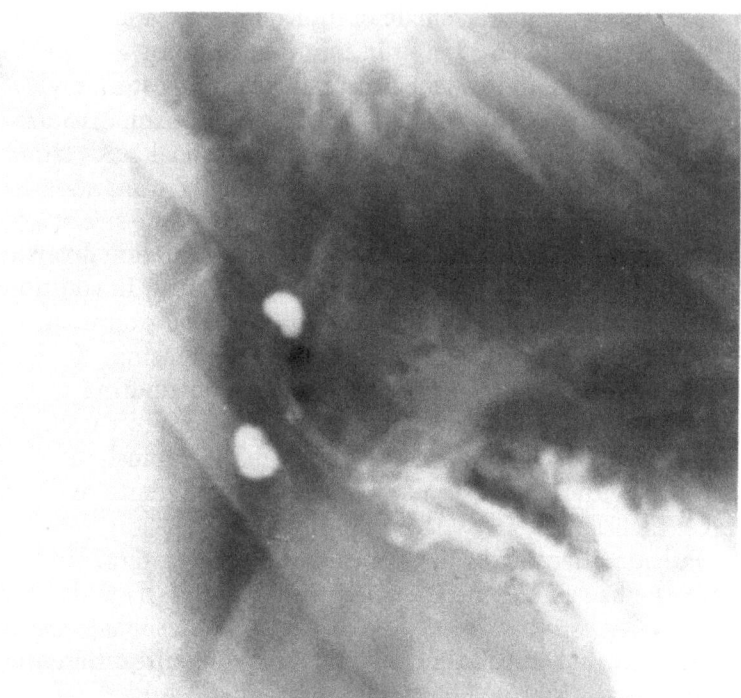

FIGURE 188
Epiphrenic diverticula, pulsion
type. From Zaino, C., et al. *The
Lower Esophageal Vestibular
Complex,* 1963. Courtesy Charles
C Thomas, Publisher,
Springfield, Illinois.

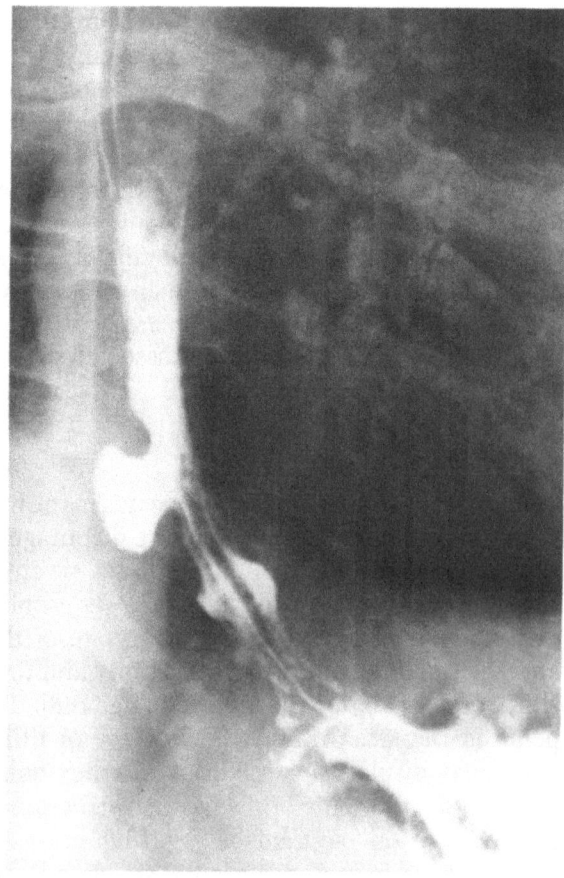

FIGURE 189
Epiphrenic diverticulum, "collar
button" type.

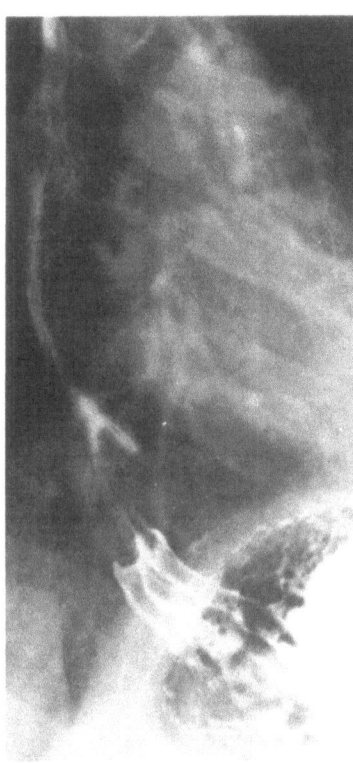

FIGURE 190
Epiphrenic diverticulum in the presence of sliding hiatal hernia with esophageal invagination.

missed on radiologic examination, particularly in the upright position or during the ingestion of a thin barium mixture. A thick barium paste, however, usually demonstrates a small retained collection of barium. Epiphrenic diverticula are best observed during fluoroscopy. On a plain chest film, an air fluid level at the right costophrenic angle is suggestive of an epiphrenic diverticulum. Although epiphrenic diverticula are commonly associated with hiatal hernia (Fig. 190) and achalasia, they may be secondary to surrounding pleural adhesions, strictures, or carcinoma of the distal end of the esophagus. An epiphrenic diverticulum must be differentiated from an ulcer niche, a redundant esophagus with saccular dilatation as in achalasia, the herniated portion of the gastric fundus in a paraeosphageal hiatal hernia, and a diverticulum of the gastric cardia.

Saccular dilatations of the lower end of a dilated esophagus are best demonstrated by following the first barium swallow before the esophagus becomes overfilled while rotating the patient into various oblique positions. A sliding esophageal hiatal hernia can be detected easily when the lower contracted sphincter zone is located above the diaphragm. Difficulty, however, may arise in differentiating a small portion of stomach herniating along the left or right lateral border of the esophagus. The direction of the flow of the barium and absence of a pedicle establish the diagnosis. Fluoroscopic and cine studies are essential for an accurate diagnosis.

A diverticulum of the gastric cardia generally is present on the left side of the gastroesophageal junction; it may resemble shelving of the cardia. Radiologic examination in the upright position generally is essential to establish the diagnosis.

A number of complications of esophageal diverticula may occur. They may become infected, hemorrhage, or perforate. A fistulous tract can develop, particularly in the traction type, associated with an adjacent neoplasm. Rarely, a carcinoma may develop within a diverticulum.

Rarely, a diverticulum develops intramurally with the sac invading the deeper muscular layers only. These intramural diverticula, which do not protrude through the connective tissue of the esophageal wall, consist of outpocketings of the mucosa. They may pose difficulty in the radiologic diagnosis.

Diverticula may be multiple and quite large (Fig. 191). A diverticulum can also be present within a large hiatal hernia (Fig. 192).

Diverticulosis

Diverticulosis of the esophagus (228, 256), also known as intramural pseudodiverticulosis (13), is a rare disorder of unknown cause. It is characterized by multiple, small flasklike, diverticula extending bilaterally beyond the borders of the esophageal lumen (Fig. 193). They are often located in the lower seg-

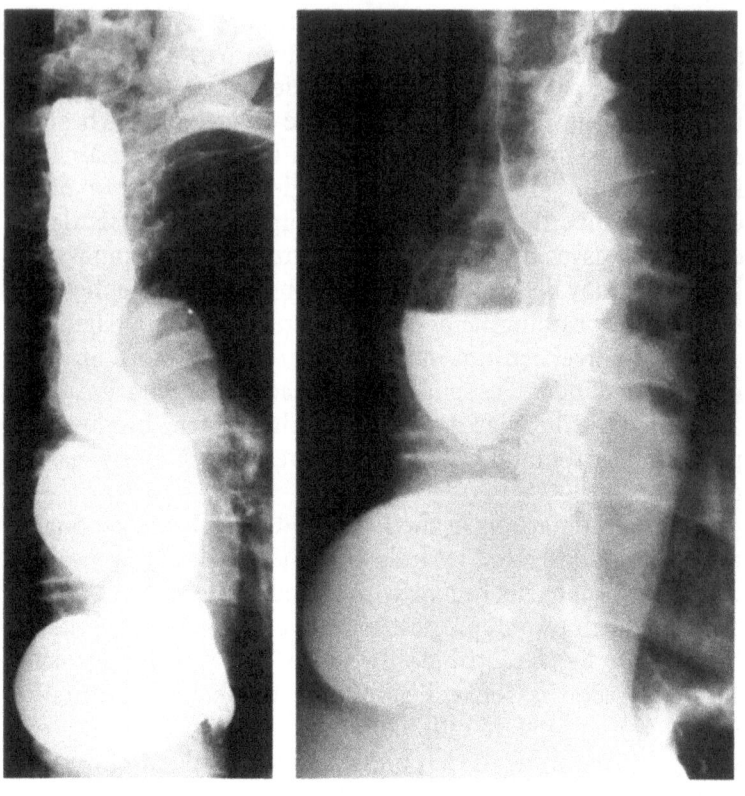

(A)   (B)

FIGURE 191
Multiple large esophageal diverticula. (A) Prone, (B) upright view.

FIGURE 192
Large diverticulum within a hiatal hernia. (A) Frontal view, (B) oblique view.

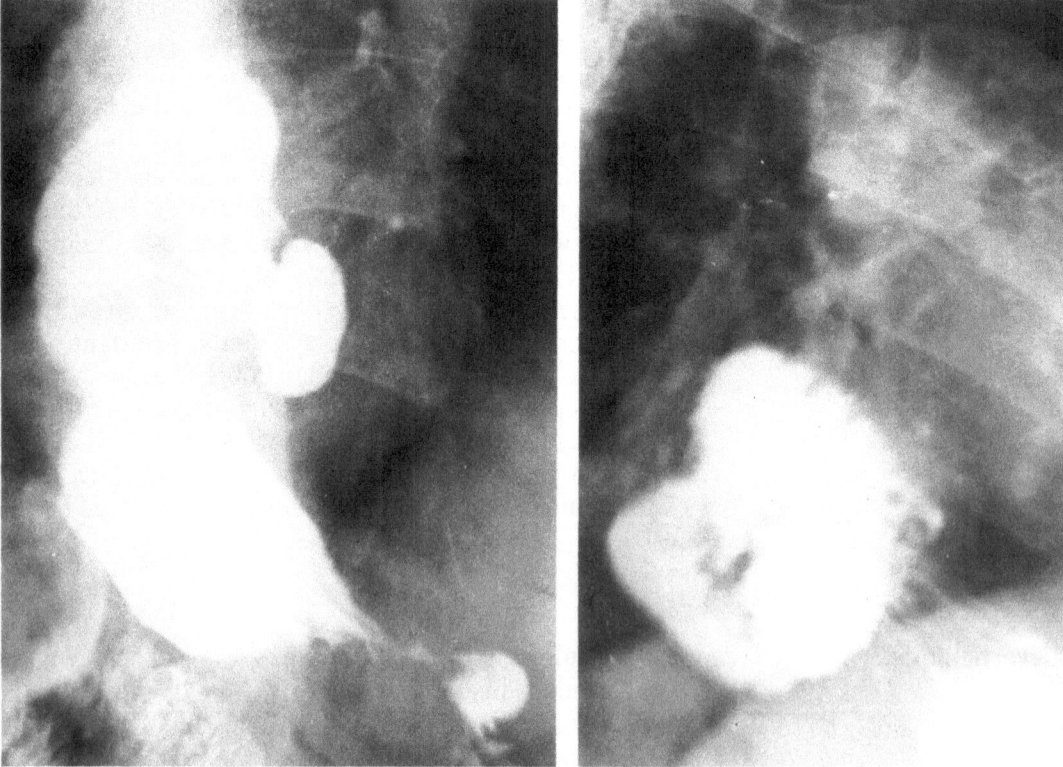

(A)   (B)

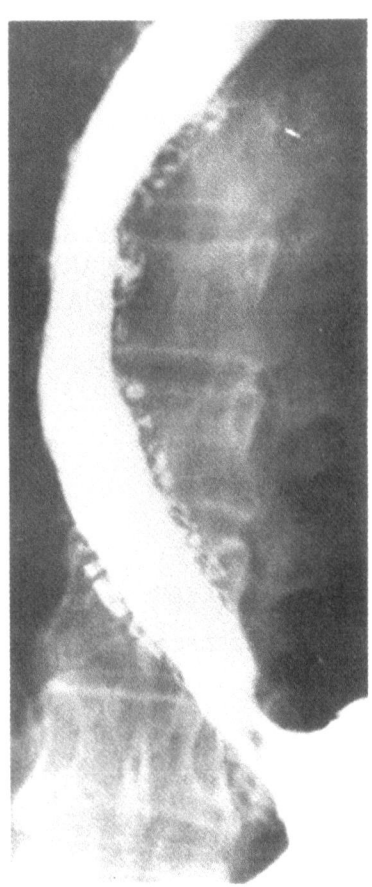

ment, although the entire esophagus may be affected. These pockets are reminiscent of the Ashoff–Rokitansky sinuses of the gallbladder or the dilated bronchial glands of chronic bronchitis (225). They have been associated with stenotic lesions of the esophagus, resulting in increased intraluminal pressure. Intramural diverticulosis has been described as hypertrophied deep mucosal glands with dilated acinar ducts. Some also suspect a congenital underlying muscular weakness and ascribe their occurence to secondary inflammatory changes. They have been frequently associated with moniliasis, although the pockets are larger and more irregular in these instances. A case of primary tuberculosis of the esophagus has been reported showing multiple small diverticula-like pockets within the area of stenosis (133) (Fig. 194). In general, esophageal diverticulosis is believed to be an acquired disorder. A case of diverticulosis of the esophagus has been reported in a child (255).

Congenital esophageal cartilagenous rings are tracheobron-

FIGURE 194
Primary tuberculosis of esophagus showing diverticular *processes* in stenotic areas. From Kolawole, T. M., and Lewis, E. A. A radiologic study of tuberculosis of the abdomen. Am. J. Roentgenol., *123*:352, 1975. Courtesy Charles C Thomas, Publisher, Springfield, Illinois.

FIGURE 193
Diverticulosis of esophagus. From Sperling, H. V., and D'Altorio, R. A. Intramural diverticulosis of the esophagus. Am. J. Dig. Dis., *18*:979, 1973. (Fig. 1B) Harper & Row Publisher.

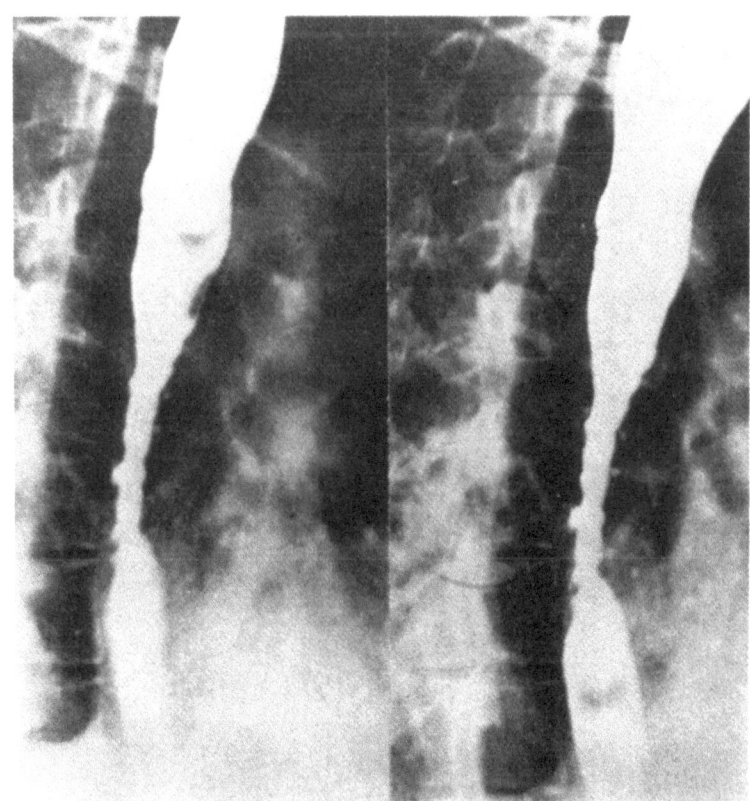

chial remnants within the esophageal wall, associated with multiple cysts similar to intramural diverticula (see Chapter 3).

Those neoplasms affecting the normal outline of the soft tissues and the barium-coated surfaces of the orohypopharynx, the esophagus, and the cardia of the stomach are reviewed here.

Benign and malignant neoplasms exist in these areas. More than 90% of the tumors originate from the squamous epithelia normally lining the surface areas. Malignant neoplasms are predominately squamous cell carcinomata. The diagnostic criteria on radiologic study generally are definitive but biopsy is, of course, required for confirmation.

PRIMARY NEOPLASMS OF THE HYPOPHARYNX AND ESOPHAGUS

Leukoplakia

Leukoplakia, particularly in the oral cavity, is presumed by some investigators to be a precancerous disorder. The entity is characterized by the presence of white, patchlike, mucosal lesions. Histologically, hyperkeratosis, acanthosis, and infiltra-

Precancerous lesions

(A)

(B)

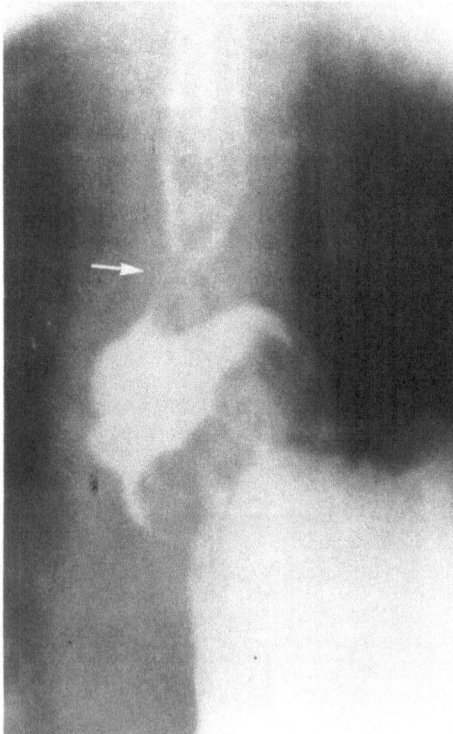 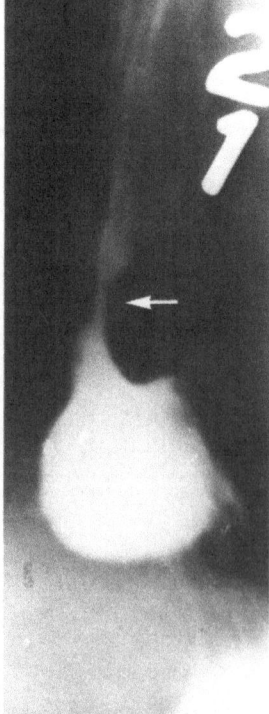

FIGURE 195
Leukoplakia (at arrow) producing an area of stenosis above a hiatal hernia. (A) Frontal view, (B) oblique view.

tion of the submucosa by round cells are observed. The esophagus may also be affected, with the development of cicatricial changes that may result in a stricture (Fig. 195).

The etiology varies but the absence of mechanical desquamation of squamous epithelium associated with lack of eating solid foods, mainly in the elderly, is a common cause.

Leukoplakia must be differentiated from glycogenic acanthosis, which is a benign epithelial hyperplasia characterized by the presence of gray–white slightly elevated mucosal plaques of unknown cause.

Plummer–Vinson syndrome

Plummer–Vinson syndrome is described in Chapter 6. It is more common in women than in men and predisposes to malignant transformation in the cervical esophagus, establishing this anatomic area as the most common site of malignant neoplastic disease in women (Fig. 196).

Classification of neoplasms

The authors have decided to discuss only a limited number of neoplasms in the oro- and hypopharynx. Totten's classification, which deals with this region, is reproduced for reference (246). A modified classification after Stout and Latter (235) is also included for lesions of the esophagus.

Selected Tumors of the Oral Cavity, Pharynx, and Larynx (from Totten, 246)
  I. Surface epithelium origin
    A. Benign
        1. Hyperplasia
        2. Papilloma
    B. Recurrent (premalignant)
        1. Leukoplakia
        2. Papillomatosis
    C. Malignant
        1. Squamous cell carcinoma *in situ*
        2. Squamous cell carcinoma, invasive
          a. Exophytic
          b. Ulcerative
          c. Verrucous
          d. With sarcoma-like stroma
        3. Undifferentiated (transitional cell) carcinoma
 II. Melanoblastic origin
    A. Benign
        1. Pigmented spot
        2. Nevus
    B. Malignant
        1. Malignant melanoma

III. Glandular epithelium origin
    A. Benign
        1. Cyst
        2. Benign mixed tumor
        3. Onkocytoma and variants
        4. Fordyce's disease
    B. Recurrent
        1. Benign mixed tumor
    C. Malignant
        1. Malignant mixed tumor
        2. Cylindromatous carcinoma
        3. Mucoepidermoid carcinoma
        4. Acinar cell carcinoma
        5. Undifferentiated carcinoma
IV. Odontogenic apparatus origin
    A. Benign
        1. Cyst
        2. Odontoma
        3. Cementoma
        4. Myxoma
        5. Other
    B. Recurrent
        1. Ameloblastoma
    C. Malignant
        1. Ameloblastoma
V. Lymphoid tissue origin
    A. Benign
        1. Lymphoid polyp
        2. Plasma cell granuloma
        3. Histiocytoma
    B. Malignant
        1. Lymphosarcoma
        2. Reticulum cell sarcoma
        3. Plasmacytoma (myeloma)
        4. Hodgkin's disease
VI. Soft tissue origin
    A. Benign
        1. Pyogenic granuloma
        2. Fibroma
        3. Hemangioma
        4. Neurofibroma–neurilemoma
        5. Angiofibroma
        6. Other
VII. Bone and cartilage origin
    A. Benign
        1. Cyst
        2. Fibroosseous lesions
        3. Giant cell granuloma
        4. Cherubism
        5. Other

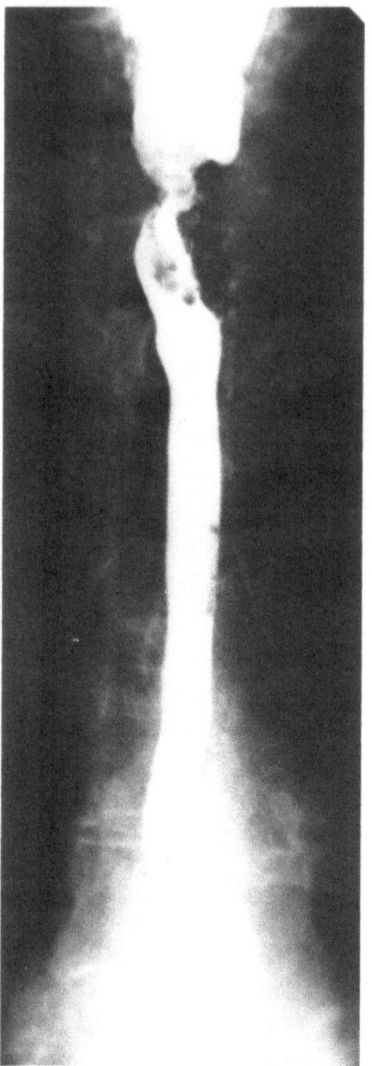

FIGURE 196
Malignant changes in patient
with *Plummer-Vinson's syndrome*.

    B. Malignant
       1. Fibrosarcoma
       2. Osteosarcoma
       3. Chondrosarcoma
       4. Ewing's tumor
       5. Malignant lymphoma
       6. Metastasis
VIII. Metastatic tumors

Orohypopharyngeal tumors in infants and children (239) present essentially the same radiologic features as in adults, although differing in location, in site and type of neoplasm, and the presence of calcification. Calcification is particularly common in teratomas and neuroblastomas. Hemangioma and polyp may be observed in the newborn. In older children, angiofibroma of the nasopharynx is encountered frequently. Sarcomas of various types and Schminke tumor (undifferentiated squamous cell carcinoma) occurs rarely in childhood but when it is encountered it must be differentiated from adenoid tissue. Cystic hygroma occurs commonly in the retropharyngeal area in childhood.

Classification of Esophageal Tumors (after Stout and Latter, 235)
A. Malignant tumors
    1. Carcinoma
       a. Squamous
       b. Undifferentiated
       c. Adenocarcinoma
       d. Secondary malignant tumors (by direct invasion or embolic metastasis)
       e. Multiple primary tumors
    2. Sarcoma
       a. Leiomyosarcoma
       b. Fibrosarcoma
       c. Rhabdomyosarcoma
       d. Reticulum cell sarcoma
       e. Hodgkin's disease
    3. Carcinosarcoma
    4. Carcinoid tumor
    5. Malignant melanoma
    6. Pseudosarcoma
B. Benign tumors
    1. Leiomyoma
    2. Fibrovascular polyp
    3. Lipoma
    4. Fibroma
    5. Hemangioma
    6. Angioendothelioma
    7. Chondroma

8. Neurofibroma
9. Papilloma
10. Granular cell myoblastoma

The most common sites for malignant lesions of the esophagus are the areas where the lumen is normally narrowed or less flexible, particularly in individuals with a tortuous or calcified aorta. Malignant neoplasms occur most often in the distal end of the esophagus and least frequently in the cervical area, particularly if malignant lesions of the gastroesophageal junction are included (204).

Pathologic considerations of malignant neoplasms

Squamous cell carcinomas

Squamous cell carcinomas arise from the squamous epithelium lining the esophagus. When the tumor growth is predominantly into the lumen, a bulky mass with obstruction is produced. When the growth is away from the lumen and penetrates into the musculature, a sclerotic lesion with irregular narrowing is produced. Obstruction in this type is less common. A lesion therefore may be described as tumefactive or infiltrating. Both types of growth may result in ulceration.

Adenocarcinomas

Adenocarcinomas arise from gastric glands in the lower end of the esophagus, by infiltration and extension from a lesion in the cardia of the stomach, or from ectopic gastric mucosa lining the upper or middle segments of the esophagus. Although such lesions are more likely to be tumefactive and ulcerating in type, they occasionally may be infiltrating.

Secondary malignancies

Secondary malignancies occur by direct extension from adjacent neoplasms, e.g., lung, or by embolic metastasis including lymphatic spread from the pancreas.

Sarcomas

Sarcomas arise from the underlying muscle and connective tissues of the esophagus. They occur more commonly in women but in general are rarely encountered. These tumors tend to be pedunculated and may even resemble benign polyps and myomas. Several pathologic varieties exist (see classification) but the radiologic criteria are not specific for any of the cell types in this group.

Carcinosarcomas

Carcinosarcomas are rare neoplasms that pathologically constitute an admixture of both carcinoma and sarcoma. This neoplasm tends to present as a bulky, intraluminal, irregularly shaped mass.

Carcinoid tumors

Carcinoid tumors of the esophagus are also rare. They are borderline neoplasms in terms of being benign or malignant. Pathologic differentiation often is difficult. This neoplasm is usually submucosal and often extends to surrounding lymph nodes (28). The blood levels of serotonin and histaminase generally are elevated—laboratory findings that often are helpful.

Malignant melanomas

Malignant melanomas are rare primary neoplasms of the esophagus (36, 169) (Fig. 197). They may be sessile or pedunculated and are histologically similar to the classical melanoma of the skin. Two main types exist: the infiltrating type and the polypoid mass lesion, which is less common. Primary melanoma of the esophagus has also been reported.

It is felt by a number of observers that most, if not all, melanomas of the esophagus represent metastases from undetected primary sources.

Pseudosarcomas

Pseudosarcomas are usually pedunculated tumors resembling sarcomas but are actually benign and nonmetastasing.

Radiologic principles in the diagnosis of malignant neoplasms

In the digestive tract, primary malignancies originate as the result of the abnormal proliferation of certain cells, which produces a local area of infiltration associated with a segmental zone of rigidity. This feature is the earliest radiologic manifestation of a malignant neoplasm and is overlooked frequently because it is often asymptomatic in the initial stage. For this reason, cineradiography is an ideal method of identifying the earliest changes of aperistalsis or rigidity in the wall of the lumen. This is particularly true of the esophagus. In the oro-

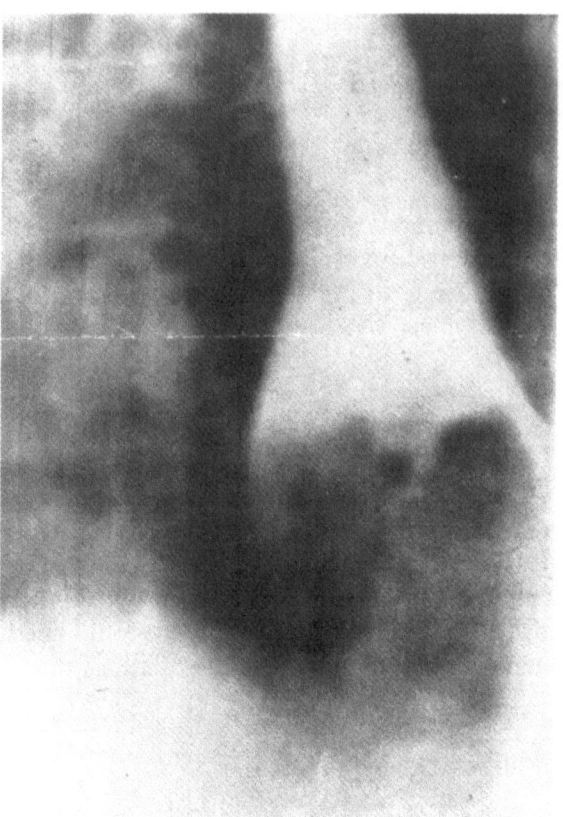

FIGURE 197
Primary melanosarcoma of the esophagus. Polypoid-type filling defect. From Burnett, J. M., and St. John, E. Primary melanosarcoma of the esophagus. Radiology, 57:868, 1951. Radiologic Society of North America, Easton, Pa.

and hypopharynx, early proliferative changes usually produce an abnormal bulge within the lumen or an abnormal thickening of the retropharyngeal soft tissues. As the malignant proliferation increases, further encroachment of the lumen of the oropharynx or esophagus takes place.

The modified Valsalva maneuver can be quite helpful in detecting tumors of the hypopharynx. As the lesions grow, progressive narrowing of the lumen occurs, with dilatation of the proximal oropharynx just superior to the site of obstruction.

In the esophagus, another important change is destruction and irregularity of the mucosa. A tubular structure is therefore involved and the mucosal pattern must be studied in all aspects and positions in order not to overlook an irregular, localized area of superficial mucosal destruction. Superimposed normal mucosal folds of the opposite esophageal wall may mask a lesion until circumferential destruction of the mucosal surface has occurred. Then a definite, irregular, rigid pattern results that can be reproduced on repeated examinations (Fig. 198).

If growth occurs within the lumen, intraluminal radiolucencies are produced. These defects must be differentiated from retained food or air bubbles (Fig. 199). On cine examina-

FIGURE 198
Infiltrating neoplastic changes of
the mid esophagus.

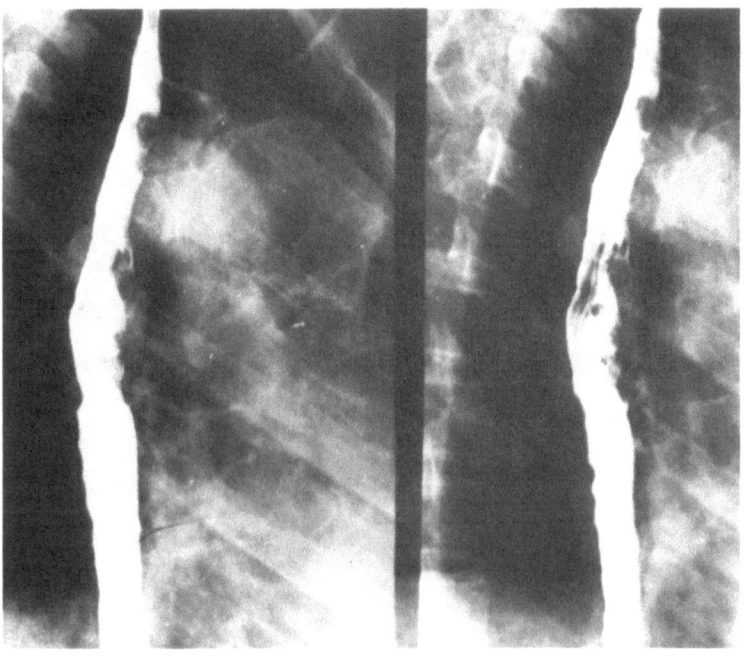

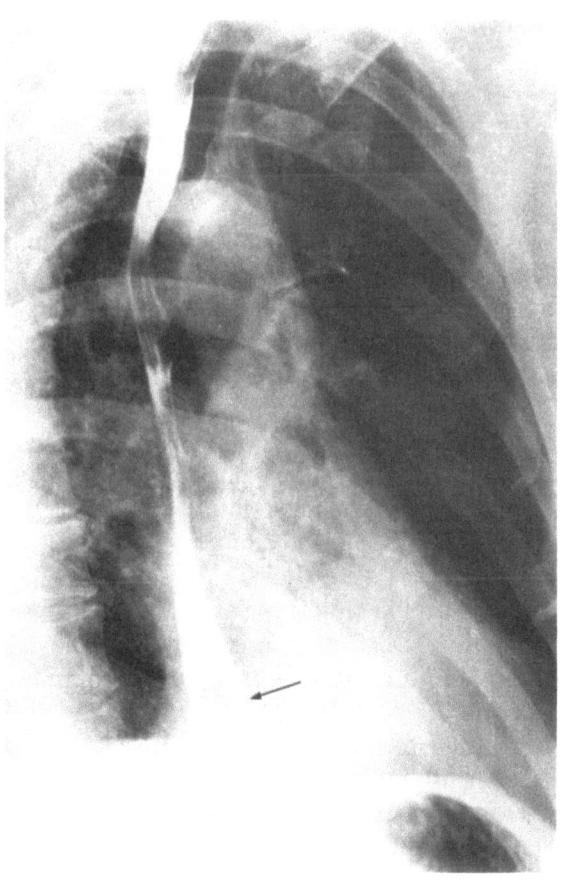

FIGURE 199
Early malignant changes, lower
esophageal mucosa (at arrow).

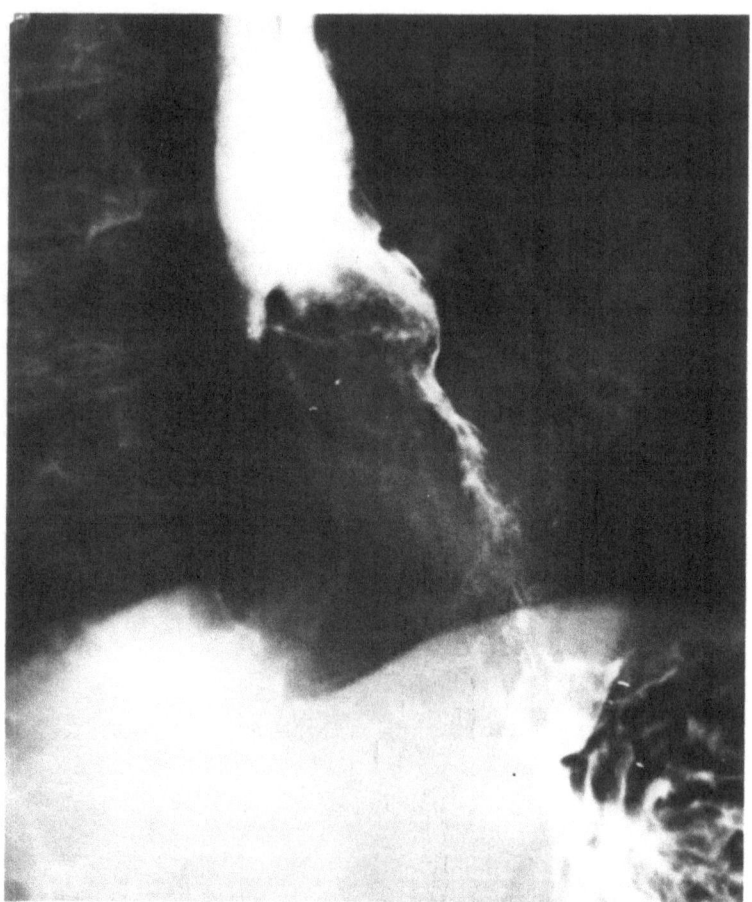

FIGURE 200
Polypoid malignant tumor of the lower end of esophagus.

FIGURE 201
Tumor mass outlined at site of lesion (squamous cell carcinoma).

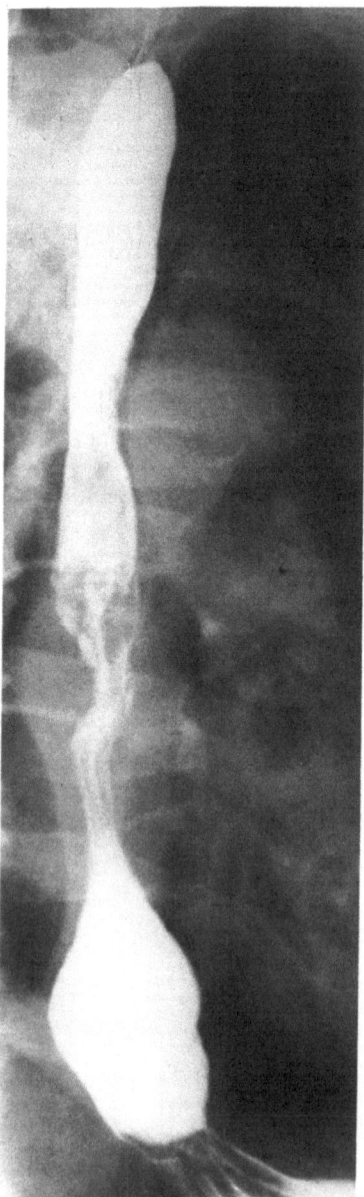

tion, this is readily accomplished because these latter defects vary in size and shape and are usually transient. A local dilatation may be produced by a polypoid neoplasm (Fig. 200).

When a tumor in the esophagus is infiltrating in character, the marginal contour of the area involved becomes ragged or nodular (Fig. 198). Although narrowing and rigidity of the area involved is present, usually little obstruction and no displacement or abnormal angulation of the esophagus occur. More extensive lesions produce fixation and abnormal angulation in the involved portion of the esophagus and irregularity of the surrounding soft tissue mass (Fig. 201).

A circumferential or "napkin-ring" type of lesion produces a cufflike defect or an annular defect with effaced or destroyed mucosal surfaces. "Napkin-ring" lesions are the most common form (Fig. 202).

Malignant ulcers (single or multiple) occur either within a localized area of neoplastic infiltration or on the surface of a tumor mass. On radiologic examination, they may be suspected when a retained barium collection is identified within

FIGURE 202
"Napkin ring" malignant lesion of the upper end of esophagus (at arrow).

FIGURE 203
Ulcerating carcinoma, mid-esophagus.

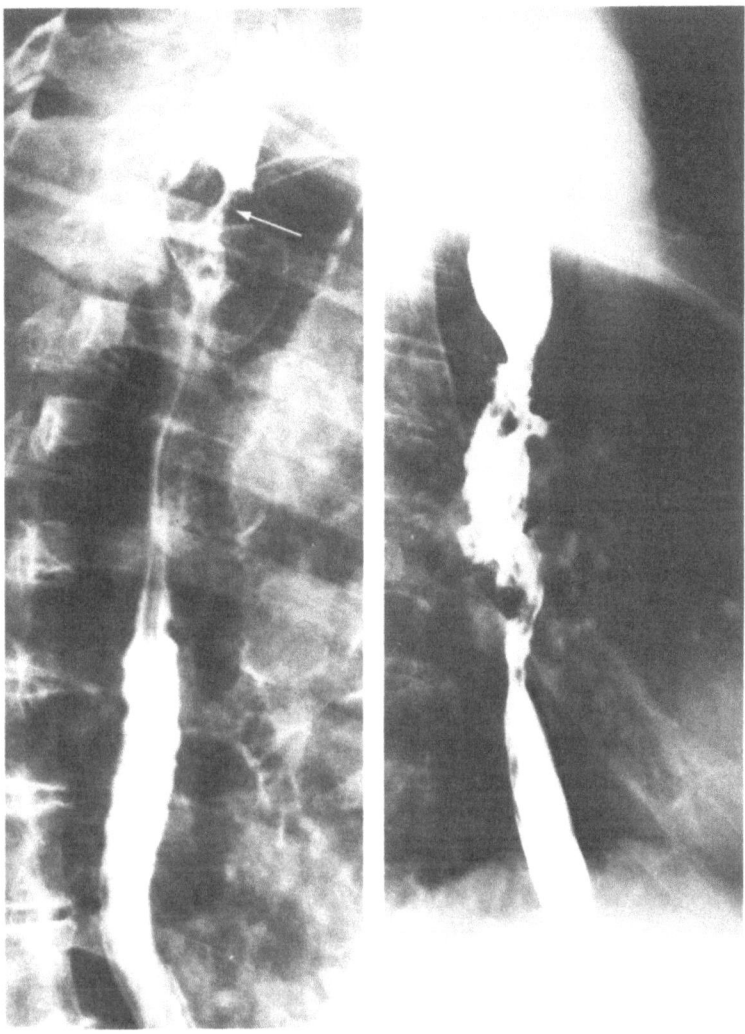

FIG. 202   FIG. 203

an area of mucosal irregularity. The bed of the ulcer niche is usually ragged and there is no neck. The crater or niche may be either superficial or deep. Shallow ulcerations may be difficult to detect because of the irregularities of the mucosal surface and scattered amounts of retained barium, which can obscure them (Fig. 203).

Obstructive lesions secondary to a primary intraluminal growth may be present with or without ulceration (Fig. 204).

Sectional lesions (malignant)

In the orohypopharyngeal area new growths are more likely to be exophytic. These appear as soft tissue masses within the lumen. Infiltrating lesions can also produce bone destruction and even bone sclerosis, as well as involvement or extension into surrounding structures of the epiglottis and larynx.

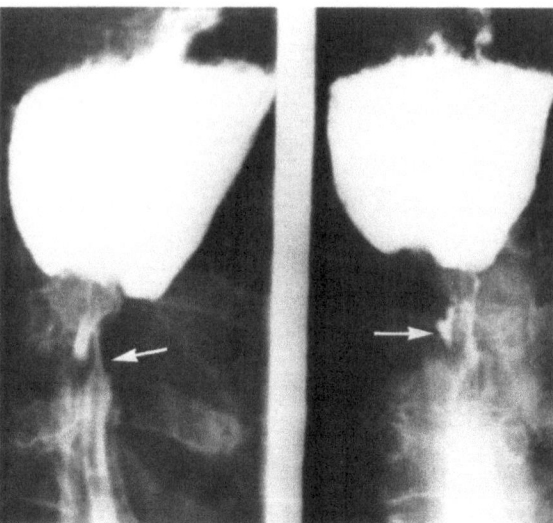

FIGURE 204

Obstructing primary lesions of esophagus. (A) Upper end of esophagus in the presence of a malignant ulcer (at arrow); (B) obstructing lesion, mid-esophagus; (C) lower end of esophagus. Note destruction of mucosal pattern at site of lesion.

(A)

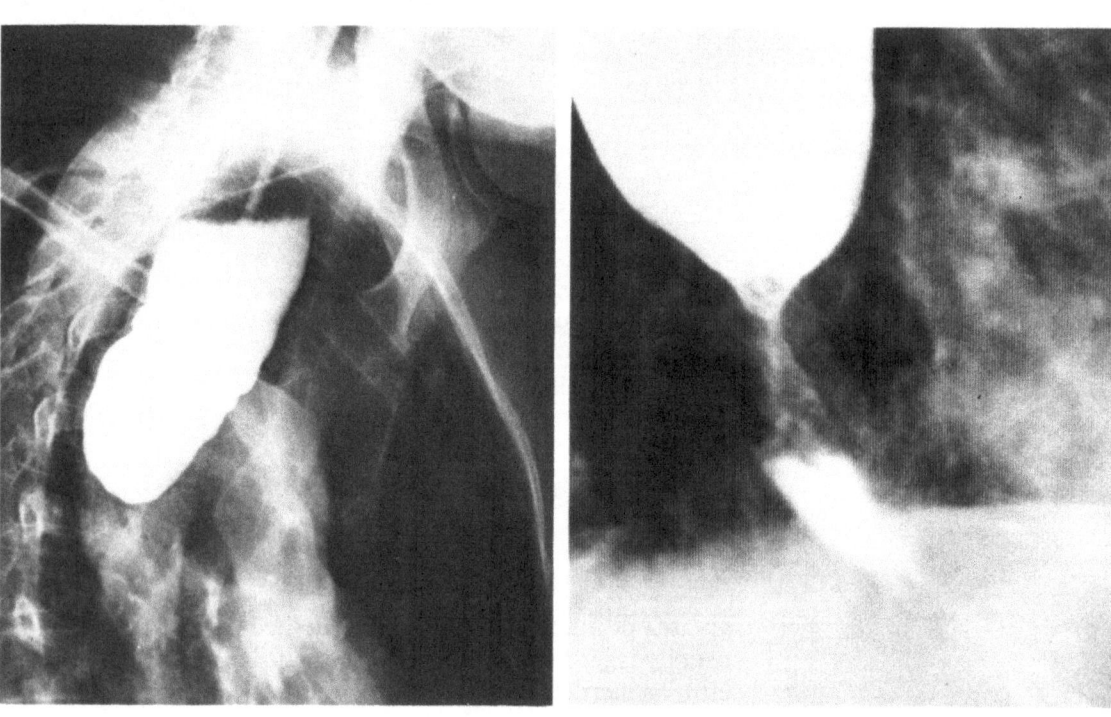

(B)   (C)

Oral cavity

In the oral cavity (57), a plain lateral film of the cervical region is basic and should precede ingestion of barium in the radiologic examination of a patient complaining of dysphagia. This is done in order to evaluate densities that may be obscured by the ingested opaque media. In the plain film, the oral cavity should be examined for erosions or sclerosis of the skeletal structures, the thickness of the soft palate and uvula, and the size of the tongue. Malignant lesions involving the mandible in the molar region do not ordinarily affect the roots of teeth in the region, in contrast to benign cystic lesions, fibrous dysphasia, and osteomyelitis. The mandibular foramen and canal may be enlarged by metastasis from an adjacent lesion. Examination of the oral cavity following ingestion of a barium bolus usually delineates the extent of any abnormal soft tissue mass or bony abnormality.

In the hard and soft palate, the radiologic appearance of irregularities of the mucosal pattern, with or without the presence of bone changes in the roof of the mouth, confirms the presence of a malignant neoplasm. In the soft palate and uvula the degree of thickening of their borders and the presence and extent of nasopharyngeal involvement can best be determined by radiologic examination.

Squamous cell carcinoma is the most frequent malignant lesion of the tongue, usually affecting older individuals. An enlarged tongue may interfere with the ingestion of a barium bolus. A barium-coated tongue best shows irregularities in its silhouette, particularly in the posterior or basal portion. An irregular soft tissue density or an ulcerating mass may be noted, confirming the presence of a carcinoma, which is also usually observed on inspection with a laryngeal mirror. Still, the extent of the lesion and the degree of displacement or involvement of surrounding structures are best determined by radiologic examination.

An enlarged tongue can also be related to such benign lesions as acromegaly, amyloidosis, or congenital muscular hypertrophy. Rarely, in younger individuals, a lingual thyroid in the region of the foramen caecum must be differentiated from a squamous cell carcinoma at the base of the tongue.

Oropharyngeal area

In the oropharyngeal area the palatine tonsils are most frequently affected by squamous cell carcinoma. On occasion, however, a lymphomatous mass or a benign papilloma may produce similar changes. Although they are detectable on oral inspection, the extent of large lesions may be difficult to determine. Their evaluation is faciliated by a barium swallow.

Posterior wall lesions of the oropharynx often produce a localized soft tissue density that is initially difficult to recognize as a tumor. Such lesions are usually exophytic growths. However, early displacement of the larynx anteriorly and encroachment on the normal pharyngeal space, as observed on a barium swallow, may be apparent. With progressive growth, an irregular shallow collection usually representing ulceration can be demonstrated radiologically. Such lesions, usually squamous cell carcinoma, can extend into the nasopharynx or hypopharynx. Rarely, benign primary retropharyngeal tumors, such as fibrolipoma and osteochondroma, grow from the underlying connective tissues or adjacent bone.

Vallecula

The vallecula may also be the site of a squamous cell carcinoma. Lesions in this area are best observed on a lateral film of the neck, in which a soft tissue mass distorts the vallecular space. The epiglottis is usually displaced posteriorly by such lesion.

Epiglottis

The epiglottis, when involved by a primary neoplasm, becomes quite shallow and protrudes into the oropharyngeal space. The clinical history and direct inspection by a laryngeal mirror help differentiate a neoplasm of the epiglottis. In advanced malignant lesions, sinus tracts can be demonstrated, following a barium swallow. Pedunculated tumors arising from the epiglottis also occur.

Hypopharyngeal area

In the hypopharyngeal area, postcricoid lesions arise in the aryepitlottic folds, in the vocal cords (Fig. 205A,B), or by extension from the pyriform sinuses or cervical esophagus. Radiologic studies show a fixed irregularity in the postcricoid region which may be confused with an irregular but normal cricoid impression (see Chapter 2). Thickening of the postcricoid soft tissue area and anterior displacement of the thyroid cartilage, as well as destruction of the underlying cricoid cartilage, may also occur. Spotty calcifications within the tumor mass should suggest a benign osterochondroma arising from an adjacent bony structure.

Postpharyngeal area

Postpharyngeal wall neoplasms are usually squamous cell carcinomas, which must be differentiated from inflammatory and posttraumatic lesions. A soft tissue mass encroaching on the hypopharyngeal area is the usual radiologic finding.

Pyriform sinuses

Neoplasms of the pyriform sinuses grow as exophytic or infiltrating lesions. When the tumor originates from the bottom of

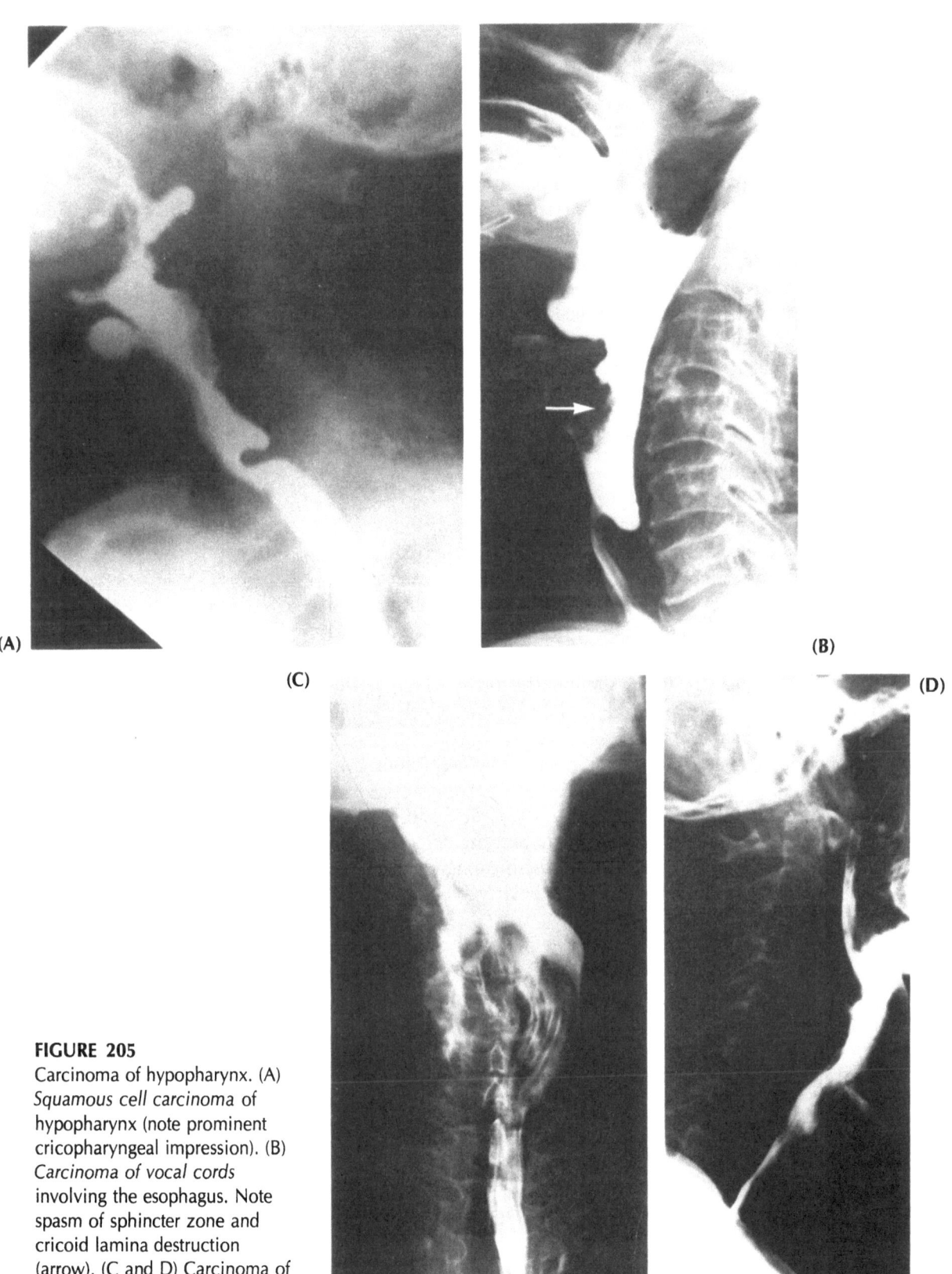

FIGURE 205
Carcinoma of hypopharynx. (A)
Squamous cell carcinoma of
hypopharynx (note prominent
cricopharyngeal impression). (B)
Carcinoma of vocal cords
involving the esophagus. Note
spasm of sphincter zone and
cricoid lamina destruction
(arrow). (C and D) Carcinoma of
right pyriform fossa. Frontal
view; (D) lateral view.

the pyriform fossa, it is usually infiltrative. When the neoplasm arises from the lateral or medial walls, it is usually exophytic and presents as a polypoid tumor. These tumors must be differentiated from invading lesions of the larynx. Anteroposterior views and tomograms of this region, as well as laryngography, are useful. Because these lesions are usually unilateral, the anteroposterior view is more helpful than the lateral film in separating the mucosal patterns of the pyriform sinuses (Fig. 205C,D). The hypopharynx is a frequent site of a diverticulum, and a squamous cell carcinoma occasionally may originate within a diverticulum. When this occurs, the early changes are reflected at the base of the diverticulum as a filling defect, which may be confused with retained food or air bubbles. Examination in various positions, including Trendelenburg and repeated studies, are usually necessary to confirm the presence of a neoplastic mass.

Cervical esophagus

In the cervical esophagus, squamous cell carcinoma may affect the sphincter zone. Carcinoma at this site is more frequent in females and is associated with atrophic mucosal changes with or without hypochromic anemia. Individuals with a Plummer–Vinson syndrome therefore should have periodic evaluations of this region, especially when a persistent web is recorded. Any alteration in contour and demonstration of irregularities in the mucosal pattern must alert the clinician to the possibility of a malignant lesion.

The cervical esophagus may be invaded by a carcinoma of the larynx or trachea, with subsequent narrowing of the lumen. Frequently, abnormal angulation and deviation of this segment of the esophagus occurs in the presence of such a lesion. Laryngograms are useful in establishing diagnosis as well as in the detection of fistulous tracts. A positive vallecular sign appears if obstruction develops.

Thoracic esophagus and the gastroesophageal junction

A common site of malignancy of the esophagus is at the level of compression by the aortic arch (Fig. 206). It is believed that this aortic compression produces stasis with repeated traumatic result to the esophagus, predisposing to abnormal cellular growth. Early neoplastic infiltration can escape notice unless this area is carefully analyzed. An increased space between the aortic arch and the esophagus should be sought. This is related to the increased thickness produced by the malignant infiltrative process. As the lesion grows, a mild degree of funneling greater than that caused by compression by the

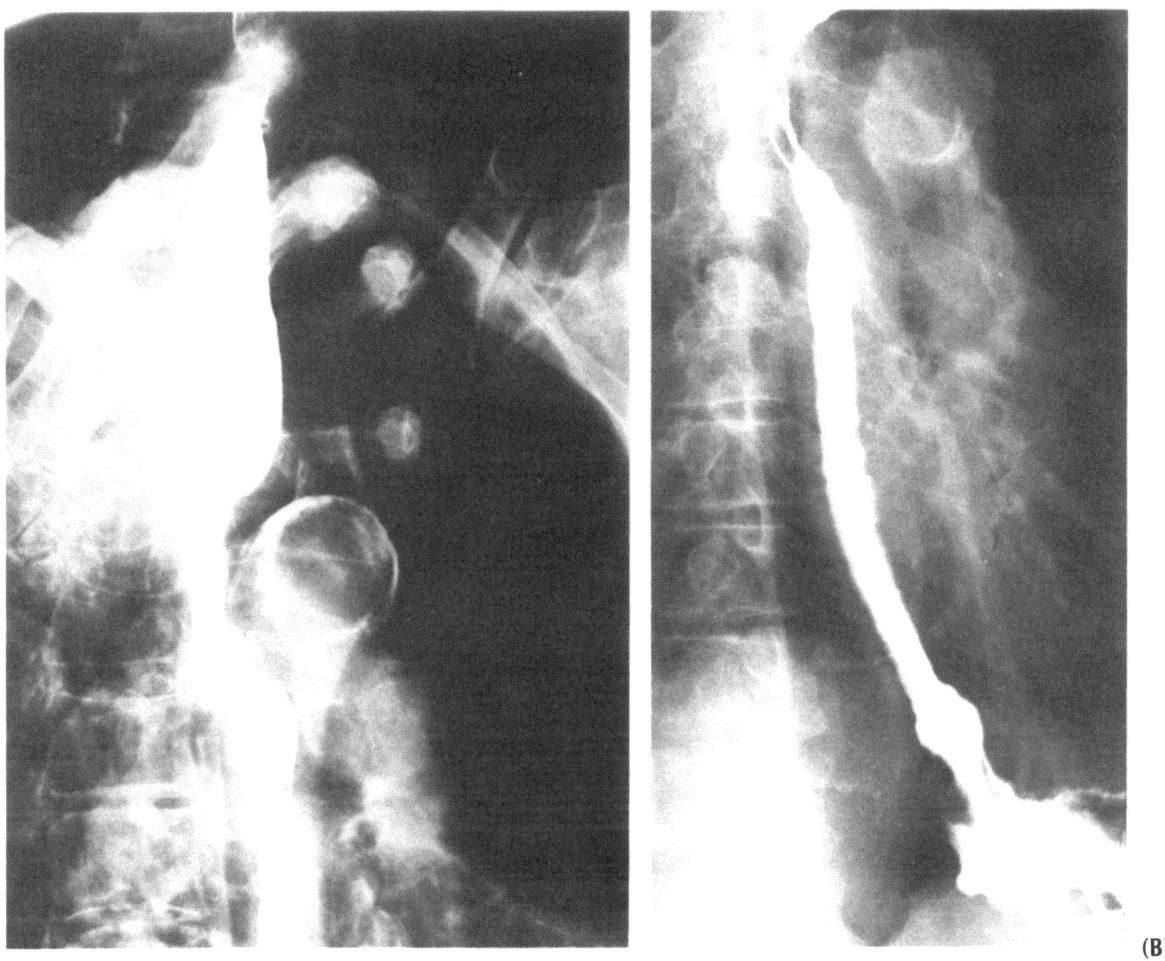

(A)

(B)

FIGURE 206
Neoplastic infiltration in region of aortic arch impression. (A and B) Two different patients.

aorta should alert the physician to malignancy. There is usually no intraluminal soft tissue tumor and obstruction is a late sign.

More distal lesions, at the level of the tracheal bifurcation, are more frequently involved secondary to extension from surrounding malignant mediastinal lymph nodes but may also be of primary origin (Fig. 207). Primary lung neoplasms may also invade the esophagus (see Chapter 3, Fig. 249A). Here, deviation and fixation, in addition to narrowing of the esophageal lumen, should be sought. The size of the surrounding tumor masses can be helpful. The larger the mass, the more likely it is to be an invading tumor. Multiple fistulae or sinuses favor a primary esophageal lesion.

The distal third of the esophagus is the most frequent site of malignant neoplasm particularly when the gastroesophageal junction is included. Here, in addition to squamous cell carcinoma, an adenocarcinoma extending from the cardia or growing from heterotopic gastric mucosa is not uncommon.

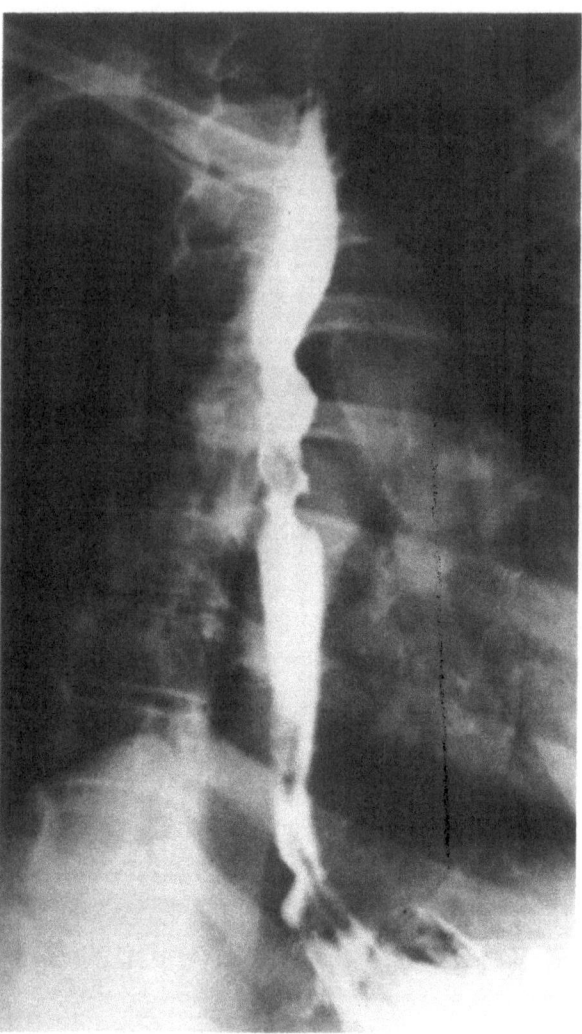

FIGURE 207
Primary malignant lesion of
mid-esophagus.

These lesions tend to be tumefactive in character. Nodulations
and irregularities of the cardia and fundus of the stomach
should be sought for in suspected neoplasms in these areas.
These significant abnormalities may be observed on plain
films of the chest or abdomen upon evaluation of the gastric
"gas bubble" in the erect position. Air contrast studies of the
cardia and fundus constitute valuable refinements of technique to visualize properly the mucosal pattern and distensibility of the cardia (Fig. 208).

The "varicoid" variety of squamous cell carcinoma resembles esophageal varices (Fig. 209). This lesion can be distinguished by its rigidity, lack of peristaltic contractions, and
abrupt demarcation. The distal end of the esophagus, which is
the most common site of esphageal varices, may be involved in
such neoplasms.

A difficult decision in radiologic differential diagnosis is the separation of achalasia from infiltrating malignancies resembling achalasia (Fig. 210), or achalasia in which a malignant neoplasm has developed. In achalasia, a beaklike contraction at the lower end of the esophagus, corresponding to the contracted lower sphincter, is observed. Prolonged stasis of barium and very weak peristaltic waves are the rule. The radiologic appearances in the upright and prone positions are essentially similar. Air in the fundus of the stomach generally is absent. In addition, in achalasia a gradual, symmetrical, tapering of the distal end of the esophagus is noted, whereas the lower segment is smooth and presents directly above the cardia. A Seidlitz test may cause the sphincter to dilate, unlike what happens in carcinoma. Mecholyl and other cholinergic drugs may also be used for momentary dilatation of the sphincter.

In the case of an infiltrating carcinoma of the sphincter zone, megaesophagus can develop from the chronic obstruction. The remainder of the esophagus is usually normal, with peristalsis initially present and quite active. With progressive obstruction distally and increased dilatation of the esophagus proximally, early depression of peristaltic activity, with stasis and dilatation reminiscent of achalasia, becomes a prominent

(A)

(B)

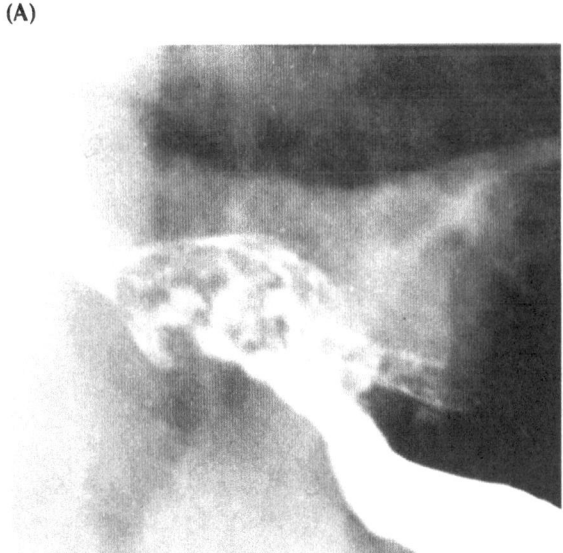
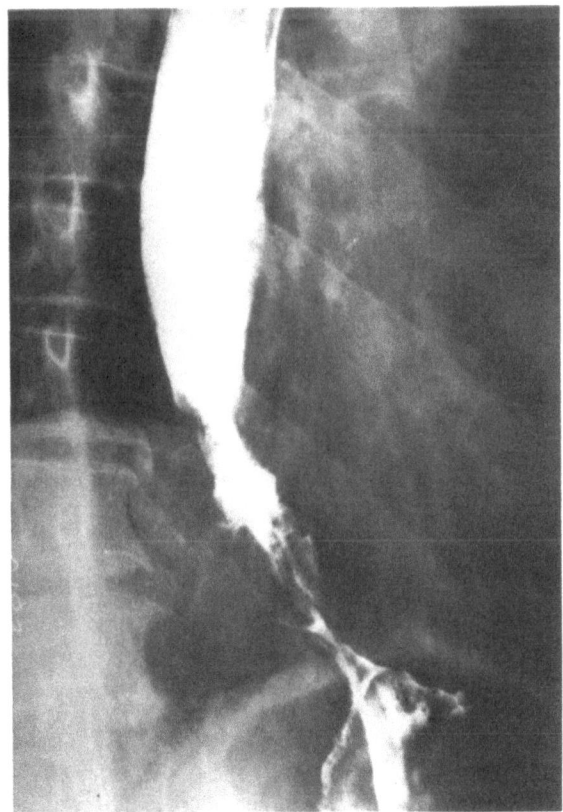

FIGURE 208

Adenocarcinoma, lower end of esophagus. (A and B) Two different patients.

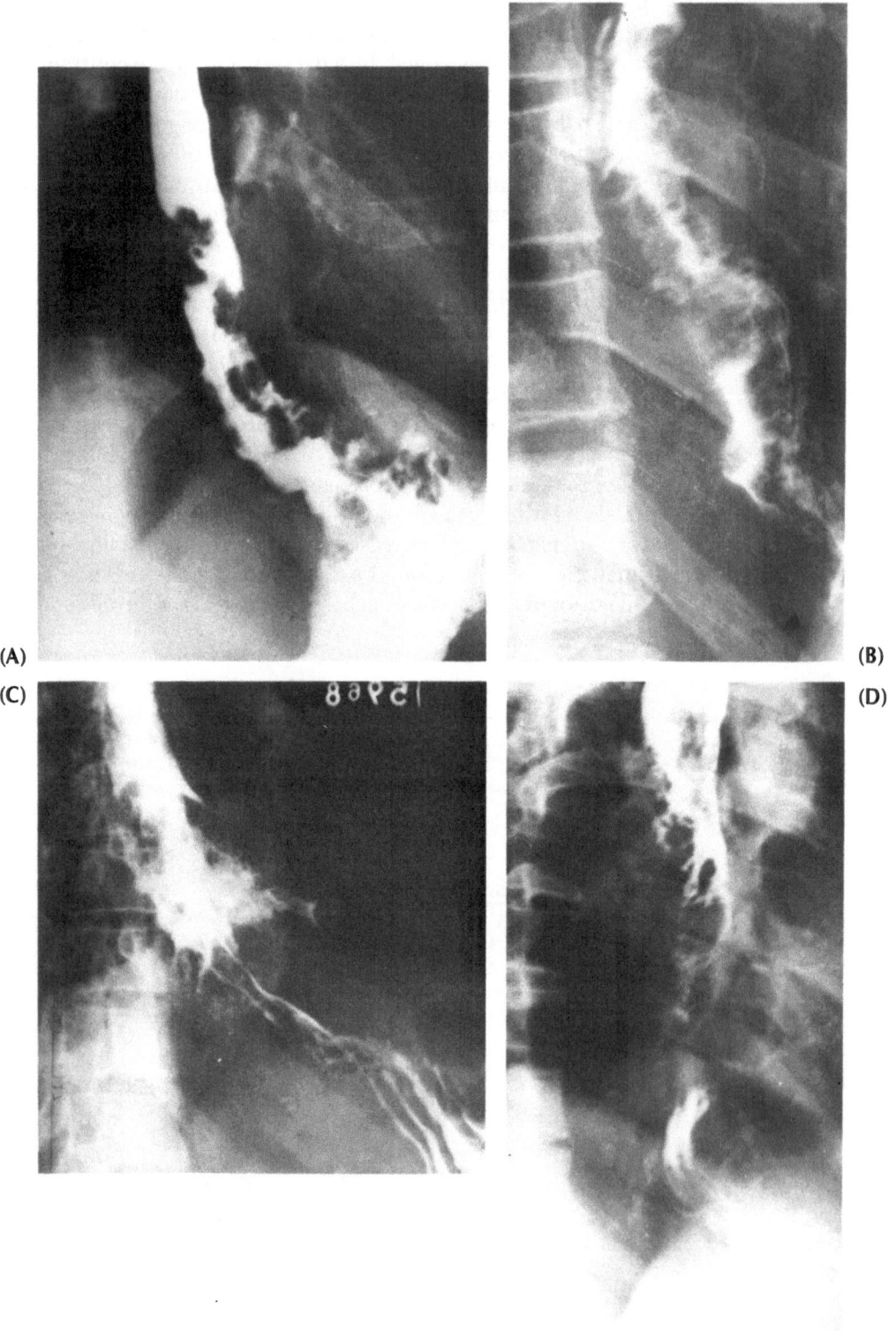

FIGURE 209
Varicoid varieties of carcinoma of the esophagus. (A and D) Four
different patients.

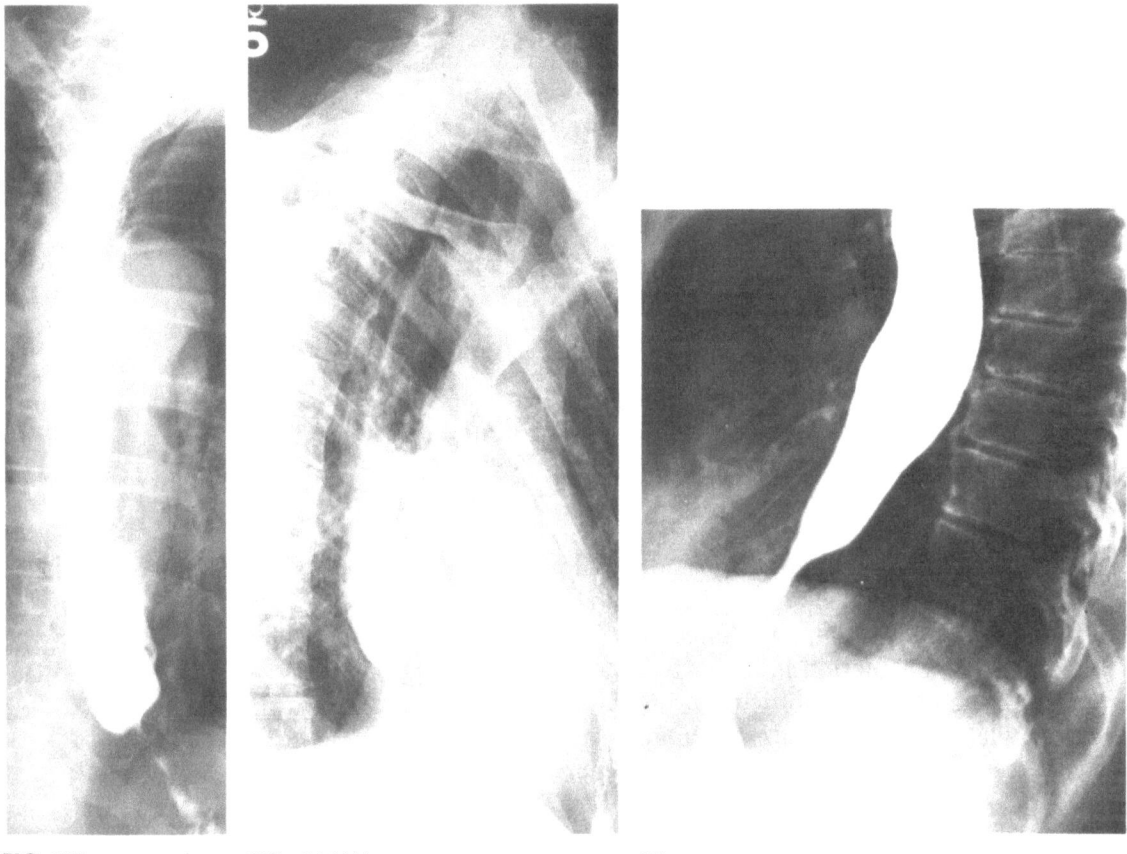

FIG. 210   FIG. 211(A)   (B)

FIGURE 210
Adenocarcinoma of the lower end of esophagus resembling achalasia. A diverticulum is also present in the lower esophagus.

FIGURE 211
Infiltrating carcinoma resembling chronic esophagitis with stricture. (A and B) Two different patients.

feature. Slight asymmetry or irregularity of the contracted lower segment may be the only clue to a malignancy. Destruction of the myenteric plexus in the sphincter zone by an invading carcinoma may also contribute to a pattern suggesting achalasia.

In established cases of achalasia of many years duration, malignant changes have been reported both in the lower and in the mid-esophageal regions. It is generally assumed that achalasia of long standing predisposes to the development of a malignant neoplasm but no definite statistical proof has been offered. In the lower end, any alteration from an established radiologic appearance (e.g., granular translucencies and asymmetry of the contracted sphincter segment) should suggest a malignant lesion. Filling defects in the mid-esophagus must be distinguished from retained food particles. This distinction is affected by aspirating and irrigating the esophagus and then repeating the examination.

Hiatal hernia may also be associated with neoplastic disease, originating in either the cardia or the lower esophagus (110). Irregularity of the lower end of the esophagus in the presence of a hiatal hernia, generally is caused by peptic esophagitis so that the appearance of the mucosal pattern and the presence and degree of rigidity of the lower esophageal segment are important in considering the development of a neoplasm. Destroyed, irregular mucosal folds of the cardia or any change from previous films, if available, should alert one to the presence of a malignant lesion. The differences in the appearance and size of an ordinary simple hiatal hernia makes it difficult to evaluate early destructive mucosal changes but fixation and rigidity not previously present should arouse suspicion.

Malignant lesions resembling chronic esophagitis with stenosis may occur (Fig. 211). Extensive lesions involving the entire esophagus are now rarely seen because of early roentgenologic detection and clinical workup (Fig. 212).

Carcinoid of the esophagus is very rare. A case has been reported (28) with the radiologic appearance of a stricture in the lower segment of the esophagus.

Benign neoplasms

Benign tumors are usually localized and mobile. In terms of location, they are divided into intraluminal and intramural varieties that must be differentiated from extrinsic lesions. The radiologic distinction between intramural and extrinsic tumors is usually not too difficult, except in advanced or very large neoplasms which invade surrounding mediastinal structures.

Intraluminal lesions

Intraluminal lesions may be sessile or pedunculated. In sessile intraluminal lesions, the mucosal pattern is primarily involved with distortion and eventually ulceration of its surface. There is no evident soft tissue mass or displacement of the esophagus, although its lumen may be narrowed without obstruction. A mucosal tumor usually shows an acute angle of encroachment at the upper and lower poles of the lesion. Sessile, benign polypoid-like tumors of inflammatory origin are usually fibrovascular.

Intramural lesions

In intramural lesions, the mucosal surface is intact, with no irregularity of the mucosa rigidity and narrowing of the esophageal lumen. At the most, only minimal stasis of ingested barium is noted. An intramural neoplasm produces a localized tumor mass which may bulge into the esphageal lumen or grow outside the esophageal wall (exophytic). The mucosal pattern over the bulging intramural mass is smooth, stretched, or effaced but not destroyed. The upper and lower poles of the lesion show an obtuse angle of encroachment of the esophageal lumen.

Extrinsic masses

Extrinsic masses affect the esophagus in a manner related to their size and degree of attachment or involvement of the esophageal wall. Such lesions usually become quite large before the esophageal wall is eroded. When direct extension into the wall of the esophagus by a relatively small lesion occurs, it is most difficult radiologically to be certain of the exact site of origin of the mass lesion.

Ectopic or heterotopic gastric mucosa

Ectopic or heterotopic gastric mucosa occasionally may resemble radiologically a polypoid tumor in the mid-esophagus. The usual appearance is that of a small, smooth, scalloped filling defect, resembling an adenomatous sessile polyp (230). This lesion is observed in young adults and is usually asymptomatic (Fig. 213).

Papilloma

A papilloma of the esophagus presents as a small, discrete, spherical mass located at the gastroesophageal junction. It may be associated with a hiatal hernia or a distal esophageal stricture. The esophageal papilloma must be differentiated from an air bubble, retained food particles, foreign body granuloma, or a small sessile adenomatous polyp (Fig. 214). A small granuloma is usually located at the level of the lower sphincter, where a foreign body usually becomes impacted in the esophageal mucosa above the level of the normally contracted lower sphincter. An area of hypertrophic gastric mucosa may be encountered, although rarely, and may be observed at the gastroesophageal junction (237) as a small, localized mass (Fig. 215).

Leiomyoma

Leiomyoma is the most common benign intramural lesion of the esophagus. Leiomyoma may be single or multiple (103), nodular, lobulated, and occasionally pedunculated and is usually located in the lower end of the esophagus. A diffuse leiomyomatosis has also been reported (80).

A leiomyoma is a slowly growing tumor and is more common in men than women. A soft tissue mass that encircles

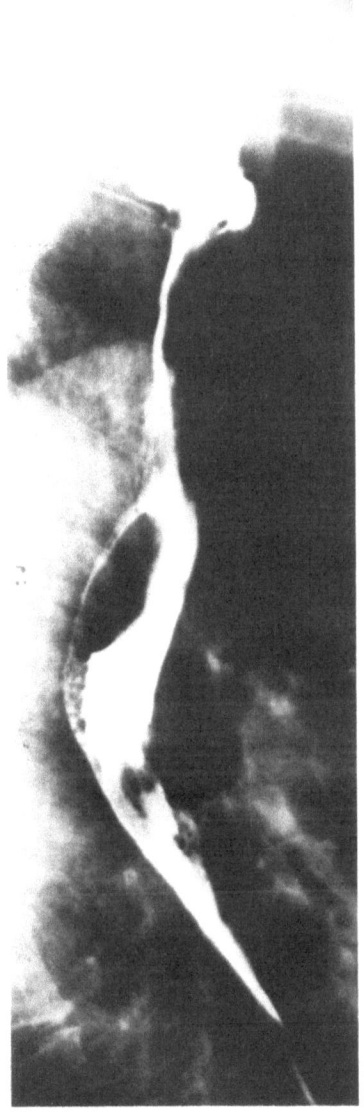

FIGURE 212
Extensive malignant changes involving the entire esophagus.

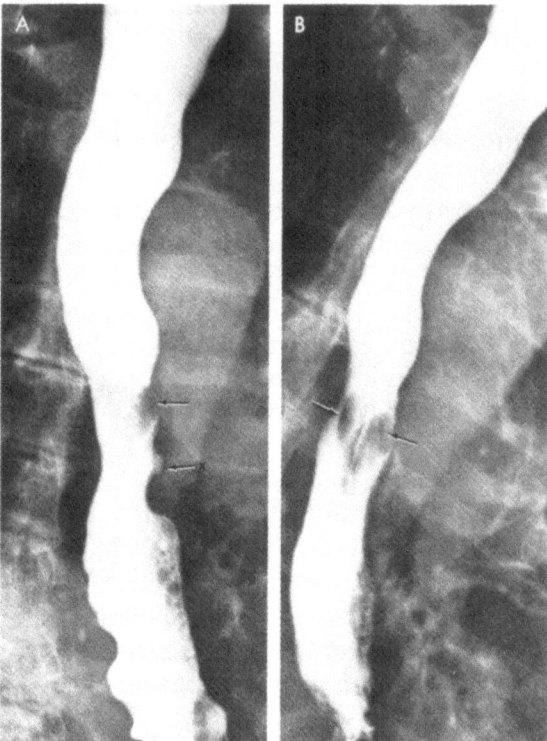

FIGURE 213
Heterotopic gastric mucosa in mid-esophagus. From Stein, G. N., and Finkelstein, A. K. The esophagus and stomach. In Hodes, P. J., ed. An Atlas of Tumor Radiology. Yearbook Medical Publisher, 1973. Fig. 21, P. 51. Permission of American College of Radiology.

FIGURE 214
Papilloma of the lower end of esophagus. From Stein, G. N., and Finkelstein, A. K. The esophagus and stomach. In Hodes, P. J., ed. An Atlas of Tumor Radiology. Yearbook Medical Publisher, 1973. Fig. 25, P. 59. Permission of American College of Radiology.

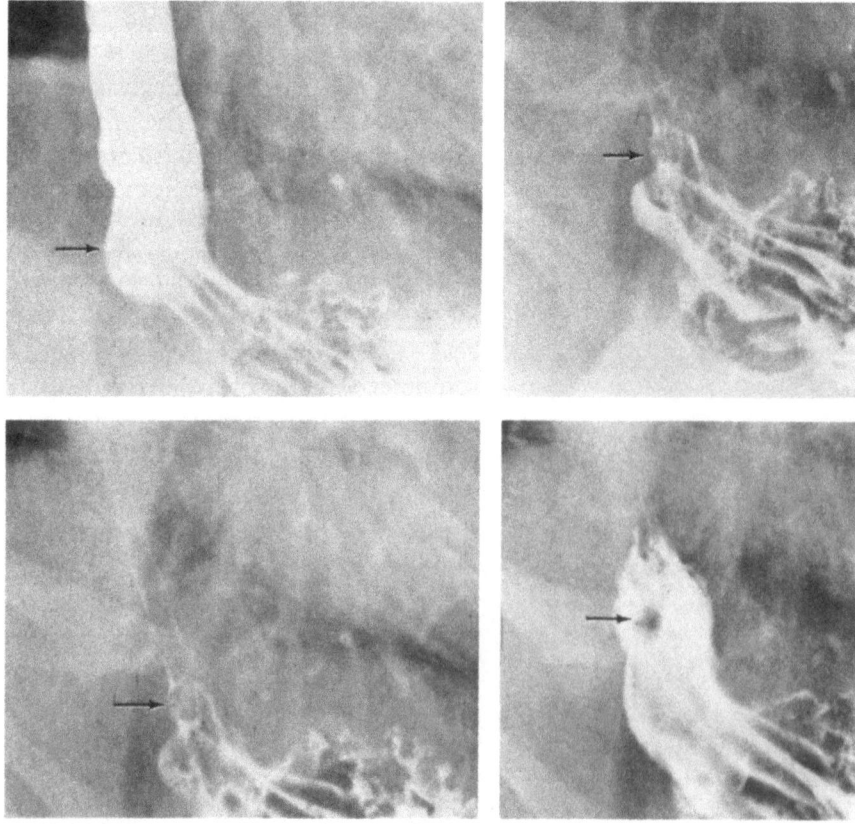

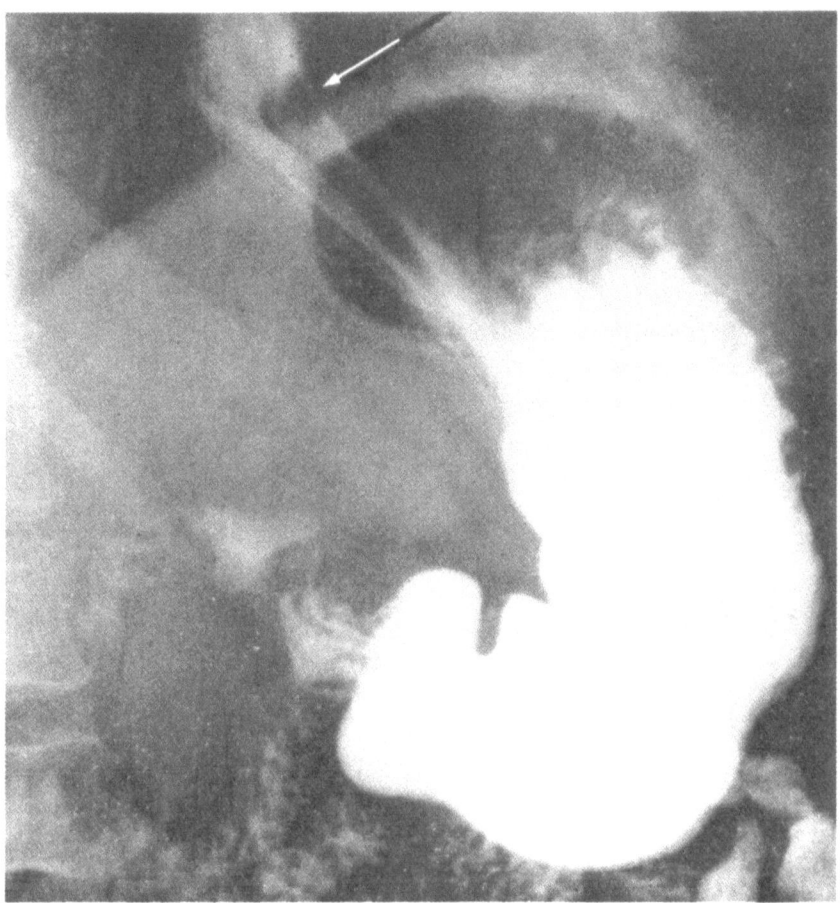

FIGURE 215

Hypertrophic gastric fold (at arrow). From Sussman, H. M. Localized gastric mucosal hypertrophy simulating tumor. Am. J. Dig. Dis., 10:711, 1965. Fig. 1. Harper & Row, Publishers.

the esophagus can occasionally be observed. The mass may grow considerably in size, with a large exophytic component even extending below the diaphragm to involve the cardia and fundus of the stomach. Esophageal leiomyomata generally do not ulcerate in contrast to gastric leiomyomata.

On radiologic examination a smoothly defined, spheroid soft tissue mass may be observed on plain films. Now here, with barium studies, an intact mucosal surface covers a localized, small, ovoid, or oblong intramural tumor without displacement, abnormal angulation, or change in mobility of the esophagus (Figs. 216 and 217). On a tangential view of the opacified esophagus, a smooth defect resembling a half moon can be seen. The upper and lower poles of the mass form a shallow obtuse angle with the inner esophageal wall. As the tumor grows, the mucosal pattern appears stretched or even obliterated, resulting in a smeared appearance of the mucosa. When a degree of obstruction develops, the barium column shows a forked–streamed appearance over the mass. Cystic degeneration of the tumor may develop and calcifications of leiomyomata are not uncommon.

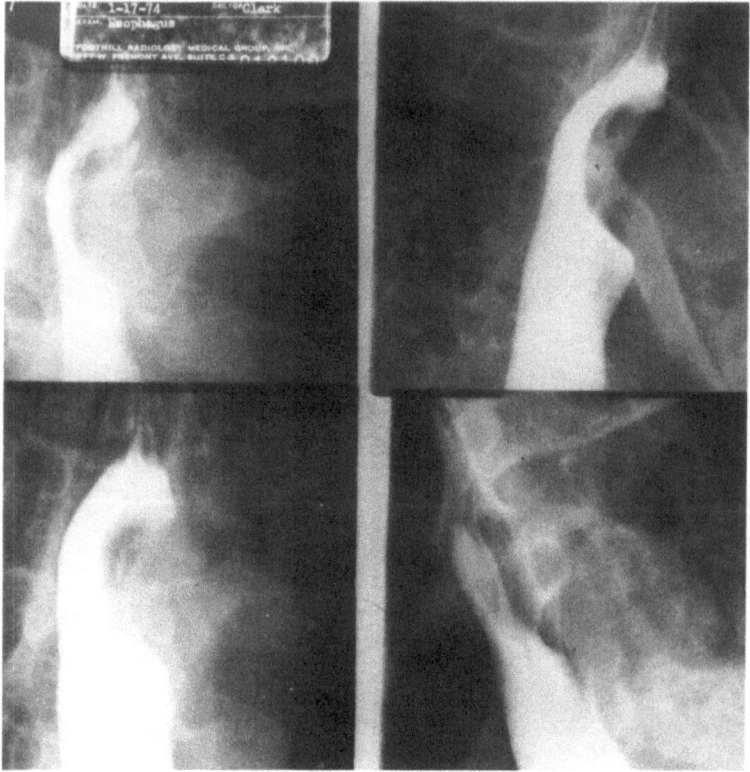

FIG. 216A

FIG. 217

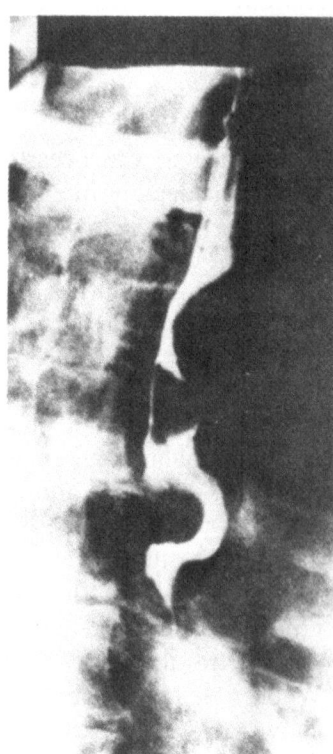

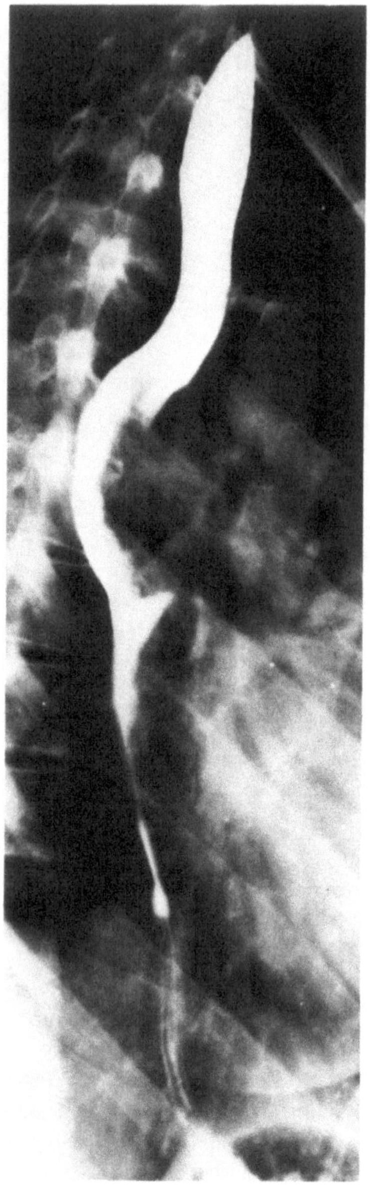

FIG. 216B

FIGURE 216
Leiomyoma in region of the aortic arch. (A) Spot films, (B) Another patient.

FIGURE 217
Leiomyoma—multiple lesions. From Haber, K., and Weinfield, A. C. Multiple leiomyomas of the esophagus. Am. J. Dig. Dis., *19*:7, 678, 1974.

Diffuse myomatosis

Diffuse myomatosis, considered a neoplasm, produces localized thickening of the esophageal wall. The smooth, circular muscle fibers of the lower third of the esophagus are particularly involved, but this disorder also may affect the stomach. This disorder is rare, occurring mainly in men. Dysphagia is the usual complaint. Irregular nodular arrangements of smooth muscle fibers are observed histologically. On endoscopy, an area of stenotic narrowing is noted, with the mucosa unaffected. On radiologic examination, the features of achalasia may be simulated, although a greater degree of funneling exists in myomatosis above the level of the lesion, extending beyond the sphincter zone. Diffuse spasm also is usually associated.

Intramural lipoma

An intramural lipoma presents radiologic features often indistinguishable from leiomyoma. Rarely, this neoplasm may appear relatively translucent. Of greater importance is the change in size and contour that may be observed in lipoma on serial films and fluoroscopy—often from a spheroid to a cigar-like configuration

Hemangioma

Hemangioma is another, less common intramural neoplasm simulating a leiomyoma. Phleboliths rarely may be present. Other even rarer benign intramural neoplasms are usually indistinguishable radiologically from the more common lesions.

Pedunculated lesions

Pedunculated tumors may be benign or malignant. Polyps are pedunculated tumors that project into the lumen (15, 116). They form about one-third of all benign tumors of the esophagus, being more common in males.

Benign polyps

Benign polyps usually arise from the pharyngoesophageal junction, have long stalks, and can develop into single, large ovoid masses (Fig. 218). They can be regurgitated into the mouth during a bout of vomiting or coughing. They are usually fibrovascular histologically but can also be composed of inflammatory, lipomatous, fibromatous, or hemangiomatous tissue. Radiologically, pedunculated polyps present as translucent,

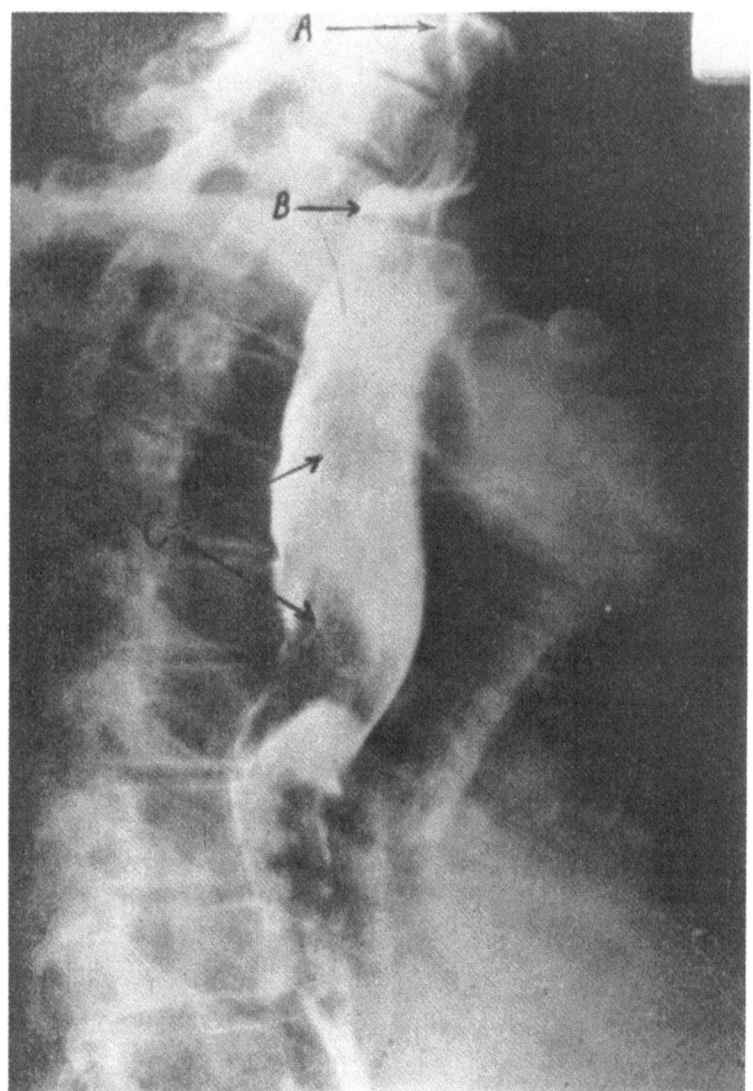

FIGURE 218
Benign pedunculated tumor, upper end of esophagus. From Beeler, R., et al. Benign pedunculated tumors of the esophagus. Am. J. Roentgenol., 60:467, 1948.

mobile masses that fill and dilatate the esophagus. A stalk is present occasionally. Swallowed air or retained food may be mistaken for a polyp. Typically, however, polyps are noted to be surrounded by a halo of barium.

Inflammatory polyps may be present in a Barrett esophagus (69), usually originating in the middle to lower esophagus. They present as ulcerating masses (147).

Polyps in the lower one-third of the esophagus tend to be malignant. Such malignant esophageal polyps are rare. They are most commonly leiomyosarcomas. The roentgenologic findings are indistinguishable from a benign leiomyoma or sessile polypoid lesion. A case of primary malignant melanoma also resembling a polypoid lesion has been reported (see Fig. 197). These are rare.

Carcinosarcoma

Carcinosarcoma is usually a pedunculated lesion (163). This neoplasm generally is large and bulky, is irregular in contour, and often is associated with a short pedicle. A mixture of carcinomatous and sarcomatous tissues is observed histologically.

Pseudo-sarcomas

Pseudo-sarcomas are polypoid or pedunculated lesions that histologically resemble sarcomas but show no infiltration or extension into the esophageal wall. They are usually smooth, rounded, intraluminal filling defects that are indistinguishable radiographically from carcinosarcoma or benign fibrous polyps.

Esophageal pseudo-tumors

Esophageal pseudo-tumors result from the retrograde prolapse of gastric mucosal folds into the lower end of the esophagus (205, 257), secondary to a redundant gastric mucosa associated

FIGURE 219
Pseudotumors in two patients. (A) Herniated gastric mucosa within a hiatal hernia. (B). From Wells, J. Herniation of gastric mucosa into the esophagus. Am. J. Roentgenol., 58:194, 1974

(A)   (B)

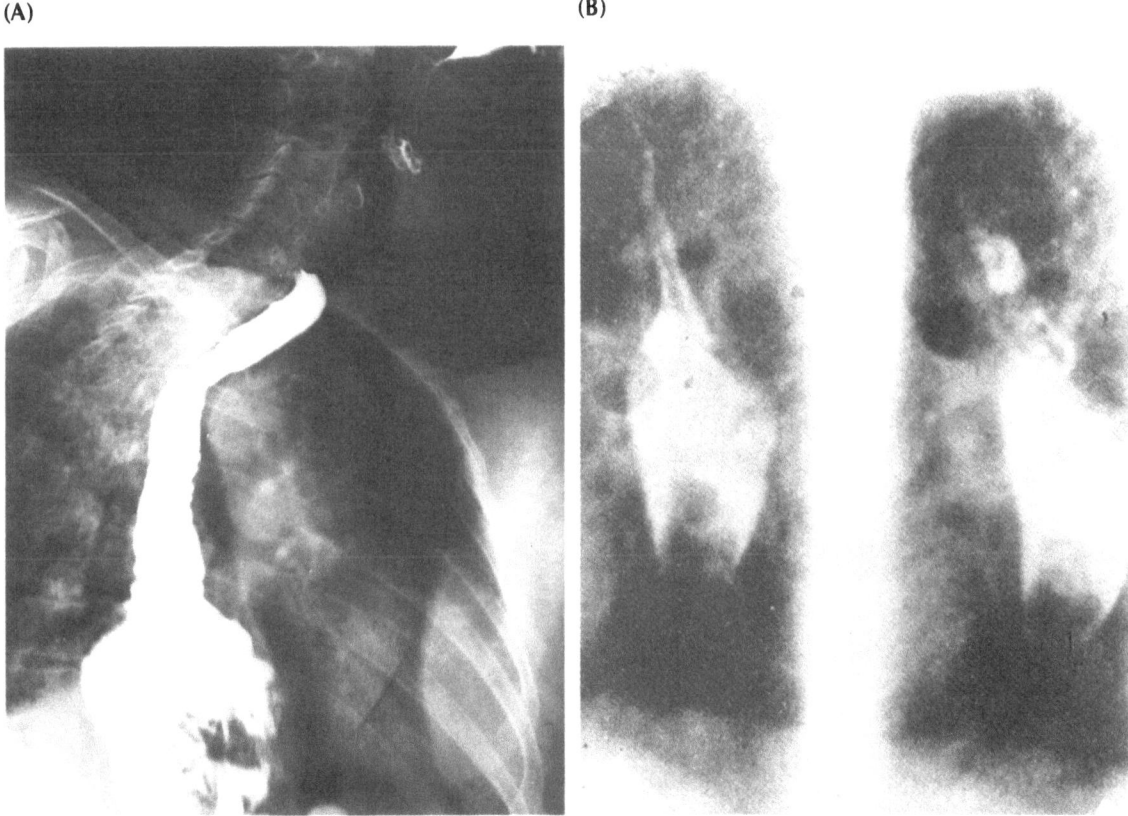

with relaxation of the lower sphincter. Retrograde herniation of a gastric fold during reverse peristalsis or regurgitation is therefore made possible.

With large hiatal hernias the herniated gastric mucosa may roll above the esophageal hiatus, producing a tumor-like mass within the herniated portion of the stomach (200) (Fig. 219). This large herniated fold occasionally may become incarcerated and even ulcerated. The radiologic findings in such instances are those of single or multiple smooth, circumscribed filling defects, best defined in the right anterior oblique position, especially with increased abdominal pressure. The filling defects tend to change in size and disappear during the emptying phase of the barium-opacified esophagus. Incomplete obstruction may occur.

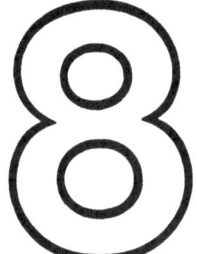

ROENTGENOLOGIC APPEARANCE FOLLOWING SURGERY AND RADIATION THERAPY

The radiologic appearance of the hypopharynx and esophagus following the surgical treatment of the more commonly encountered lesions (and their complications) are considered here. The radiologic appearance of the esophagus as a result of radiation therapy is also presented.

RADIOLOGIC CHANGES FOLLOWING SURGERY
Radiologic changes following surgery for repair of hiatal hernia and esophageal reflux

In an individual with a symptomatic hiatal hernia that is not responsive to medical treatment, surgical management becomes a consideration. Chronic esophagitis is usually present in such instances so that surgical intervention is frequently necessary to prevent an esophageal stricture. An attempt is made in such surgical procedure to reestablish the normal structural anatomy and to insure the normal function of the lower sphincter.

Surgical procedures

In general, the esophagus and the weakened phrenoesophageal membrane are attached to the under surface of the diaphragm. The widened esophageal hiatus is closed by suturing the right diaphragmatic crus posteriorly, in order to reestablish the snug esophageal hiatus. In this connection, Nissen's fundoplication is presently popular, particularly for the correction of uncontrolled reflux (201). A posterior gastropexy or a Belsey (Mark IV) procedure is also used for correction of a hiatal hernia with or without reflux.

271

FUNDOPLICATION In fundoplication, when the abdominal approach is used, the stomach is freed of all its diaphragmatic attachments. Then the gastric fundus is wrapped around the distal end of the esophagus and the free anterior end is sutured to the anterior wall of the stomach. A snug cuff of stomach is thus produced around the sphincter zone of the lower end of the esophagus. The esophageal hiatus is also repaired posteriorly. The resultant gastric cuff mechanically restrains the distal end of the esophagus, actually retaining it in the abdomen. The gastric cuff also increases pressure in the sphincter zone, minimizing reflux as well as reducing the hiatal hernia. In the presence of a short esophagus, a thoracic approach is indicated, with the placement of the cuff in the thoracic cavity directly above the diaphragm.

Several other modifications of this type of surgical procedure exist. Such operations may be used in infants and children or after surgical recurrences of previous unsuccessfully repaired hiatal hernias.

When reflux esophagitis is present without a hiatal hernia, repair of the esophageal hiatus is usually not necessary. Therefore, pyloroplasty or a vagotomy occasionally is carried out, especially when an active or chronic duodenal ulcer with hyperacidity is present.

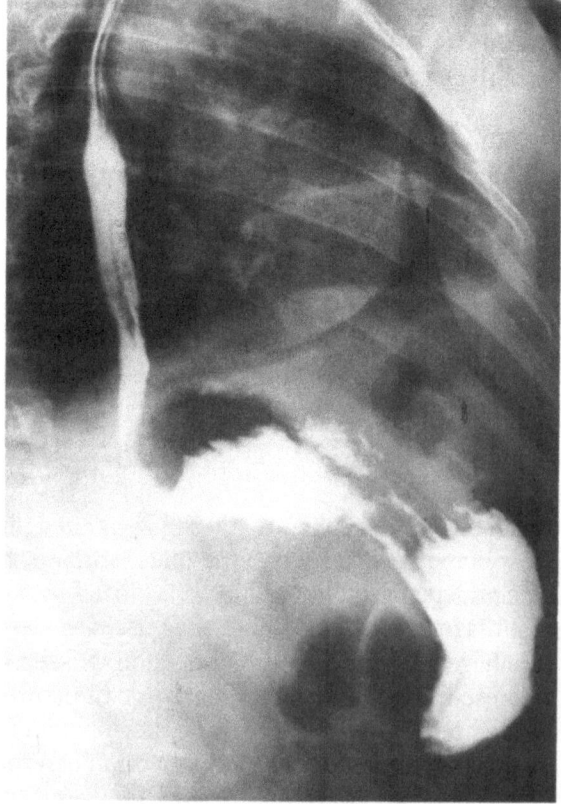

FIGURE 220
Postoperative repair of hiatal hernia.

GASTROPEXY Several other types of surgical repair for hiatal hernia exist. In the posterior gastropexy procedure, an abdominal approach is used. The lower end of the esophagus is sutured to the posterior abdominal wall and the phrenoesophageal membrane is divided and pulled down, thus reducing the hernia. The esophageal hiatus is repaired and the stomach rotated anteriorly. The stomach is fixed by suturing the connective tissue at the gastroesophageal junction to the aortic fascia. If a duodenal ulcer or hyperacidity is present, a vagotomy may be done at the same time (see section on vagotomy).

An anterior gastropexy is performed in debilitated patients or in instances when a hiatal hernia is discovered incidently during a laporatomy. In anterior gastropexy the greater curvature of the stomach is pulled down and sutured to the anterior wall of the abdomen, preventing upward migration of the stomach. This procedure reduces the hernia partly or completely.

BELSEY PROCEDURE A Belsey procedure through a thoracic approach is more complex. Both the diaphragm and the gastric fundus are utilized to produce an abdominal esophageal segment, following reduction of the hernia. The fundus and esophagus are sutured together and maintained below the diaphragm by additional sutures to the right crus of the diaphragm.

Radiologic appearance

The radiologic appearance of the lower esophagus following some of these operative procedures is illustrated next (76, 241). After a successful operation that reestablishes the normal anatomic structures of the area, the hernia is no longer demonstrable. However, some difficulty may exist in visualizing the lower sphincter, which has been anchored intraabdominally (Fig. 220). The reduced size of the esophageal hiatus is evaluated by the degree of narrowing, stasis, or invagination of the supradiaphragmatic esophagus.

In the Nissen procedure or fundoplication operations, the appearance of the lower esophagus resembles a filling defect of the cardia (Fig. 221). Cine studies may be performed to determine the efficacy of esophageal reflux correction, the size of the repaired esophageal hiatus, and the occasional recurrence of the hiatal hernia. When the hernia is not completely reduced or has been changed from a sliding to a paraesophageal type, an abnormal residual angulation at the esophagogastric junction, which is secondary to the surgery, may be observed. Following a posterior gastropexy, a long intraabdominal segment of esophagus is identified with straightening of the distal end of the esophagus (Fig. 222A).

In the Mark IV procedure, a long segment of the lower end of the esophagus is noted to be intraabdominal, with a double

(A)

(B)

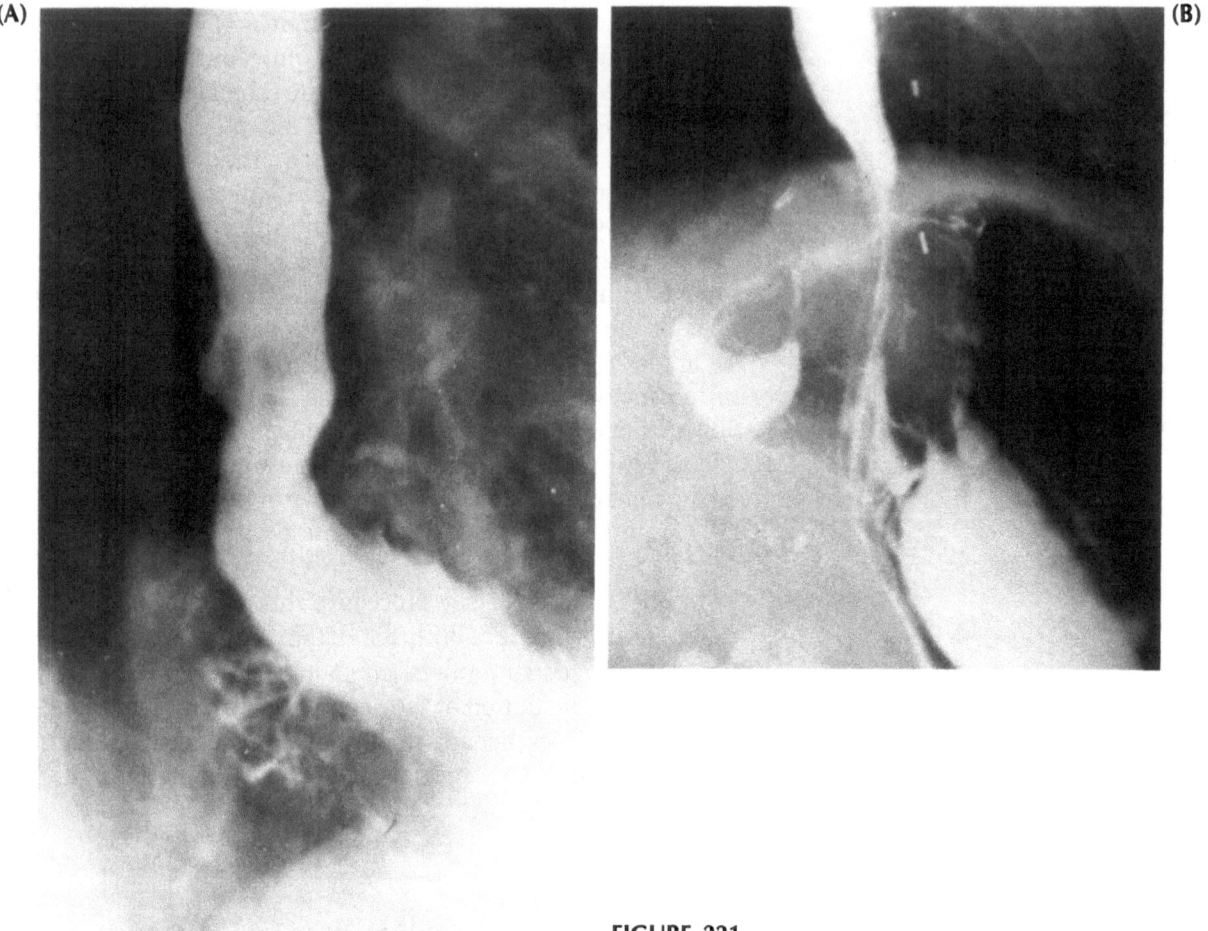

FIGURE 221
Nissen procedure: fundoplication repair of hiatal hernia.
(A) Preoperative, (B) postoperative.

angulation, one at the upper end of the diaphragm and fundus and the other at the lower end of the esophagus and fundus, close to the gastroesophageal junction (Fig. 222B).

The surgical management of paraesophageal hiatal hernia is quite different. In this type of hernia the esophagus normally is anchored posteriorly. The gastric fundus rolls through the esophageal hiatal, carrying with it the greater curvature and producing eventually an inverted stomach in the thoracic cavity. The stomach is enclosed within a peritoneal sac. This type of hernia is subject to the complications of ulceration, incarceration, strangulation, and volvulus, the last three requiring immediate surgery (8). The abdominal approach is usually preferred. The esophageal hiatus is repaired and the lesser curvature of the stomach is anchored posteriorly. A normal appearance is reestablished radiologically when the hernia has been completely reduced and the esophageal hiatus repaired. Incomplete reduction or recurrences are not unusual. In volvulus, a closed loop obstruction of the herniated stomach occurs. Suc-

FIGURE 222

(A) Gastropexy procedure, (B) Mark IV procedure for repairs of hiatal hernia. From Feigen, D. S., et al. Radiologic appearance of hiatal hernia repairs. Radiology, *110*:73, 1974.

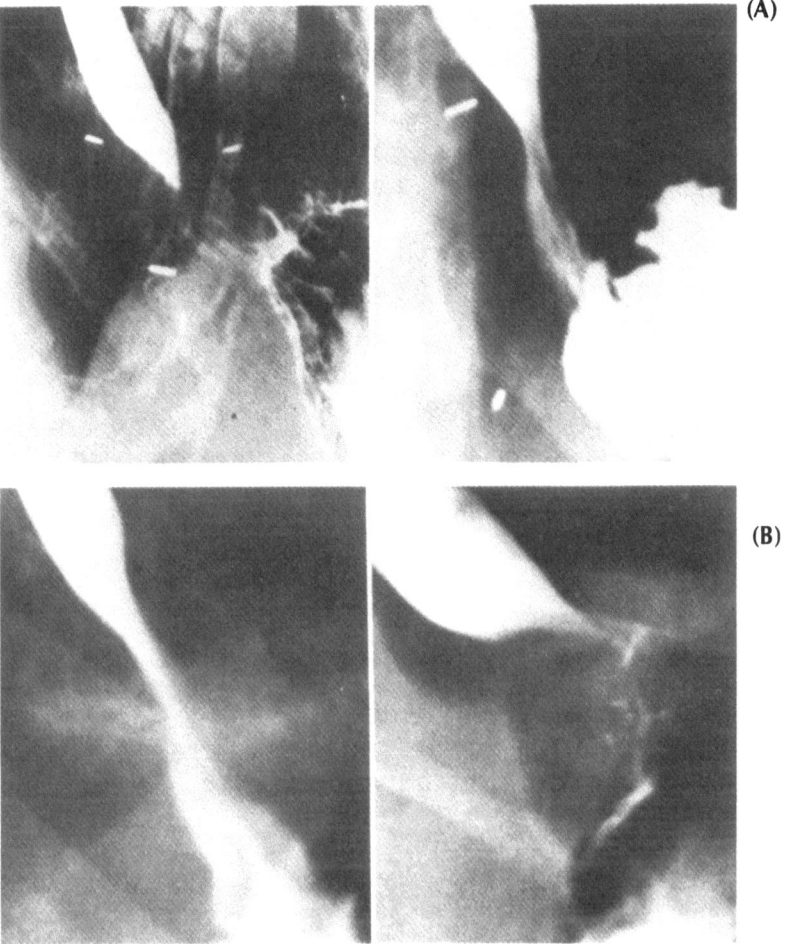

(A)

(B)

cessful surgical repair depends on the blood supply and integrity of the gastric wall. Occasionally, only an anterior gastropexy can be done. The radiologic examination becomes of marked importance in the followup of the surgical results (Fig. 223).

Radiologic changes following myotomies and pneumatic dilatation

Myotomies

Myotomies are performed by incising the outer muscular layers down to the mucosa (70). These procedures are usually carried out to relieve dysphagia secondary to localized or generalized muscular hypertrophy.

As an example, myotomy performed for symptomatic hypertrophy of the cricopharyngeus muscle usually results in relief of the dysphagia. Myotomy may also be affective in instances of hypertensive sphincters with chronic dysphagia.

In this connection hypertrophy of the transverse fibers of

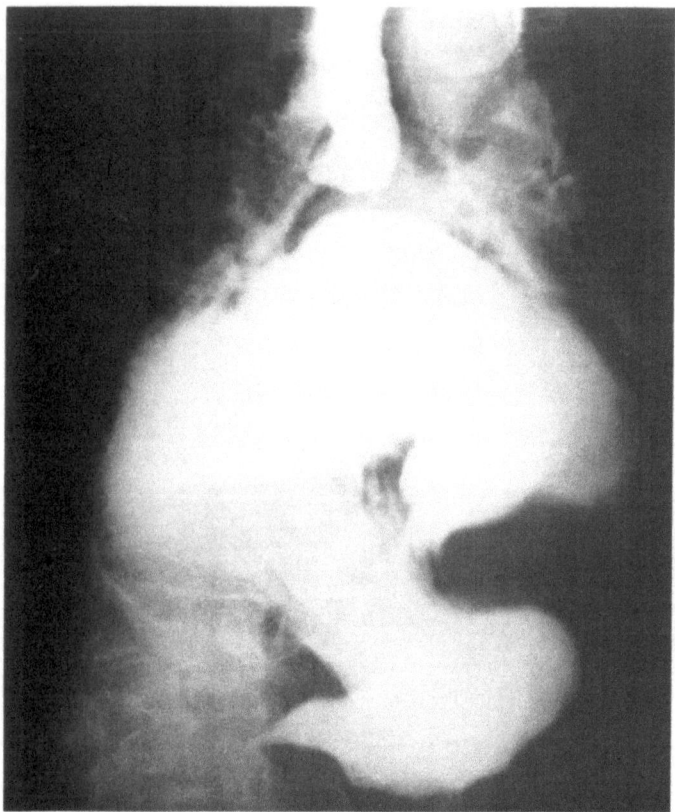

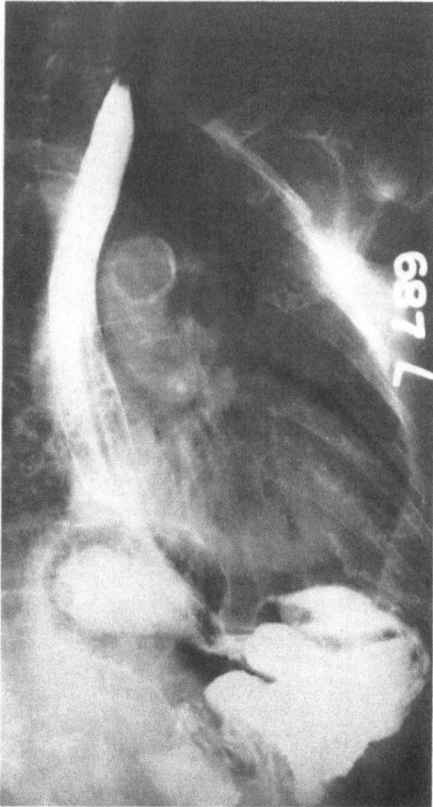

(A)

(B)

FIGURE 223
Partial volvulus of a thoracic stomach. (A) Preoperative, (B) postoperative following anterior gastropexy.

the cricopharyngeus muscle may be associated with a Zenker's diverticulum. The hypertrophy itself may be the causative factor in the production of the diverticulum. When the size of the diverticulum is less than 5 cm and the patient has dysphagia, a myotomy relieves the symptoms, often permitting the diverticulum to become smaller or even disappear without resection (72) (Fig. 224). In larger diverticula, a one-stage diverticulectomy has become the operation of choice.

In instances of hypertrophy of the cricopharyngeus muscle with dysphagia, a myotomy cuts not only through the transverse fibers of the cricopharyngeus muscles but also through the sphincter muscles. Such a procedure produces a considerable drop in the sphincter pressure.

HELLER OPERATION The Heller operation, which has been used for the surgical relief of achalasia unresponsive to bouginage or dilatation by a balloon, is a myotomy of the musculature of the lower sphincter, with extension slightly below the level of the gastroesophageal junction. This operation currently is the procedure of choice, particularly in children with achalasia, in preference to bouginage or hydrostatic dilatation.

Myotomy of the upper sphincter is performed following extensive resections of the hypopharynx in order to prevent the dysphagia that usually results from the persistent spasm of this sphincter after such resections. Extensive myotomy of the greater portion of the lower end of the esophagus is also used to relieve the hypertrophy secondary to diffuse spasm of the lower third of the esophagus.

The radiologic appearance of the sphincters following myotomy usually is one of improved motility and relief of the antecedent obstructive findings observed with the barium esophagogram. In achalasia, the esophagus is smaller in size and the dilatation is less marked than before myotomy. The atonia usually persists, however, in spite of the relief of the dysphagia (Figs. 225 and 226). The aftereffects of myotomy of the lower end of the esophagus may be radiologically confused with other operative procedures, e.g., fundoplication.

BOUGINAGE Bouginage is usually the initial form of treatment

(A)

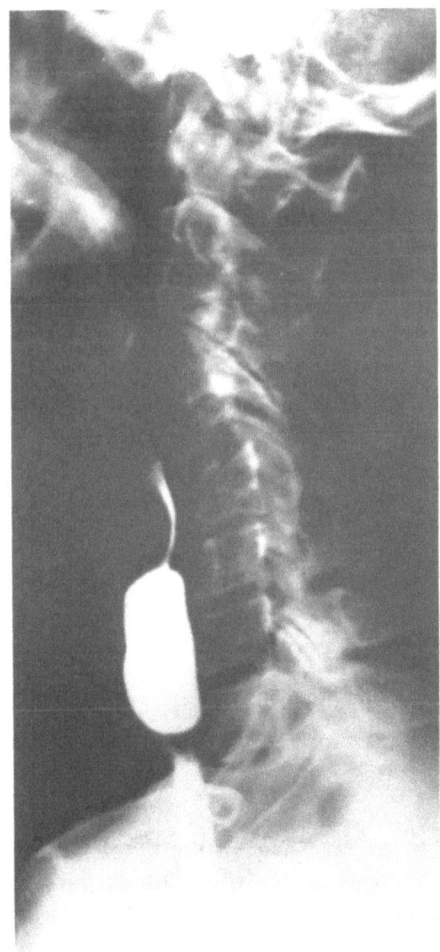

FIGURE 224
Myotomy. (A) Preoperative, Zenker diverticulum; (B) following myotomy.

(B)

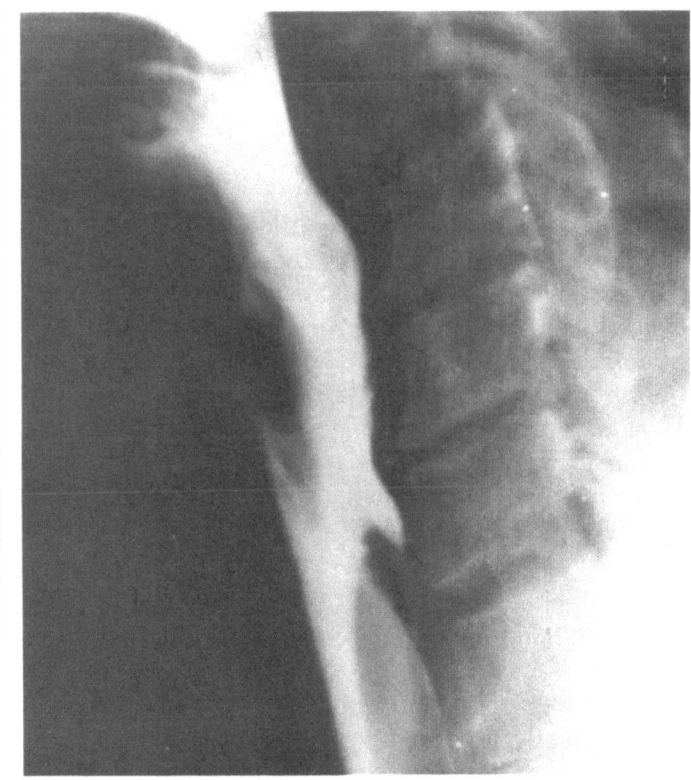

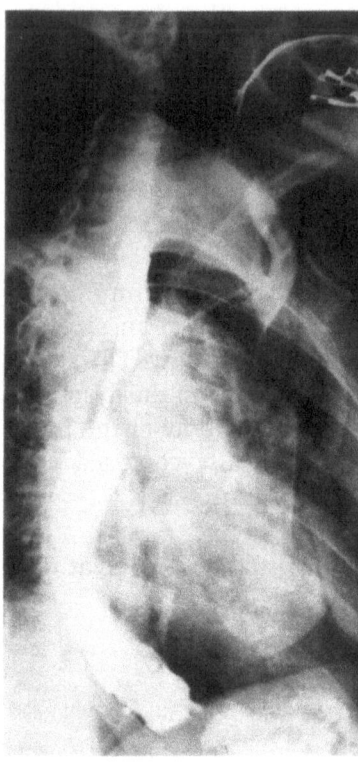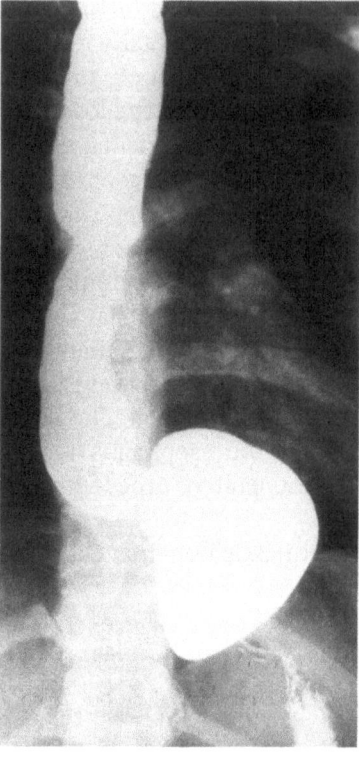

FIGURE 225
Heller operation for advanced
achalasia (postoperative results).

FIGURE 226
Postoperative diverticulum
following Heller operation for
advanced achalasia.

FIG. 225   **FIG. 226**

in strictures of the lower end of the esophagus. This procedure
is facilitated by fluoroscopic monitoring, in marked preference
to "blind" dilatations and positioning of dilators.

Pneumatic dilatation

Pneumatic dilatation is used in the treatment of webs, rings,
and early cases of achalasia in order to relieve dysphagia (210).
On radiologic examination following dilatation, the webs and
rings (including Schatski's ring) can be eradicated. In this
examination, the pneumatic dilator is positioned under
fluoroscopic control and then inflated with air to a pressure of
15 pounds per square inch. Following deflation, the process is
repeated (Fig. 227). In achalasia pneumatic dilatation of the
lower end of the esophagus appears to be the initial treatment
of choice (Fig. 228).

Congenital atresia and tracheoesophageal fistulae

Radiologic examination following the surgical treatment of
congenital atresia, with or without tracheoesophageal fistulae,
is essential in order to evaluate the results of the various

**Radiologic Changes
following surgery of
benign lesions**

FIGURE 227
Pneumatic dilation with a Mosher bag in achalasia.

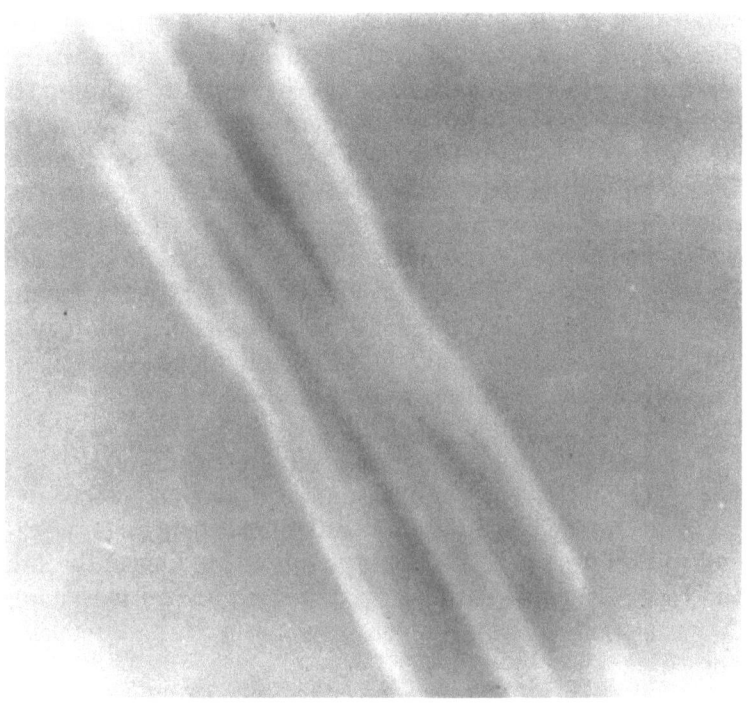

FIGURE 228
Hydrostatic dilatation, lower end of esophagus, for achalasia. Followup films (A) original film (B) 7 years after dilitation, (C) 19 years after dilitation. From Olsen, A. M., et al. Esophageal motality in achalasia (cardio spasm) after treatment. J. Thoracic Cardiovascular Surg., 34:615, 1957. C. V. Mosby Co., St. Louis, Mo.

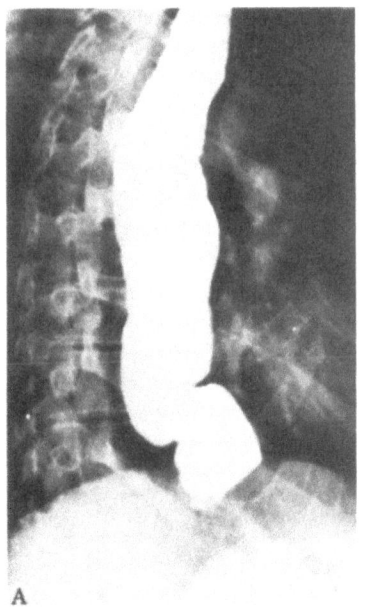
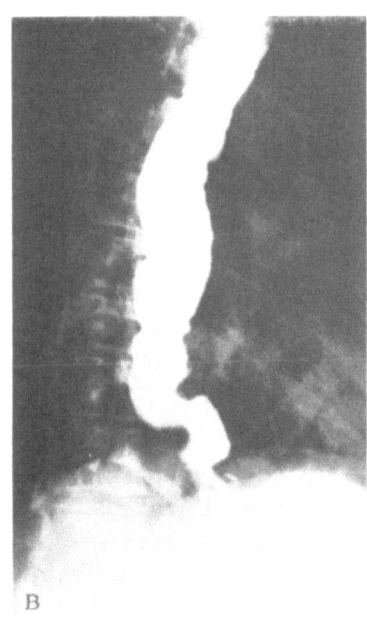
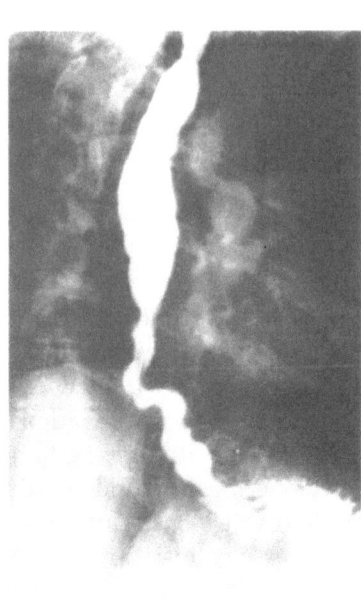

A

B

C

surgical procedures. The radiologic study is usually performed several days after operation with the ingestion of a thin barium mixture. Evidence of leakage of the opaque medium is searched for carefully. An area of narrowing or a defect at the site of the surgical procedure and the manifestations of motor dysfunction often are observed. However, these abnormalities usually return to normal as healing occurs. Localized leaks reflected in opacified fistulous tracts may extend to the pleura or skin. Such postoperative fistulae are usually associated with superimposed infection and local fibrosis. Frequent acute pulmonary infection and choking episodes following esophageal surgery should raise the suspicion of recurrent fistula. These tracts usually heal spontaneously when the patient's nutrition is maintained with a temporary feeding gastrotomy. A stricture occasionally may result from the surgical procedure, leaving permanent anatomic and functional changes. Serial radiologic studies reveal a variable picture depending on the site and type of surgery. Although postoperative fistulae are rare, they can occur months after surgery and necessitate reoperation.

After surgical repair of esophageal atresia, peristalsis abnormalities may persist for years. The primary wave often will stop at the site of the operative anastomosis, permitting food to collect. This temporary stasis will eventually be cleared by strong esophageal contractions. Foreign bodies may impinge above a residual area of stenosis at the site of the surgical repair (see Fig. 96 in Chapter 4). Aspiration may occur, resulting in recurring pulmonary infections.

Esophageal cysts or duplications

Surgical treatment of esophageal cysts or duplications is simple excision. The esophagus should return to normal radiologically relatively quickly after such a procedure.

Strictures

Surgical intervention for acquired lesions most commonly deals with the treatment of strictures. In children, extremely long strictures are treated in much the same fashion as congenital atresia. Bypass operations with colonic interposition (151) are often effective (151). In adults, the procedure used varies with the location and length of the stenotic esophageal segment. Bypass operations are highly successful here, also. The transverse colon is preferred in such procedures because of its mobility, length, viable blood supply, and resistance to gastric secretion (Fig. 229). The colon is used in an isoperistaltic configuration, placed through the anterior mediastinum or in an

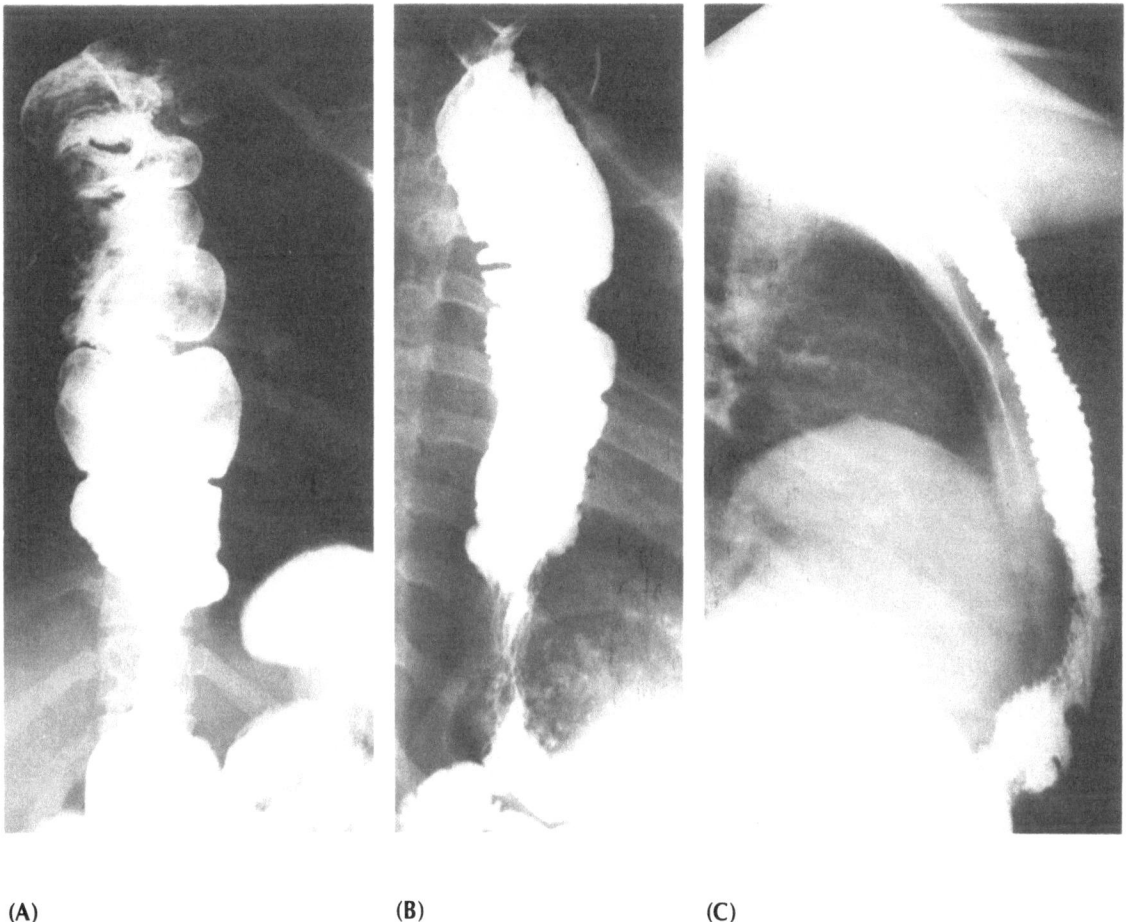

(A)   (B)   (C)

FIGURE 229

Colon bypass operation. (A, B, and C) Different views of same patient.

extrathoracic subcutaneous position. The ascending colon or other portions of the mobile large bowel also may be used in such procedures (105). Swallowing does not seem to be impaired by such operations (171).

Roentgenologic studies after such bypass procedures show absent peristalsis throughout the colonic segment, which serves only as a conduit. Gravity plays an important role in the passage of ingested food. Leakage, abnormal angulation, compression, or obstruction occasionally may occur. The development of a diverticulitis and other pathologic processes in the transplanted colonic segment also has been reported.

FUNDUS FLAP OPERATION The fundus flap operation (Thal) is a procedure used to repair lower esophageal strictures accompanied by peptic esophagitis and esophagogastric reflux. In this procedure, the lower esophageal wall is incised full thickness through the sphincter area in a longitudinal fashion. The incision is carried upward for 4 to 5 cm as well as to a point below the esophagogastric junction for approximately 2 cm. The longitudinal incision is triangulated with sutures at the esophagogastric junction and the fundus of the stomach is used to close the resulting triangular defect. The fundus of the stomach is then sutured over the defect, effecting a serosal patch to the newly widened esophageal lumen. This serves to dilate the lumen of the esophagus and produces a flap valve at the esophagogastric junction (176). Additional fundoplication is sometimes added to augment the prevention of esophagogastric reflux.

The barium swallow demonstrates the corrected esophageal lumen as well as an apparent "para esophageal hernia" (Fig. 230). This "paraesophageal hernia" represents the portion of gastric fundus that has been surgically brought into the thorax to be sutured into the linearly incised esophagus. No lumenal communication at the esophageal incision site and the serosal surface of the gastric fundus remains. A radiologic "clear space" can be demonstrated, representing the thickness of gastric wall serving to patch the newly widened esophageal lumen.

HEIMLICH'S PROCEDURE Another very successful operation is the design of a stomach tube constructed from the greater curvature of the stomach, as described by Heimlich (107). The procedure offers an excellent blood supply. The tube can be placed intrathoracically or subcutaneously anterior to the sternum (Figs. 231 and 232). The cervical anatomy is preserved at the upper esophageal sphincter so that normal swallowing is maintained. The esophagus may or may not be resected as part of the procedure.

OTHER PROCEDURES More difficult surgical problems deal with the relief of strictures of the lower esophageal segment, secondary to peptic esophagitis or following previous operations involving the lower sphincter (183). In this connection, many surgical procedures have been attempted. The treatment requires the correction of the underlying cause of gastric hyperacidity while the esophageal obstruction is relieved. In cases of esophageal hiatal hernia, the hernia is first reduced, following which a vagotomy is performed and a partial gastrectomy with a gastrojejunostomy is constructed. In cases with a short esophagus, paralysis of the left diaphragm is induced and the esophagogastric junction is reimplanted into the dome of the diaphragm. Radiologic examinations are important to evaluate the functional as well as the structural results of the surgical procedures. Cine studies are valuable after such procedures.

Mid-esophagus and epiphrenic diverticula

Mid-esophagus and epiphrenic diverticula require special and sometimes difficult surgical approaches, depending on the un-

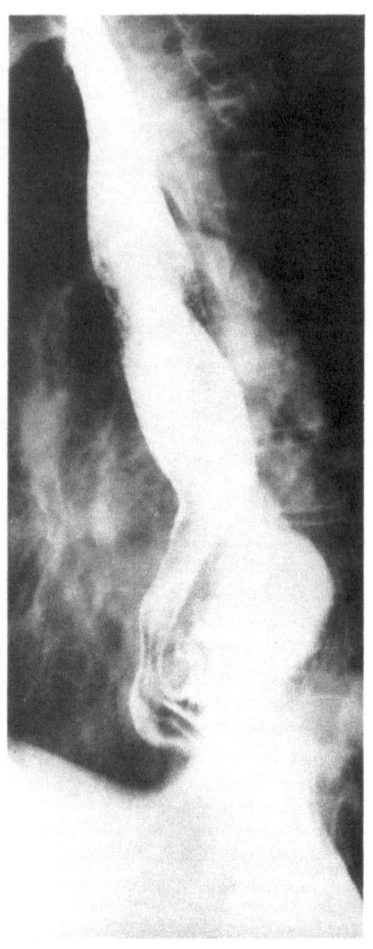

FIGURE 230
Thal procedure for the surgical treatment of a stricture in the lower end of the esophagus.

FIGURE 231
Heimlich's procedure. Stomach tube bypass for carcinoma of the upper third of the esophagus.

FIGURE 232
Heimlich's procedure. Stomach tube replacement of resected lower esophageal segment.

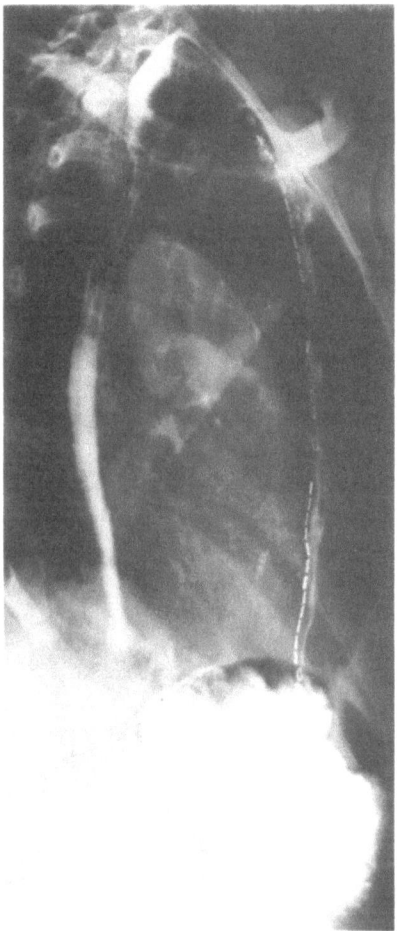
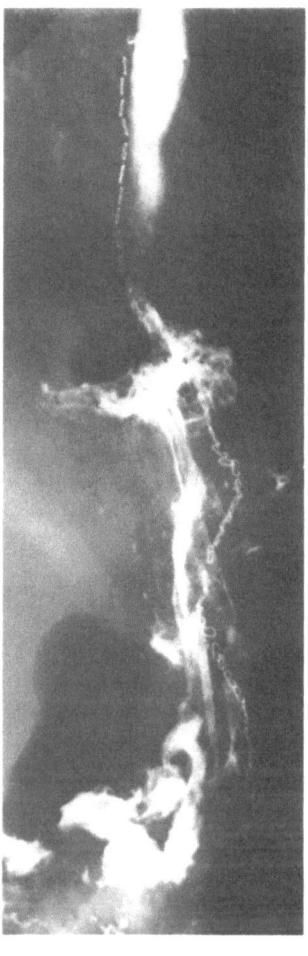

FIG. 231   FIG. 232

derlying causes. A transthoracic diverticulectomy or invagination of the diverticulum may be required following exploration and removal of surrounding adhesions. For epiphrenic diverticula a diverticulopexy or an esophagogastrostomy may be needed. Radiologic postoperative studies are mandatory to exclude surgical complications. Specifically, cine studies are important to evaluate the underlying motor abnormalities in determining the results of operative intervention.

The radiologic examination of the esophagus following the surgical removal of benign esophageal tumors usually reveals the reappearance of a normal esophagus.

The surgical treatment of malignant lesions is discussed in the section on malignant lesions. However, strictures and other complications can also result from surgical removal of a malignant lesion. In this connection, operations such as jejunal interposition (245) (Figs. 233 and 234), esophagogastrotomy (Fig. 235) and esophagojejunostomy (Fig. 236) are still being performed.

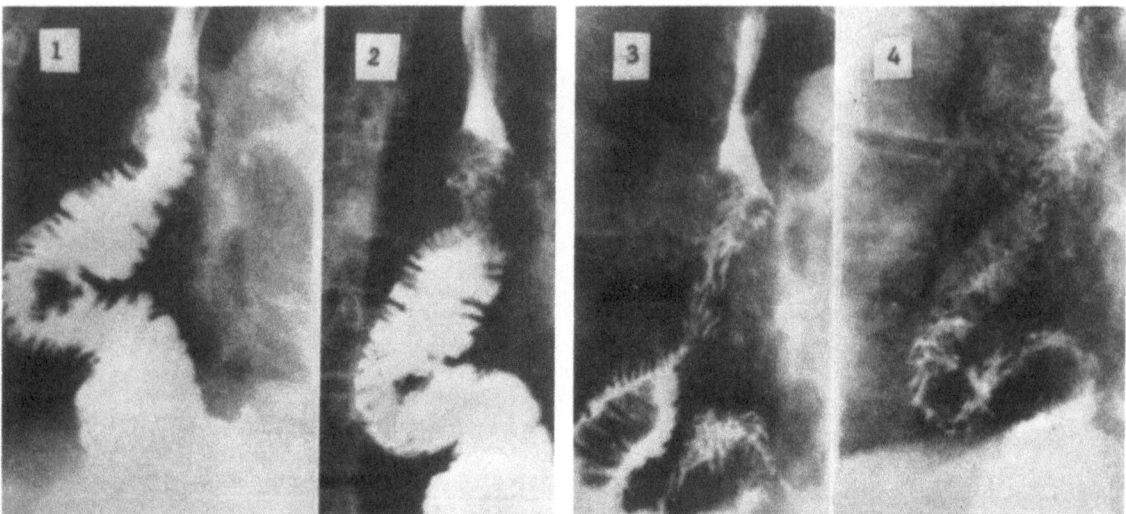

FIG. 233

FIG. 234

FIG. 235

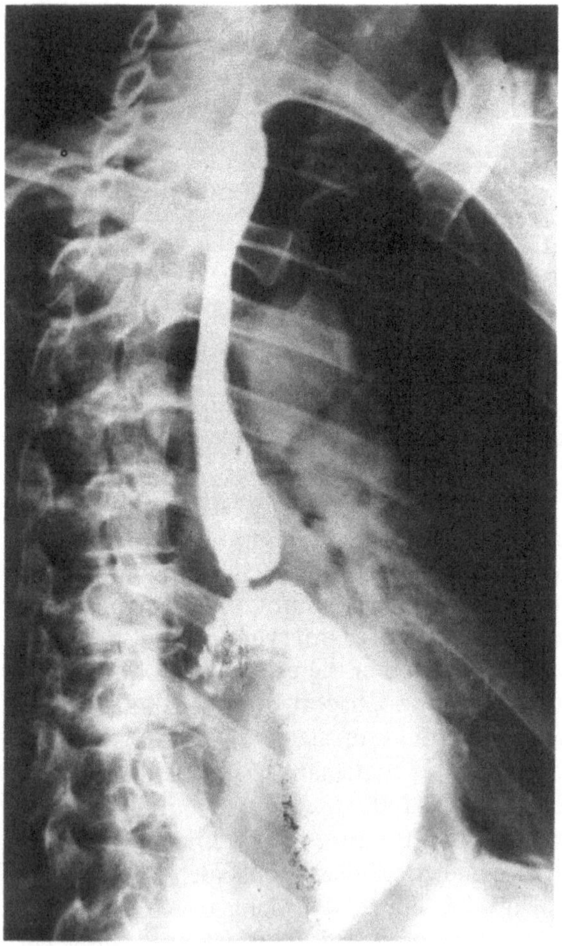

FIG. 236

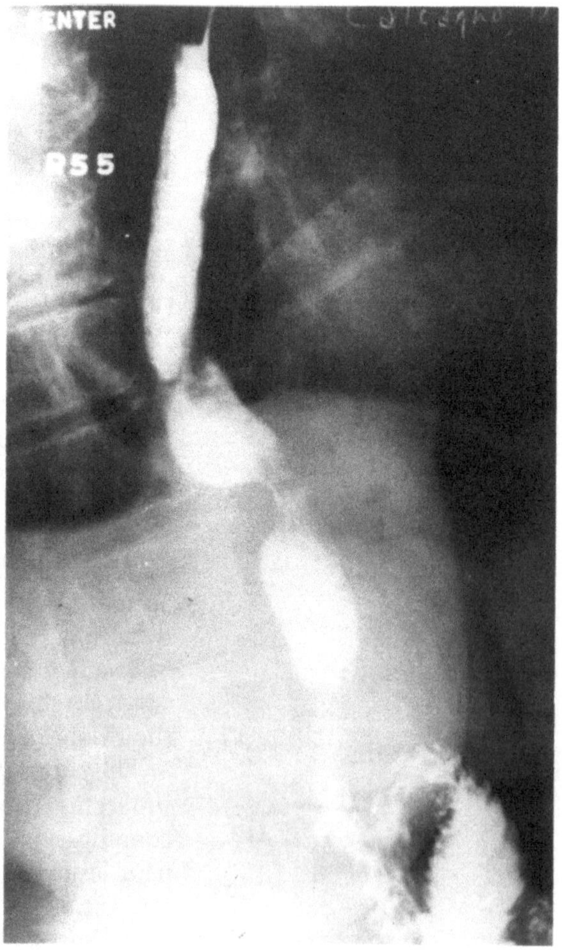

Radiologic changes following perforations

The surgical treatment of hypopharyngeal and esophageal perforations depends on the site and extent of extraesophageal involvement. The higher the level of perforation, the simpler the treatment becomes.

Hypopharynx

In the hypopharyngeal area, cellulitis followed by a localized abscess usually requires only surgical drainage. On radiologic examination, a pharyngeal abscess produces a temporary straightening of the normal cervical lordosis, which returns to normal with resolution of the abscess. Postsurgical radiologic evaluation, therefore, generally demonstrates the efficacy of treatment.

Esophagus

Perforation of the esophagus may produce a localized mass, widespread mediastinitis, pyothorax (pleural cavity), purulent pericarditis and even seepage into the upper abdomen with abscess formation. Other complications secondary to esophageal perforation include pneumothorax, pneumoperitoneum, and subcutaneous and/or mediastinal emphysema. Surgical intervention in such instances is obviously necessary.

Spontaneous rupture of the esophagus is a more serious condition. The esophagus usually ruptures in the lower left lateral wall above the level of the sphincter zone. Rupture may also occur above the level of a hiatal hernia (Fig. 237) or diverticulum (Fig. 238). A pleural effusion usually develops as well as mediastinitis. When pleural contamination is present, serious complications follow. Esophageal obstruction may also be present when the rupture is secondary to a neoplasm. If a fistulous tract or extravasation of the barium is noted following a barium swallow, immediate surgery is indicated. A jejunostomy or gastrostomy may be necessary for nutritional reasons. When obstruction, whatever the cause, or hiatal hernia is also present, such abnormalities are corrected in addition to the existing esophageal tear. In weakened or toxic patients, only a local drainage is carried out (24). Perforations may also follow any surgical procedure (Fig. 239). Postsurgical roentgenologic studies are again used to follow the progress of leaking and the state of surgical repair.

Permanent lung changes can result, following rupture or tear of the esophagus. In an unusual case, orally ingested barium was observed to fill a large pulmonary cavity in addition to opacifying the lower end of the esophagus and stomach. Clinical manifestations were related to a period several weeks before the radiologic studies, when the esophagus apparently

FIGURE 233
Jejunal interposition. Dilated jejunal segment.

FIGURE 234
Jejunal interposition. Jejunal mucosal pattern. Reprinted from Thomas, G. I., and Merendino, K. E. Jujunal interposition operation, analysis of thirty-three clinical cases. Jama, 168:(73), 176, 1958. Copyright 1958, American Medical Association.

FIGURE 235
Esophagogastrostomy following removal of an adenocarcinoma of lower esophagus.

FIGURE 236
Esophagojejunostomy following removal of an adenocarcinoma of the lower esophagus.

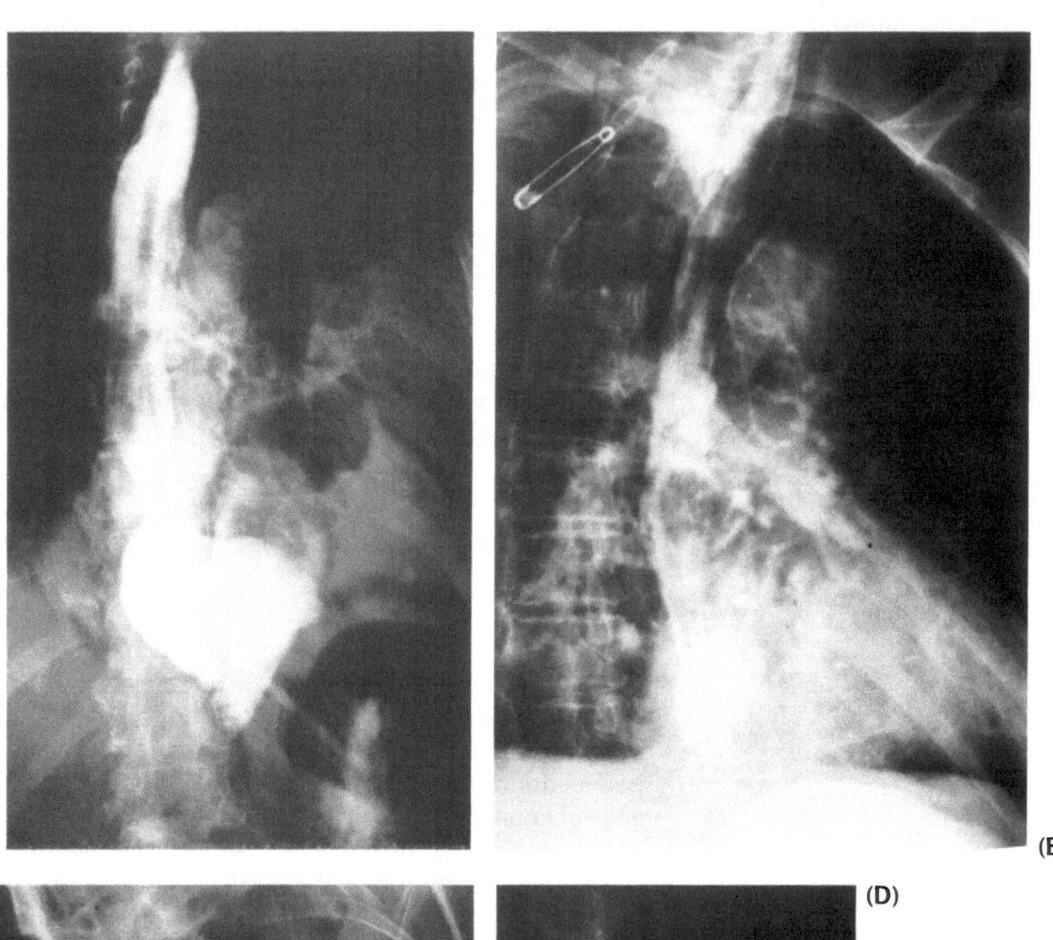

FIG. 237(A)

(B)

(C)

(D)

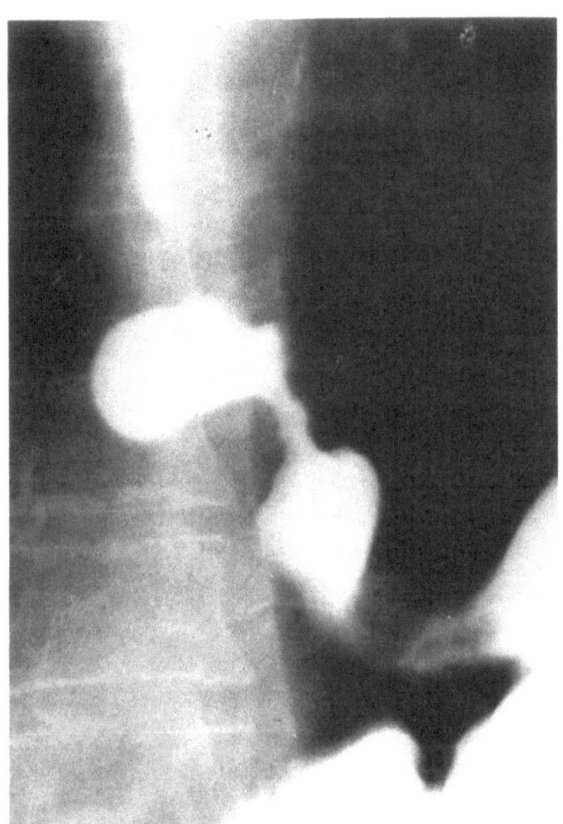

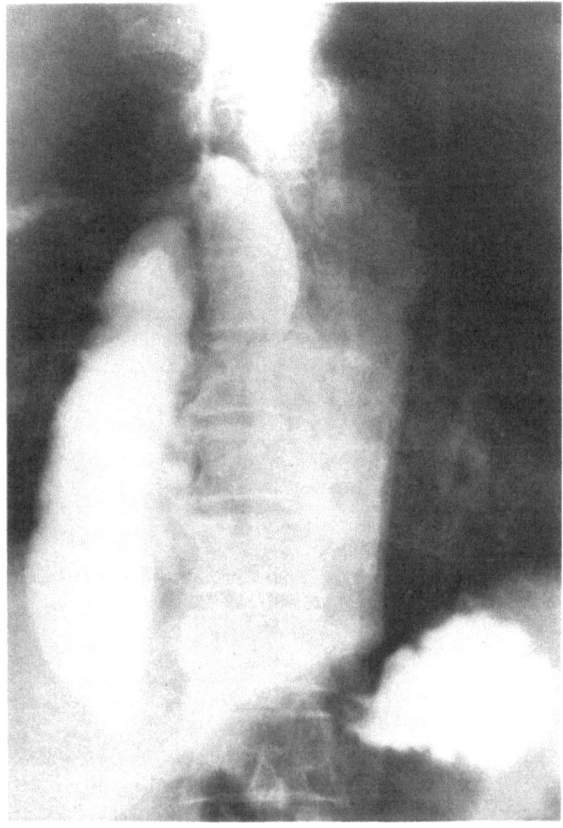

FIG. 238(A)

(C)

(B)

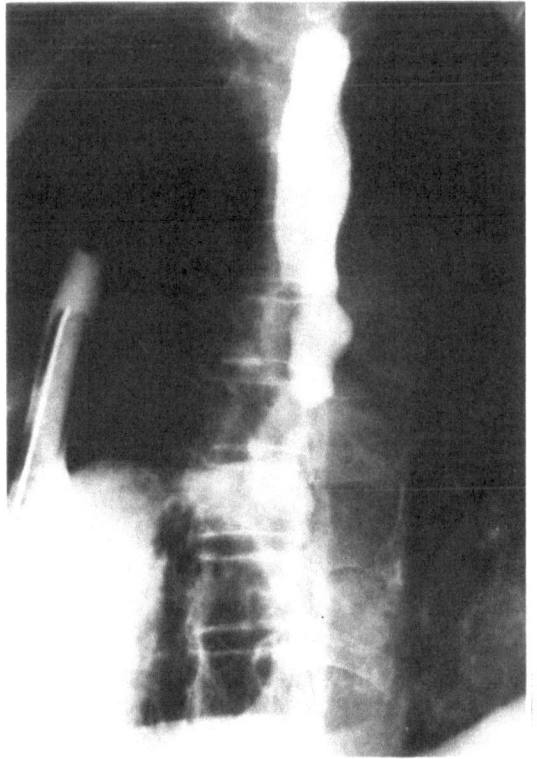

FIGURE 237
Spontaneous rupture of the esophagus in the presence of a hiatal hernia. (A) Immediate films following rupture showing the hiatal hernia, (B) first postoperative film (C) subsequent postoperative film showing pseudodiverticulum, at site of perforation, (D) final film, after recovery from surgery.

FIGURE 238
Spontaneous rupture of the esophagus above the level of a diverticulum. (A) Before rupture, (B) at time of rupture, (C) following surgical repair.

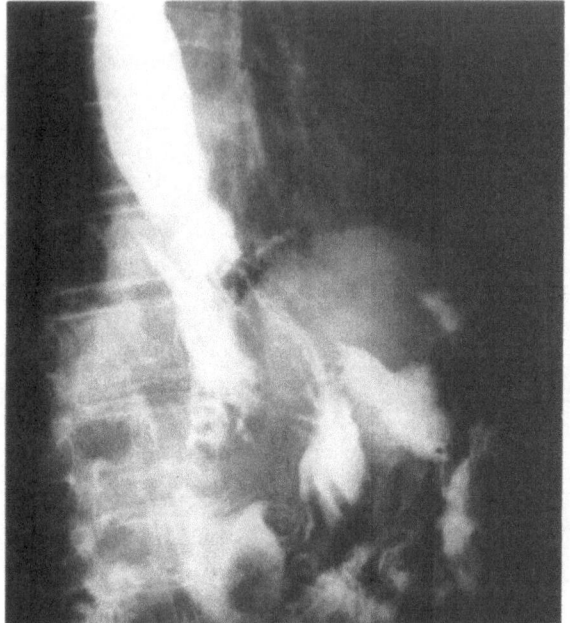

(A)

FIGURE 239
Postoperative fistulae at site of esophagogastric
anastomosis following partial gastric resection for
carcinoma. (A and B) Different levels.

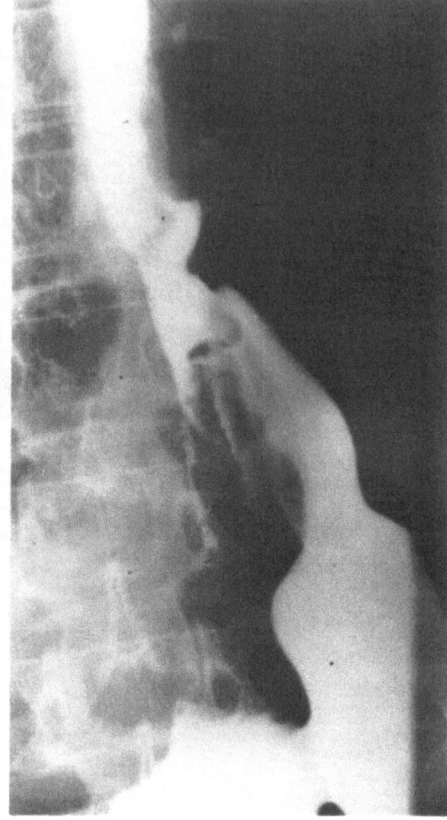

(B)

ruptured spontaneously above the level of a large hiatal hernia.
The patient refused surgery (Fig. 240).

The type of repair of a tracheoesophageal fistula depends on
the cause. Ordinarily, a retropleural approach is preferred to a
transpleural repair. Radiologic examination following operation is essential to insure that no additional leak at the site of
the repair exists.

Vagotomy

The purpose of such an operation, which is performed mainly
in those individuals with chronic duodenal ulcer, is to reduce
gastric acidity. However, vagotomy is not an operation to be
considered lightly because of possible complications, including
esophageal motor changes. The variable anatomic distribution
of the right and left gastric branches of the vagus nerve, and
even occasionally the presence of a plexus of nerves, makes
operative denervation difficult regardless of the surgical approach (transabdominal, transthoracic). However, in order to
achieve satisfactory clinical results, all branches of the vagus
nerve reaching the stomach must be severed (25). Usually,

**Radiologic changes
following vagotomy and the
Zollinger–Ellison syndrome**

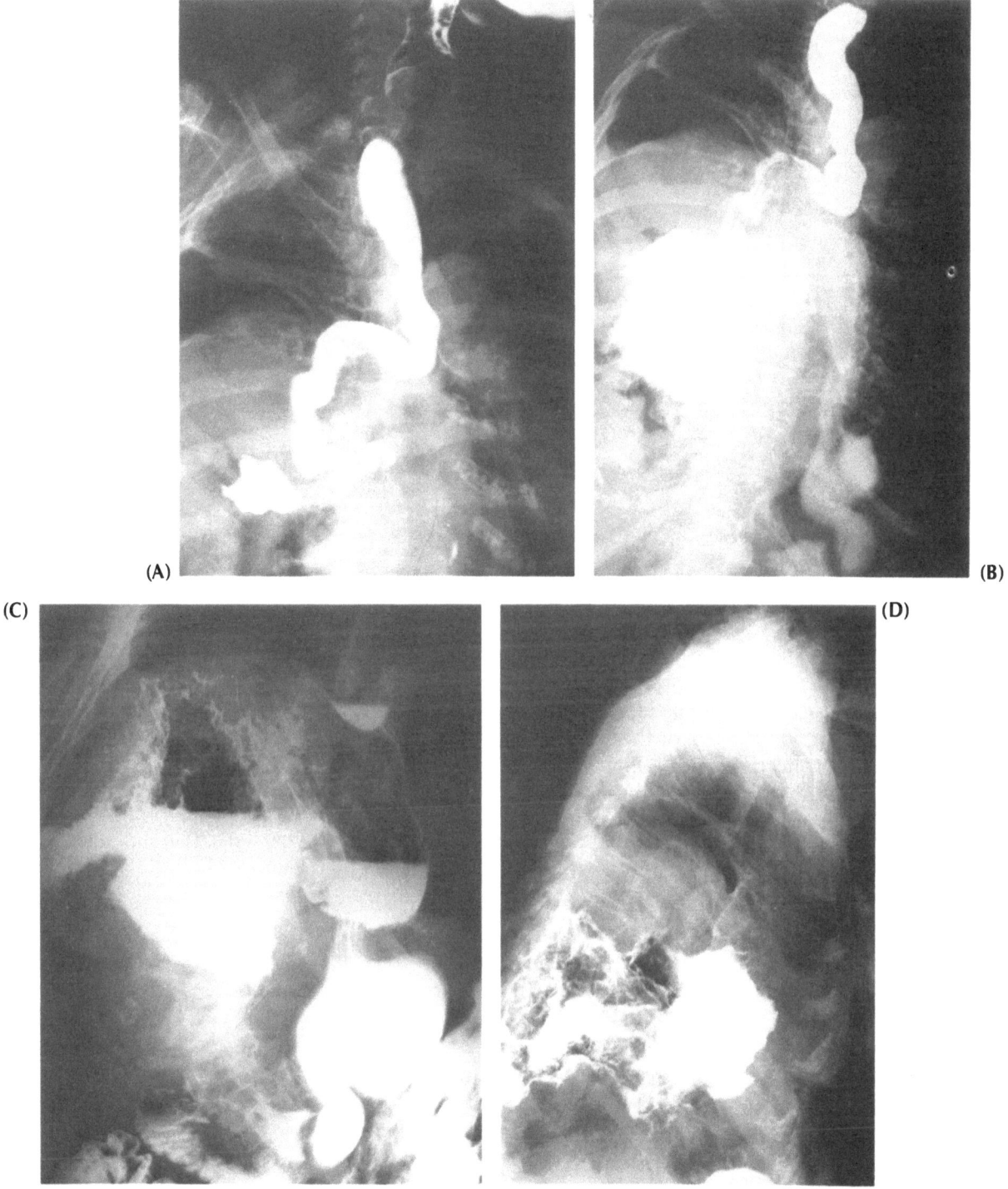

FIGURE 240

Neglected spontaneous rupture of the esophagus in the presence of a large hiatal hernia. (A and B) Barium filling a chest cavity during barium swallow. (C) Upright film also showing filling of lower end of esophagus and stomach. (D) Lateral view of the chest cavity filled with barium.

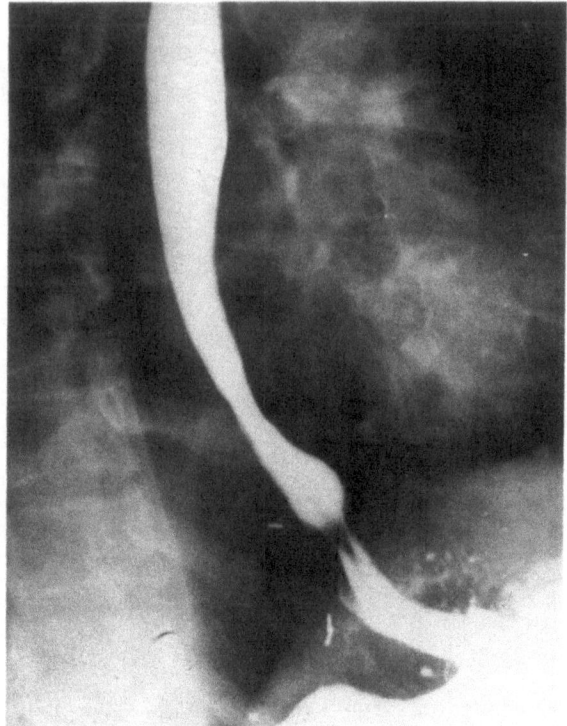

(A)

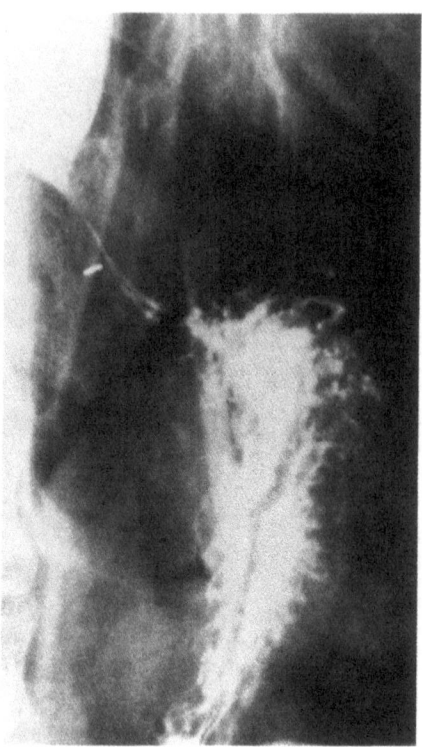

(B)

FIGURE 241
Vagotomy in two patients. (A) Metal clips at site of surgery; (B) complicating hematoma following a vagotomy. From Rabiah, A. F., and Elliot, H. B. Intramural hematoma of the esophagus. Am. J. Dig. Dis., *13*:925, 1968. Harper & Row, Publishers.

metal clips that can readily be identified on radiologic examination are placed at the site of the severed nerves (Fig. 241A).

Various complications may follow a surgical vagotomy (84). Operative injury can produce perforation of the esophagus, hemorrhage, or occasionally an intramural esophageal hematoma. Robiah (193) has reported the radiologic findings in a patient which suggested a transient achalasia with obstruction, except that the contracted distal end of the esophagus appeared longer than in a true achalasia (Fig. 241B).

Ordinarily, no changes in the functioning of the lower sphincter occur, although the alterations in the circulatory levels of gastrin and gastric pH often affect its tone. As a result, chronic spasm of the sphincter may occur, with resultant radiologic findings appearing reminiscent of achalasia and requiring dilatations for treatment. Distinct motor changes immediately following vagotomy, especially noted on cine, may be observed. These include loss of esophageal muscle tone and diminished motility, usually transient. Gastroesophageal reflux and even subsequent development of hiatal hernia are late complications if the phrenoesophageal membrane has been compromised. When reflux is present and the vagotomy has been insufficient to reduce the gastric acidity, esophagitis, luminal cicatricial changes, and actual strictures may develop. The administration of cholinergic drugs to patients after vagotomy and antrectomy raises the pressure in the lower sphincter area, thus preventing reflux (111).

Zollinger–Ellison syndrome

Before any surgical procedure involving the lower esophageal sphincter is contemplated, the Zollinger–Ellison syndrome, the result of an islet cell tumor of the pancreas, must be excluded. In this syndrome, which includes the presence of marked gastric hyperacidity and peptic ulcerations of the stomach and duodenum, the esophagus generally is not involved initially. An operation that compromises the function of the lower esophageal sphincter often results in severe esophagitis which is unresponsive to vagotomy and/or partial gastrectomy (58). Total gastrectomy is considered currently to be the treatment of choice.

Radiologic changes of the crippled laryngopharynx

The crippled laryngopharynx (49) results from trauma or operation for disorders of the tongue, mandible, pharynx, and larynx. Both the respiratory and swallowing mechanisms may be affected with their functions compromised as much as 50% of normal without serious impairment. Because the functions of respiration and swallowing usually are altered, compensatory factors come into play. These depend on the type of operation and the skill of the surgeon in preserving and/or repairing the important muscular attachments and nerve structures. The degrees of functional and structural impairment are best studied by the detailed analysis of cine films or tapes during and following a barium swallow.

Radiologic changes following surgery of malignant lesions

Oropharynx

Some lesions of the oropharynx are treated by radical resection (48). As a result, because of the compromise of the neurogenic pathways, interference with the normal functioning of the pharyngoesophageal sphincter produces failure of relaxation and spasm. The spasm may be severe enough to produce dysphagia, on occasion requiring a myotomy. As a consequence, some surgeons routinely include myotomy as a part of the operative procedure.

Larynx

Following radical resection of a lesion in the hypopharynx or cervical esophagus a laryngectomy usually is performed. Reconstruction of this area has been attempted, using a penile

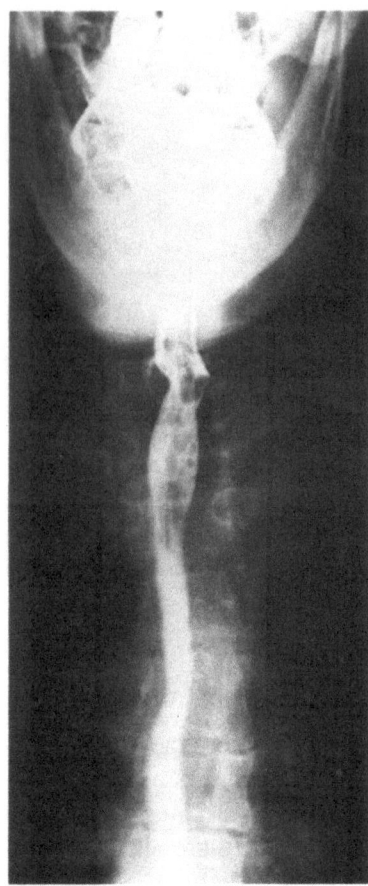 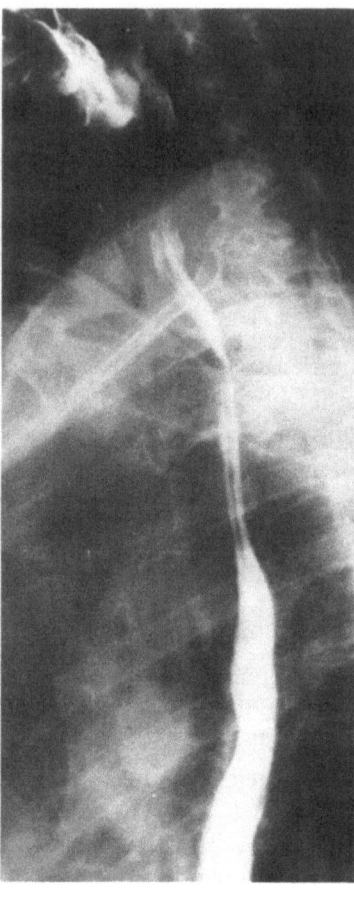

FIGURE 242
Total laryngectomy. (A) Frontal view, (B) oblique view of esophagus.

(A)   (B)

skin graft (216), other types of skin grafts, and plastic tubes, with some success.

Following *total laryngectomy* for a lesion not involving the posterior pharyngeal wall, with the sphincter zone preserved, a proper repair is essential for a normal swallowing function as well as for the future development of alaryngeal speech (Fig. 242). Radiologic studies following laryngectomy are to evaluate the speech mechanism and help with corrective measures. As an example, various types of phonation produce different degrees of distension of the pharyngoesophageal segment. The effects of mechanical muscular assistance can also be studied (129).

A negative pressure exists normally in the esophagus and a positive pressure is observed in the oropharynx. Muscle action can be a controlling factor in overcoming the upper sphincter zone pressure, permitting varying amounts of air to be ingested in the esophagus, thus affecting the laryngeal speech. It has also been determined that when the residual sphincter zone pressure is elevated sufficient air swallowing needed for laryngeal speech can be prevented. Therefore, the sphincter zone repair should not be too tight. The sphincter zone seg-

FIGURE 243

The Pharyngoesophageal spincter following a total laryngectomy during esophageal speech. (A) At beginning of speech, (B) at end of speech. Reprinted from Pancoast, H. K., Pendergrass, P. E., and Shaeffer, J. P. The Head and Neck in Roentgen Diagnosis, p. 863. Charles C. Thomas publisher, New York, 1940. (Arrow shows soft tissue density representing the contracted sphincter.

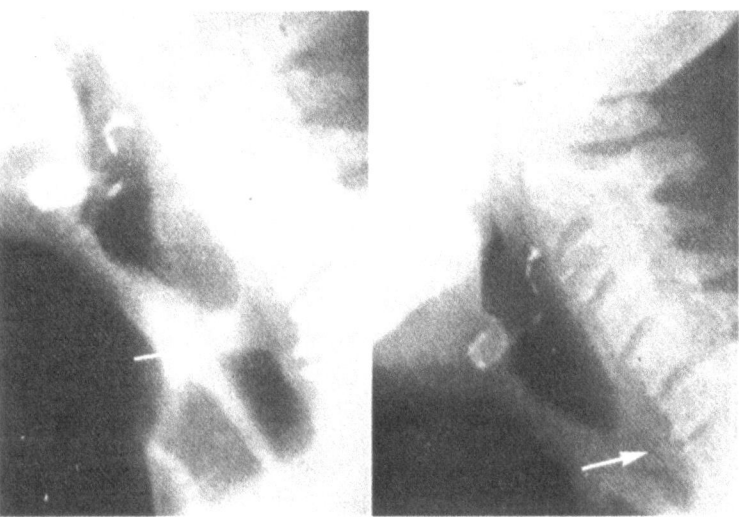

ment is observed on radiologic examination as a contracted soft tissue density between the hypopharynx and cervical esophagus (Fig. 243).

The pressure of a tracheotomy tube acts as an irritant and may be responsible for spasm of the pharyngoesophageal sphincter. In Figure 244, the tracheotomy was performed because of respiratory distress, associated with neoplasm of the epiglottis. Spasm of the sphincter is noted.

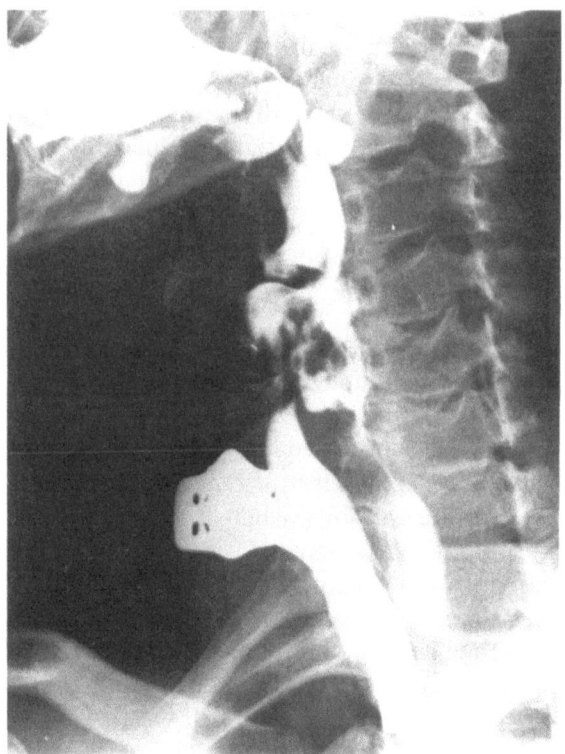

FIGURE 244

Tracheotomy tube in position in the presence of a malignancy of epiglottis.

Esophagus

RADICAL EXCISION Primary and secondary malignant lesions of the cervical esophagus may warrant radical surgical excision, particularly in the early stages (223). Partial esophagostomy, total laryngectomy, thyroid lobotomy, and neck dissection of lymph nodes all may be necessary. Palliative treatment is usually confined to bypass operations, such as esophagogastrostomy or retrosternal, extrapleural esophagojejunostomy. Radiation therapy generally is the treatment of choice, particularly with advanced neoplasms (see section on radiation therapy). Operation is attempted only when adequate removal of the entire lesion is possible.

Surgical cures of malignant neoplasm of the lower two-thirds of the esophagus are uncommon. Esophagogastrostomy seldom produces satisfactory results. Most neoplasms in this area, when detected, already involve surrounding structures. A number of palliative measures exist for nonresectable lesions that are causing obstruction.

PALLIATIVE OPERATIONS Palliative operations are used to bypass inoperable malignancies without resorting to esophageal resection, as previously described in the surgical treatment of strictures. Segmental replacement by a plastic tube has been tried. Holes at each end of the plastic tube are used to secure the prosthesis in place. A fibrotic sheath eventually develops around the tube, occasionally permitting removal of the tube after several months. However, recurrences of the tumor, leaks, perforations, and necrosis may also result, all demonstrable on radiologic examination.

INTUBATION Intubation has been used to maintain patency in an obstructing lesion (19) (Fig. 245). Originally, plastic tubes were pushed through the area of obstruction from above. Perforations, however, were a common complication. Later, push and pull methods via a gastrotomy were used more successfully in placing the tube. The size and patency of the tube were also found to be important, because soft tubes collapsed as the pressure of the growing tumor increased. Adaptability to varying length and size, with simple insertion and retention of the tubes, is important in the choice of tubes and in the methods that have been developed by Macker, Soutler, Moussen-Barden, Haering, and Celestin. Some tubes can be placed directly without gastrotomy, whereas others require both a laparotomy and esophagoscopy.

Intubations not requiring a laparotomy are of many types. A nylon tube prosthesis in the shape of a rigid screw can be inserted perorally over the bougie without previous dilatation. A metal rod is used to place the tube and is removed after the tube is in position. The length of the tube will vary with the

FIGURE 245
Intubation in the presence of a primary carcinoma of the esophagus.

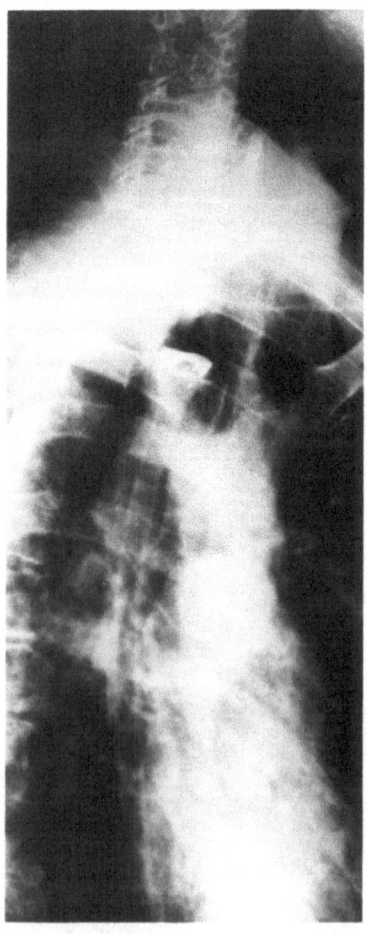

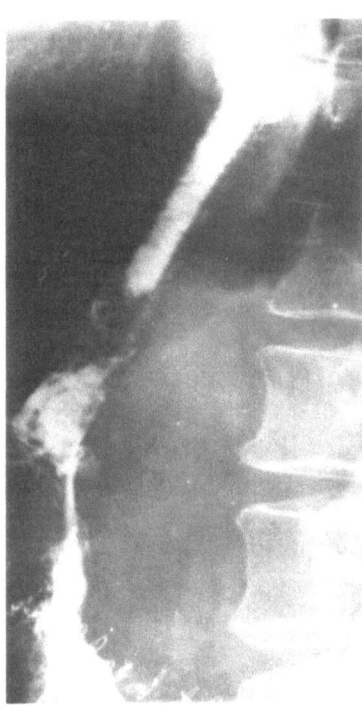

FIGURE 246
Machler tube in the lower end of esophagus in the presence of a carcinoma.

length of the tumor as observed on radiologic examination. A polyethelene tube can be slipped over a filiform bougie under direct endoscopic control and positioned across the site of the tumor. The lesion holds the tube in position via flanges at its proximal end and a beveled distal end. A Haering tube (142) made of latex reinforced with a stainless steel coil can also be inserted without a laporatomy by the use of a lumen finder and dilators. The Soutlar tube is made of gold-plated nickel wire embedded in a coil spring and has a special bougie and plunger for its placement. Dilatation with a bougie may be necessary before placement endoscopically (274).

Tubes requiring a laporatomy are more accurately and permanently fixed. A Mackler tube (51) has holes at its upper and lower ends for attachment of sutures used in its positioning. A special Tucker dilator requires traction from below via a gastrotomy. The tube is positioned accurately in the tumor area and then anchored in position after the dilator has been removed (Fig. 246).

A Moussen–Barden tube (19) is 100 cm long and 10–16 cm in diameter in its first 3 cm of length, tapering gradually. The upper end is funnel shaped. Traction is applied to the tube by its lower end via a gastrotomy until the upper end is positioned at the site of the lesion. The excess tubing is then cut from below, as needed.

The Celestin-type tube (240) was, at first, made of stiff polyethylene, of latex, or silastic coated with steel. More recently, a flexible latex and nylon tube with a radiopaque line in its shaft (207) has been employed. Under direct endoscopic direction, a pilot bougie is passed and grasped by the surgeon via a gastrotomy. The tube is pushed from above into the bougie and positioned from below. Excess length of the tube is resected and the tube is anchored high along the lesser curvature of the stomach.

These tubes are now used infrequently because they may loosen and be regurgitated from the esophagus or passed into the stomach. The upper or lower end can become obstructed by the growing tumor. Perforation may take place, resulting in a tracheal fistula with its associated complications.

Most of these tubes are opaque to insure visualization on radiologic examination in order to better determine their position and function.

Radiologic changes following surgery for esophageal varices

Following shunt operations, esophageal varices previously demonstrated on radiologic examination usually persist and become reduced in size (181). A fluctuating portal pressure is not unusual even after surgical decompression. This procedure affects the degree of engorgement of these varices, permitting varying degrees of visualization of the enlarged veins. Occasional spontaneous recurrences of esophageal varices can also occur in patients with cirrhosis of the liver following surgery.

In infants and children with bleeding esophageal varices, a shunt operation usually yields poor results. Here, intrathoracic replacement of the esophagus by the colon is a more successful operation (151). The level of the upper anastomosis is not necessarily connected to the cervical region. The radiologic appearance of this reconstruction has been previously described.

Thorocoplasty

Although thorocoplasty was performed frequently in the past to treat a unilateral chronic tubercular lesion, this operation today is done infrequently. The esophagus is seldom affected. Esophageal displacement, particularly, after thoracoplasty is encountered rarely.

Lobectomies

Lobectomies are usually employed to exterpate a small localized lesion. Depending on the site of the surgical procedure, displacement of the mediastinal structures, including the esophagus, may occur, often to the ipsilateral side of the operative procedure. A compensatory expansion of the remaining lung, however, may develop, reestablishing the generally normal midline position of the esophagus.

Pneumonectomy

Pneumonectomy usually produces a shift of mediastinal structures to the side of the removed lung. The esophagus is thus displaced laterally but interference of the normal swallowing function generally does not occur.

Thoracotomy

Thoracotomies for mediastinal surgical procedures, e.g., the repair of hiatal hernia, myotomy, or ruptured esophagus, may result in scarring, retraction, displacement, and abnormal angulation or obstruction of the esophagus. Postoperative changes must be differentiated from recurrence of the original lesion or postsurgical complications, such as involvement of the surrounding pleura, pericardium, or other nearby structures. Partially removed ribs will usually be the clue to previous operations on the chest.

Radiologic appearance of the esophagus following surgical procedures of the chest

Thoracocentesis

Thoracocentesis for the relief of pleural effusion permits the return of a displaced esophagus to its normal position, because massive effusion generally displaces the mediastinal structures to the contralateral side. Repeated thoracocentesse may produce complications, including pneumothorax, pleural adhesions, and loculation of fluid. All these complications can indirectly affect the position of the esophagus.

Cardiac and vascular surgery

Open-heart surgery, cardiac transplants, repair of thoracic aneurysms, and other cardiac and vascular surgical procedures may also produce some displacement and abnormal angulations of the esophagus.

RADIOLOGIC CHANGES FOLLOWING RADIOTHERAPY FOR NEOPLASMS

Radiation therapy is now used extensively both as an adjunct to operation or even as the definitive treatment in the therapeutic approach to esophageal tumors (202). The form and extent of therapy depend on the location, size, and degree of extension of the neoplasm. Determination of the extent of tumor growth requires an accurate radiologic evaluation.

In the treatment of malignant esophageal and hypopharyngeal lesions, radiation therapy often is preferred over surgical removal. (Fig. 247). With radiotherapy, fewer complications are likely to result, the patient is more comfortable, and the possibility of a more prolonged period of survival without significant disfigurement is greater.

In the oral cavity, evidence of bone involvement of the mandible excludes radiation therapy. In the orohypopharynx, lesions of the pyriform sinuses, the postcricoid area, and the posterior pharyngeal wall are less responsive to radiation therapy than laryngeal tumors except in the early stages. If radiation fails to cure or palliate, radical surgery may be possible. However, if radical surgery is first attempted, then radiation treatments as a rule are less effective. Late-appearing radiation-induced carcinomas can occur. If both radiation and attempted surgical extirpation are contemplated, the radiation dose administered is usually less than when radiation therapy alone is used. Results of the radiation therapy may be evaluated by periodic radiologic studies, usually employing a barium swallow.

During the treatment of a malignant neoplasm of the esophagus by radiation, the effects may be followed by a barium swallow. Initially, inflammatory changes and edema are noted. At the end of the treatment, the primary lesion usually has di-

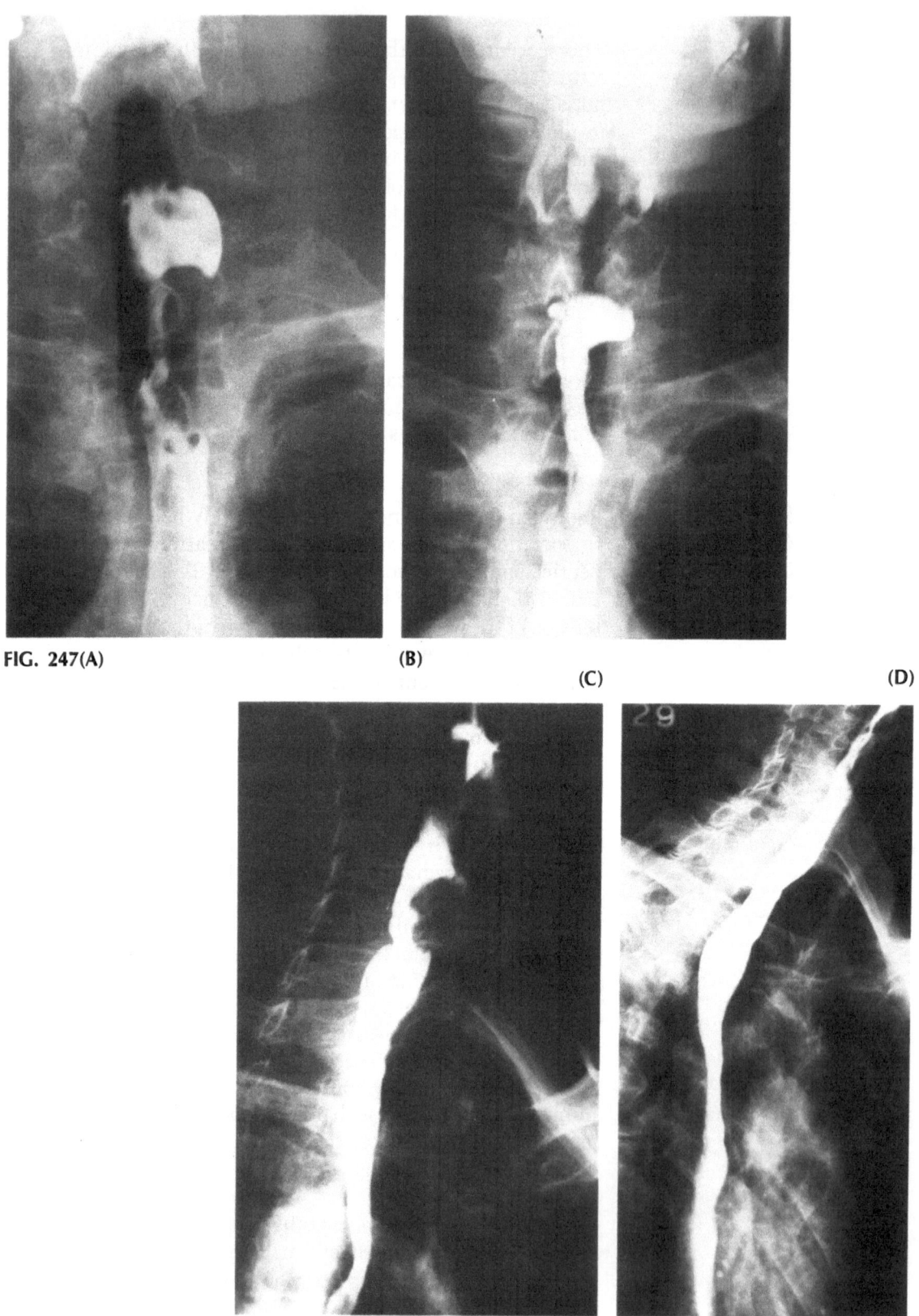

FIG. 247(A)   (B)

                                                        (C)   (D)

FIGURE 247
Radiation (cobalt) therapy.
Carcinoma of the cervical
esophagus in two separate patients.
(A and B) Pre- and postradiation
therapy; (C and D) Pre- and
postradiation therapy.

minished in size considerably, diminishing the dysphagia. Occasionally, as a sequela of radiotherapy, a stricture results. This complication can be treated with bouginage. A residual loss of the normal distensibility of the esophagus at the site of the treated tumor can persist for years after treatment.

Radiation injury to the esophagus secondary to the treatment of other mediastinal lesions is not uncommon. These injuries can be reversible if the esophagus previously has been normal. Radiologic examination during the peak period of therapy will show serrated esophageal projections associated with acute radiation-induced ulcerative esophagitis (Fig. 248). This change is followed by thickening of the esophageal wall caused by edema, resulting in reduced motility. Perforation may also occur at the site of the lesion (Fig. 249). Gradually, these findings resolve and within a period of 6 months, no abnormality may be detected on radiologic examination. If the radiation has been excessive fibrosis usually occurs, with the gradual formation of a stricture that can be confused with the reappearance of an infiltrating neoplasm.

Another complication of a radiation-damaged esophagus is the late appearance of a radiation-induced carcinoma. This occurrence is more common in the hypopharyngeal and cervical regions. The radiologic appearance of such a neoplasm is generally grossly similar to a malignancy arising *de novo.*

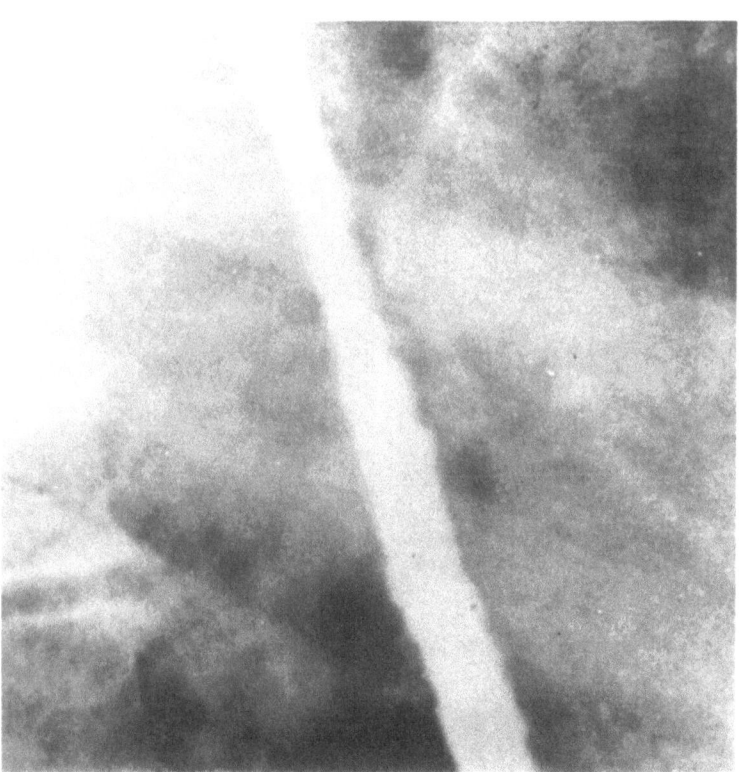

FIGURE 248
Acute radiation esophagitis. From
Seaman, W. B., and Ackerman, L. V.
The effect of radiation on the
esophagus. Radiology, *68*:535,
1957. Radiologic Society of North
America, Easton, Pa.

In a recent report following the use of supervoltage medistinal therapy (4,500 to 6,000 rads, 6 to 8 weeks), chiefly used for the treatment of bronchogenic carcinoma in which the esophagus initially was normal, increased functional changes in the esophagus were described. Following the acute phase of radiation damage, disturbed esophageal motility consisted of inpaired peristalsis, tertiary contractions, spasm of the lower esophageal sphincter, and delayed emptying of the esophagus.

(A)   (B)

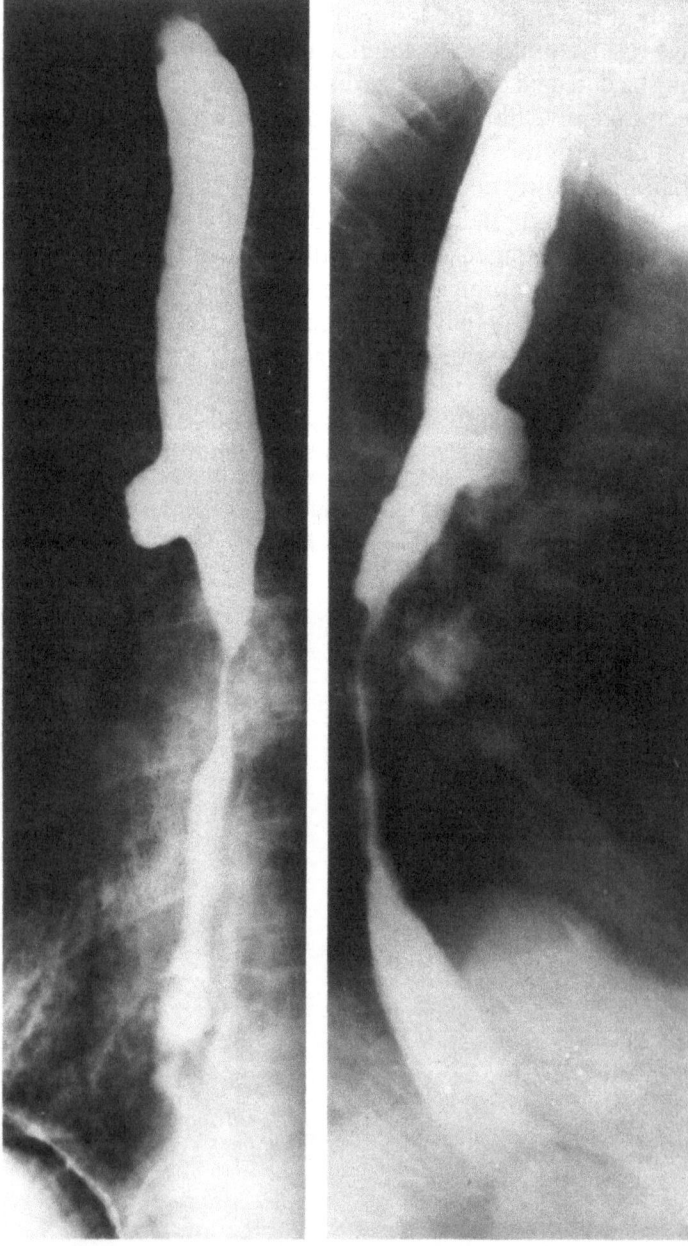

FIGURE 249
Radiation for bronchogenic carcinoma involving the esophagus. (A) Initial film, (B) Posttherapy film, showing presence of fistulous tract. A traction diverticulum in the upper esophagus is also present.

These changes may be responsible for some degree of dysphagia. However, in a more severely damaged esophagus an organic stricture may still eventually develop (98b).

CONCLUDING REMARKS

We have attempted to illustrate the importance of the barium swallow as a diagnostic procedure. Its value has been greatly enhanced by cineradiography, which is particularly helpful in the recognition of functional disturbances.

Based on recent anatomicoroentgen studies we have emphasized the radiographic appearance of the esophageal sphincters in order to illustrate their importance in evaluating abnormalities of the hypopharynx and esophagus.

REFERENCES

1. Adams, H. D. Amyenteric achalasia of esophagus. Surg. Gynecol. Ostet., *119:*251, 1964.

2. Adler, D. C., Haverback, J. B., and Meyers, H. I. Cineradiography of esophageal varices. JAMA *189*(2):77, 1964.

3. Albers, D. G. Branchial anomalies. JAMA, *183*(6):399, 1963.

4. Anderson, L. S., Shackelford, G. D., Mancilla-Jimenez, R., and McAllister, W. H. Cartilaginous esophageal ring: a cause of esophageal stenosis in infants and children. Radiology, *108*(3):665, 1973.

5. Antonio, J. M. T., Hunter, C. H., and Dobbins, W. O. Mallory-Weiss Syndrome. Am. J. Dfg. Dis., *15*(11):1043, 1970.

6. Ardran, G. M., and Kemp, F. H. The nasal and cervical airway in sleep in the neonatal period. Am. J. Roentgenol., *108:*3, 1970.

7. Arey, L. B. *Developmental anatomy.* Philadelphia, Saunders, 1926.

8. Babb, R. R., Peck, O. C., and Jamplis, R. W. Gastric volvulus and obstruction in paraesophageal hernia. Am. J. Dig. Dis., *117*(2):119, 1972.

9. Babka, J. C., and Castell, D. O. On the genesis of heartburn. Am. J. Dig. Dis., *16:*5, 1973.

10. Bao-Shan-Jing. Roentgen examination of larynx and hypopharynx. Rad. Clinic NA, *8*(3):361, 1970.

11. Baronofsky, I. D., Krell, I., Steinfeld, L., and Grishman, A. Vascular ring in infancy. N.Y. State J. Med., *60:*1246, 1960.

12. Bartels, J., and Mazzia, V. D. B. Familial dysautonomia. JAMA, *212*(2):318, 1970.

13. Beauchamp, J. M., Nice, C. M., Belanger, M. A., and Neitzschman, H. R. Esophageal intramural pseudodiverticulosis. Radiology, *113*(2):273, 1974.

14. Becker, M. H., and Swingard, C. A. Epidermolysis bullosa dystrophica in children. Radiology, *90:*124, 1968.

15. Beeler, R. C., Collins, J. N., and Hall, M. F. Benign pedunculated tumors of the esophagus. Am. J. Roentgenol., *60*(4):466, 1948.

16. Berenbaum, S., and Meyers, P. H. *Special procedures in roentgen diagnosis.* Springfield, Ill., Thomas, 1964.

17. Berenberg, W., and Neuhauser, E. B. D. Cardio esophageal relaxation (chalasia) as a cause of vomiting in children. Pediatrics, *5:*414, 1950.

18. Berdon, W. E., and Baker, D. H. Vascular anomalies and the infant lung. Sem. Roentgenol., *7*(1):39, 1972.

19. Berg, D. C., Jackson, B. A., Nanson, M. D., and Robinson, C. L. N. Intubation of obstructed esophagus. Surg. Gynecol. Obstet., *116:*705, 1963.

20. Bernstein, I. M., and Baker, I. A. A clinical test for esophagitis. Gastroenterology, *34:*760, 1958.

21. Berquest, T. H., Nolan, N. G., Stephens, D. H., and Carlson, H. C. Radioisotope scintinography in diagnosis of Barrett's esophagus. Am. J. Roentgenol., *123*(2):401, 1975.

22. Birnholz, J. C., Ferrucci, J. T., Jr., and Wyman, S. M. Roentgen features of dysphagia aortica. Radiology, *111*(1):93, 1974.

23. Bosma, J. F., Graykowski, E. A., and Tryostad, C. W. Chronic ulcerative pharyngitis. Arch. Otolaryngol., *87:*85, 1968.

24. Boyd, D. P., and Wittmann, C. J. Some principles in

treating perforation of esophagus. Surg. Clin. N.A., 51(3):567, 1971.

25. Bradley, W. F., Small, J. T., Wilson, J. W., and Walters, W. Anatomic considerations of gastric neurectomy. JAMA, 133(7):459, 1947.

26. Bragg, D., and Hussar, A. L. Cine-radiographic evaluation of the swallowing act in schizophrenic patients. XII International Congress of Radiology, Tokyo. 1969, Book of Abstracts, Paper 0417, 224.

27. Brean, H. P., and Neuhauser, E. B. D. Syndrome of aberrant right subclavian artery with patent ductus arteriosus. Am. J. Roentgenol., 58(6):708, 1947.

28. Brenner, S., Heimlich, H., and Widman, M. Carcinoid of esophagus. N.Y. State J. Med., 69:1337, 1969.

29. Brombart, M. Clinical radiology of the esophagus (translated by Sheila Kenny). Wright & Sons, Bristol, 1961.

30. Brown, J. W., and McKee, W. M. Acute monilial esophagitis occurring without underlying disease in a young male. Am. J. Dig. Dis., 17(1):85, 1972.

31. Brown, R. E., Madge, G. E., and Howell, T. R. Congenital short esophagus in the newborn. Am. J. Dig. Dis., 15(9):863, 1970.

32. Bruggeman, L. I., and Seaman, W. B. Epiphrenic diverticula. Am. J. Roentgenol., 119(2):266, 1973.

33. Brunton, F. J., and Eban, R. E. Sideropenic webs in men. Clin. Radiol., 11(1):65, 1960.

34. Buckstein, J. The digestive tract roentgenology, Vol. I. Philadelphia, Lippincott, 1953.

35. Buckstein, J., and Reich, S. Lateral pharyngeal diverticula as a cause of dysphagia. JAMA, 144:14, 1950.

36. Burnett, J. M., and St. John, E. Primary melanosarcoma of the esophagus. Radiology, 57:808, 1951.

37. Burns, W. A., Flores, P. A., Moshyedi, A., and Albacete, R. A. Clinical conditions associated with columnar lined esophagus. Am. J. Dig. Dis., 15(7):607, 1970.

38. Caffey, J. Pediatric x ray diagnosis. Chicago, Year Book Publ. Co., 1956.

39. Capetanio, M. A., and Kirkpatrick, J. A. Nasopharyngeal lymphoid tissue. Radiology, 96(2):389, 1970.

40. Caruso, R. D., and Berk, R. N. Lymphoma of the esophagus. Radiology, 95(2):381, 1970.

41. Chandrahasan, J. A. "Indian serpent eater" Cine film shown at XII International Congress of Radiology, Tokyo, 1969. Book of abstracts, page 543.

42. Chin, P., Lebowitz, R., and Lewicki, A. M. Spontaneous hematoma of the esophagus. Radiology, 100(2):281, 1971.

43. Chin, J. T. T., Lester, R. G., and Peter, R. N. Posterior wedging sign in mitral insufficiency. Radiology, 113(2):451, 1974.

44. Chittinaud, S., Patheja. S. S., and Wisenberg, M. J. Barium Nasopharyngography. Radiology, 98(2):387, 1971.

45. Christopher, N. L., and Watson, D. W. Relationship of chronic ulcerative esophagitis to ulcerative colitis. Ann. Inter. Med., 70:971, 1969.

46. Chung I Liu. Enhanced visualization of esophageal varices by Buscopan. Am. J. Roentgenol., 121(2):232, 1974.

47. Code, C. F., Schlegel, J. F., Kelley, M. L., Olsen, A. M., and Ellis, F. H. Hypertensive gastrointestinal sphincter. Proc. Staff meetings Mayo Clinic, 35:391, 1960.

48. Conley, J. J. One stage radical resection of cervical esophagus, larynx, pharynx and lateral neck. Arch. Otolaryngol., 58:645, 1953.

49. Conley, J. J., and Seaman, W. Function of the crippled laryngopharynx. Am. J. Otol. Rhinol. Laryngol., 72(2):441, 1963.

50. Cross, F. S. Esophageal diverticula related neuromuscular problems. Am. J. Otol. Rhinol. Laryngol., 77:914, 1968.

51. Culligan, J. A., Jensen, K., and Schmidt, R. W. Palliation in esophageal cancer. Abstr. Mod. Med.—Minnesota Med. J., 44:6, 1961.

52. Degradi, A. E., Broderick, J. T., Juler, G., Walinsky, S., and Stempien, S. J. The Mallory–Weiss syndrome and lesion. Am. J. Dig. Dis., 11(9):710, 1966.

53. Dalinka, M. K., Smith, E. H., Wolfe, R. D., Goldengerg, D., and Langdon, D. E. Pharmacologically enhanced visualization of esophageal varices by Pro-Banthine. Radiology, 102(2):283, 1972.

54. Darling, D. Hiatal hernia and gastroesophageal reflux in infants and children. Am. J. Roentgenol., 123(4):724, 1975.

55. Davenport. H. W. The first Walter Bradford Cannon lecture before the society of gastrointestinal radiologists. Am. J. Roentgenol., 119(2):235, 1973.

56. DeLorimer, A. A., and Warren, J. P. Prolapse of the mucosa of the esophagogastric junction. Am. J. Roentgenol., 84:1061, 1960.

57. Dockerty, M. D., Parkhill, E. M., Dahlin, D. C., Woolner, L. B., Soule, E. H., and Harrison, E. G. Tumors of the oral cavity and pharynx. Washington, D.C., Armed Forces Institute of Pathology, 1968.

58. Dodds, W. J., Dehn, T. G., Hogan, W. J., Worman, L. W., and Wilson, S. D. Severe peptic esophagitis in a patient with Zollinger-Ellison syndrome. Am. J. Roentgenol., 113(2):237, 1971.

59. Dodds, W. J., McGlaughlin, P. S., Goldberg, H. I., and Dehn, T. G. Esophageal roentgenography using Tantalum paste. Radiology, 102:204, 1972.

60. Donner, M. W. Swallowing mechanism and neuromuscular disorders. Sem. Roentgenol., 9(4):273, 1974.

61. Donner, M. W., and Siegel, C. I. The evaluation of pharyngeal neuromuscular disorders by cinefluorography. Am. J. Roentgenol., 94(2):299, 1965.

62. Donner, M. W., Silbiger, M. L., Hookman, P., and Hendrix, T. R. Acid-barium swallows in the radiographic evaluation of clinical esophagitis. Radiology, 87:220, 1966.

63. Doub, H. P. Mediastinal cysts of embryologic origin. J. Faculty Radiologists, 2:302, 1951.

64. Dotter, C. T., and Steinberg, I. "Angiocardiography. Annals of Roentgenology," Vol. XX. New York, Haeber, 1951.

65. Dreyfuss, J. R., and Willock, R. G. The elevator esophagus. Radiology, 75:914, 1960.

66. Dunbar, S. J. Upper respiratory tract obstruction in infants and children. Am. J. Roentgenol., *109*(2):227, 1970.

67. Durham. R. H. *Encyclopedia of medical syndromes.* New York, Hoeber, 1949.

68. Eckardt, V., Degradi, A. E., and Stempien, S. J. The esophagogastric (Schatzki) ring and reflux esophagitis. Am. J. Gastroenterol., *58*(5):525, 1972.

69. Eller, J. L., Ziter, F. M. H., Zuck, F. T., and Brott, W. Inflammatory polyp—a complication in esophagus lined by epithelium. Radiology, *98*(1):145, 1971.

70. Ellis, H. F. Upper esophageal sphincter in health and disease. Surg. Clin. N.A., *51*(3):553, 1971.

71. Ellis, H. F., Jr., and Olsen, M. A. Achalasia of the esophagus. Philadelphia, Saunders, 1969.

72. Ellis, H. F., Schlegel, J. F., Lynch, V. F., and Payne, S. W. Cricopharyngeal myotomy for pharyngoesophageal diverticulum. Ann. Surg., *170*:340, 1969.

73. Ennis, J. T., and Lewicki, A. M. Mecholyl esophagography. Am. J. Roentgenol., *119*(2):241, 1973.

74. Evans, W. "The course of the esophagus in health, and in disease of the heart and great vessels." Special report series No. 208. London, His Majesty's stationary office, 1936.

75. Everette, J., Montall, R., Chaffer, V., Streker, E. P., and Vesal, K. Barium or gastrografin which contrast media for diagnosis of esophageal tears. Gastroenterol., *68*:1163, 1975.

76a. Farman, J., Laster, W., Rose, J. S., and Faegenburg, D. Bronchogenic cysts involving the esophagus. N.Y. State J. Med., *76*(9):1507, 1976.

76b. Feigin, D. S., Everette, A. J., Jr., Stitik, F. P., Donner, M. W., and Skinner, D. B. The radiological appearance of hiatal hernia repairs. Radiology, *110*(1):71, 1974.

77. Feldman, M. D. Retrograde extension of prolapse of gastric mucosa into the esophagus. Am. J. Med. Sci., *222*:54, 1951.

78. Fellows, K. E., Sigmann, J., Stern, A. M., and Bookstein, J. D. Coronary sinus enlargement in infants. Radiology, *94*(2):347, 1970.

79. Felson, B., and Palayew, M. J. The two types of right aortic arch. Radiology, *81*(5):745, 1963.

80. Fernandes, J. P., Mascarenhas, M. J., Celestino da Costa, J., and Correia, J. P. Diffuse leiomyomatosis of the esophagus. Dig. Dis., *20*(7):684, 1975.

81a. Fleischner, F. G. The esophagus and mediastinal lymphadenopathy in bronchial carcinoma. Am. J. Roentgenol., *58*:48, 1952.

81b. Foerster, A., Bliesener, J. A., and Runge, K. A new method of localization of a tracheoesophageal fistula in the thorax. Z. Kinderchir., *16*(4):445, 1975.

82. Forrest, J. V., and Lester, P. D. Roentgenographic evaluation of lingual tonsillitis. Arch. Otolaryngol., *97*:482, 1973.

83. Forrester, H. D. Laryngocele. Am. J. Roentgenol., *81*(2):321, 1958.

84. Fostlethwait, R. W., Seuk, K. K., and Dillon, M. I. Esophageal complications of vagotomy. Surg. Gynecol. Obstet., *128*:481, 1969.

85. Frank, M. M., and Gatewood, B. M. O. Transient pharyngeal incoordination in the newborn. Am. J. Dis. Child., *111*:178, 1966.

86. Franken, E. A. Caustic damage of the gastrointestinal tract: roentgen features. Am. J. Roentgenol., *118*(1):77, 1973.

87. Fraser, R. C., and Pare, J. A. P. *Diagnosis of diseases of the chest.* Philadelphia, Saunders, 1970.

88. Friedland, G. W., Dobbs, W. J., Sunshine, P., and Zboralski, F. F. The apparent disparity in incidence of hiatal hernia in infants and children in Britain and the United States. Am. J. Roentgenol., *120*(2):305, 1974.

89. Friedland, G. W., and Filly, R. The postcricoid impression masquerading as an esophageal tumor. Am. J. Dig. Dis., *20*(3):297, 1975.

90. Gallina, F. Mass survey for neoplasm of digestive system. Book of Abstracts. XII Internal Congress of Radiology, Tokyo, Japan, Oct. 1969. Abst. 50049, p. 28.

91. Geffan, N. Rumination in man. Am. J. Dig. Dis., *11*(12):963, 1966.

92. Ghabreman, G. G., Heck, L. L., and Williams, J. R. A pharmacologic aid in radiographic diagnosis of obstructive esophageal lesions. Radiology, *103*(2):289, 1972.

93. Giedion, A. Pacifer nipple (dummy) in pediatric radiology. Am. Radiol., *11*(5-6):437, 1968.

94a. Giedion, A., and Nolte, K. The nonobstructive pharyngoesophageal cross roll. Ann. Radiol., *16*(3-4): 129, 1973.

94b. Gignoux, F. H. M., Fourre, P. P. D., LeRoquais, P., and LeSaint, J. N. L'azygographic dans l'etude radiologigne des tumeurs malignes de l'oesophage. J. Radiol. Electrol., *56*(3):227, 1975.

95. Girdany, B. R. The esophagus in infancy; congenital and acquired diseases. Radiol. Clin. N.A., *1*(3):557, 1963.

96. Givler, R. L. Esophageal lesions in leukemia and lymphosema. Am. J. Dig. Dis. (new series), *15*(1):31, 1970.

97. Goldberg, I. H., and Dodds, J. W. Cobblestone esophagus due to monilial infection. Am. J. Roentgenol., *103*(3):608, 1968.

98a. Goldstein, H. M., and Dodd, G. D. Double contrast examination of the esophagus. Gastrointest. Radiol., *1*:3, 1976.

98b. Goldstein, H. M., Rogers, L. F., Fletcher, G. A., and Dodd, G. D. Radiologic manifestations of radiation including injury to the normal upper gastrointestinal tract. Radiology, *117*(1):135, 1957.

99. Gonzalez, G. Diffuse esophageal spasm. Am. J. Roentgenol., *117*(2):251, 1973.

100. Gonzalez, G. Esophageal moniliasis. Am. J. Roentgenol., *113*(2):233, 1971.

101. Goyal, R. K., Bauer, J. I., and Spiro, H. H. The nature and location of lower esophageal ring. N. Eng. J. Med., *284*(21):1175, 1971.

102. Grunebaum, M., and Moskowitz, G. The retropharyngeal soft tissues in young infants with hypothyroidism. Am. J. Roentgenol., *108*(3):543, 1970.

103. Haber, K., and Winfield, A. C. Multiple leiomyomas of the esophagus. Am. J. Dig. Dis., 19(7):678, 1974.

104. Harell, G. S., Friedland, G. W., Daily, W. J., and Cohn, R. B. Neonatal Boerhaave syndrome. Radiology, 95:665, 1970.

105. Haupt, G. J., Templeton, J. X., and Amadeo, J. H. Retrosternal placement of ascending colon for esophageal substitution. JAMA, 167(7):832, 1958.

106. Healy, R. J. Bronchogenic cysts. Am. J. Roentgenol., 57:200, 1951.

107. Hemlich, H. J. Peptic esophagitis with stricture treated by reconstruction of the esophagus with a reversed gastric tube. Surg. Gynecol. Obstet., 114:673, 1962.

108. Heitmann, P., Cseudes, A., and Struszer, T. Esophageal strictures and lower esophagus lined with columnar epithelium. Am. J. Dig. Dis., 16(4):307, 1971.

109. Heitzman, E. J., Heitzman, G. C., and Elliott, C. F. Primary esophageal amylordosis. Arch. Intern. Med., 100:141, 1962.

110. Hellemans, N., and Julius, J. Hiatal hernia associated with malignancy in the region of the cardia. Am. J. Dig. Dis. (new series), 10(5):467, 1965.

111. Higgs, R. H., and Castell, D. O. Cholinergic stimulation of the lower esophageal sphincter in patients with vagotomy and antrectomy. Am. J. Dig. Dis., 20(3):195, 1975.

112. Hollinshead, W. H. Anatomy for Surgeons. New York, Haeber-Harper, 1954, Vols. I and II.

113. Hutton, C. F. Plummer–Vinson syndrome. Br. J. Radiol., 29:338, 1955.

114. Jacobson, G. H., Poppel, M. H., Hanenson, I. B., and Dewing, S. B. Left atrial enlargement. Am. Heart J., 43(3):423, 1952.

115. Jaffe, N., and Millan, V. G. Post-traumatic dissection intramural hematoma of the esophagus. Radiology, 95(2):379, 1970.

116. Jang, G. C., Clouse, M. E., and Fleischner, F. G. Fibrovascular polyp—a benign intraluminal tumor of the esophagus. Radiology, 92(6):1196, 1965.

117. Jorup, S. Congenital esophageal varices. Acta. Ped., 48(35):247, 1959.

118. Johnstone, H. S. Diffuse spasm and diffuse muscle hypertrophy or lower esophagus. Br. J. Radiol., 33:723, 1960.

119. Johnstone, H. S. Radiology of the oesophagus. In Jones, A. F., ed. Gastroenterology. New York, Haeber, Modern trend series, 1952, Chapter II.

120. Jullen, P. J., Goldberg, H. I., Margulis, A. R., and Belzer, F. O. Gastrointestinal complications following renal transplantation. Radiology, 117(1):37, 1975.

121a. Kaufmann, S. A. Epiphrenic diverticula of the esophagus. Am. J. Dig. Dis., 3(4):38, 1958.

121b. Kaye, M. D. Dysfunction of the lower esophageal sphincter in disorders other than achalasia. Am. J. Dig. Dis., 18(9):734, 1973.

122. Keats, T. E., Berclon, W. E., Kirkpatrick, J. A., and Young, L. W. Pediatric Disease Syllabus. Chicago, Ill., Am. Coll. of Radiol., 1974.

123. Keats, T. E., and Smith, T. H. Air esophagogram. Am. J. Roentgenol., 120(2):300, 1974.

124. Kendall, B. E., Asheroft, K., and Whiteside, C. G. A physiological variation in the barium filled gullet. Br. J. Radiol., 35:769, 1962.

125. Khoo, F. Y., Chea, K. B., and Nalpon, J. A new technique of contrast examination of the nasopharynx with cinefluorography and roentgenography. Am. J. Roentgenol., 99(1):238, 1967.

126. Killian, G. Ueber den mund der speiscröhre. Ztsch. Ohrenh. Wiesh., 55:1, 1908.

127. Kinsbourn, M. Hiatus hernia with contortions of the neck. Lancet, 1:1058, 1964.

128. Kirkpatrick, J. A., Capitanio, M. A., and Pereira, R. M. Immunologic abnormalities—roentgen observations. Radiol. Clin. N.A., 10(2):250, 1972.

129. Klinger, H. Concept of mechanical asset in esophageal speech. Arch. Otolaryngol., 92:244, 1970.

130. Klinkheimer, A. C. Esophagography in Anomalies of the Aortic Arch System. Baltimore, Md., Williams and Wilkins, 1969.

131. Knudsen, K. B., and Sparberg, M. Letter to JAMA on ulcerative esophagitis and ulcerative colitis. JAMA, 201(2):154, 1967.

132. Koberle, F. Enteromegaly and cardiomegaly in Chaga's disease. Gut, 4:399, 1963.

133. Kolawale, T. M., and Lewis, E. A. A radiologic study of tuberculosis of the abdomen (gastrointestinal tract). Am. J. Roentgenol., 23(2):348, 1975.

134. Krain, S., and Rabinowitz, J. G. Radiologic features of myotonic dystrophy with presentation of new findings. Clin. Radiol., 22:462, 1971.

135. Labowreau, J. P., LeTouze, P., and Caldera, R. Neonatal herpes. Exc. Med., 30(3):163, 1006, 1974.

136. Lacroix, L. Sulla visualizazione radiologica della tiroide. Minerva Med., 48:1, 1957.

137. Ladd, W. E., and Scott, H. W. Esophageal duplications or mediastinal cysts of enteric origin. Surgery, 16:815, 1944.

138. Legge, D. A., Carlson, H. G., and Judd, E. S. Roentgenologic features of regional enteritis of the upper gastrointestinal tract. Am. J. of Roentgenol., 110(2):355, 1970.

139. Leigh, T. F., Abbott, O. A., and Hopkins, W. A. Roentgenologic considerations in tracheoesophageal fistula without esophageal atresia. Radiology, 57:871, 1951.

140. Lerche, W. The Esophagus and Pharynx in Action. Springfield, Ill., Thomas, 1950.

141. Levene, G., and Kaufman, S. A. The roentgen diagnosis of pericardial effusion. Am. J. Roentgenol., 57:373, 1951.

142. Lewis, R. J. Tube helps patients with cancer of esophagus. JAMA, 223(13):1445, 1973.

143. Lichter, I., and Borrie, J. Intramural oesophageal abcess. Br. J. Surg., 52(3):185, 1965.

144. Lieber, A., Mandelstan, F., Siegal, G. I., and Siegal, N. Disordered esophageal function in diabetes mellitis. XII International Congress of Radiology, Tokyo,

Japan, Oct. 6–11, 1969. Book of Abstracts, Paper 0420, p. 225.

145. Liebowitz, H. R. *Bleeding Esophageal Varices—Portal Hypertension.* Springfield, Ill., Thomas, 1959.

146. Linsman, J. F. Gastroesophageal reflux elicited while drinking water (water siphonage test). Am. J. Roentgenol., *94*(2):325, 1965.

147. Li Voisi, V., and Perzini, K. M. Inflammatory pseudo-tumors (Inflammatory fibrous polyps) of the esophagus. Am. J. Dig. Dis., *20*(5):475, 1975.

148. Lockard, V. M. Lesions of the upper gastrointestinal tract in infants and children. Am. J. Roentgenol., *58*:696, 1952.

149. Logan, W. J., and Bosma, J. F. Oral and pharyngeal dysphagia in infancy. Ped. Clin. N.A., *14*(1):47, 1967.

150. Longemann, J. A., Blousky, R. E., and Boshes, B. Editorial on dysphagia in Parkinsonism. JAMA, *231*(1):69, 1975.

151. Longino, L. A., Woolley, M. D., and Gross, R. F. Esophageal replacement in infants and children with use of segment of colon. JAMA, *171*(9):1187, 1959.

152. Lorber, S., and Shay, H. Roentgen study of esophageal transport in patients with dysphagia due to abnormal motor function. Gastroenterology, *28*(5):697, 1955.

153. Lowman, R. M., Goldman, R., and Stern, H. The roentgen aspects of intramural dissection of the esophagus. Radiology, *93*(6):329, 1969.

154. Lubert, M., Epstein, H. C., Mendelsohn, H., and Freedlander, S. O. An unusual variant of double aortic arch. Am. J. Roentgenol., *67*(5):763, 1952.

155. Macfie, D. D. Asymptomatic laryngoceles in wind instrument bandsmen. Arch. Otolaryngol., *83*:270, 1966.

156. Maclean, A. D., and Houghton, A. Upper esophageal web in childhood. Ped. Radiol., *3*:240, 1975.

157. Madden, J. I., Ravid, J. M., and Haddock, J. R. Regional esophagitis: a specific entity simulating Crohn's disease. Ann. Surg., *170*:351, 1969.

158. Margulis, S. I., Brunt, P. W., Donner, M. W., and Silbiger, M. L. Familial dysautonomia. Radiology, *90*:107, 1968.

159. Marchese, G. S., and Grassi, E. Congenital nonfistular atresia of the esophagus. Notes from Regina Margherita Hospital, Torino, Italy, 1965.

160. Marks, I. N., and Keert, A. D. Instrumental rupture of the esophagus. Br. Med. J., *3*:536, 1968.

161. Martel, W. Radiologic features of esophagitis secondary to extremely caustic agents. Radiology, *103*(1):31, 1972.

162. Mata, R. M., Reyes, P. A., Segovia, D. A., and Garza, R. Esophageal mobility in systemic lupus erythematosus. Am. J. Dig. Dis., *19*(2):132, 1974.

163. McCort, J. J. Esophageal carcinosarcoma and pseudo-sarcoma. Radiology, *102*(3):519, 1972.

164. McCort, J. J., and Robbins, L. L. Roentgen diagnosis of intrathoracic lymph node metastasis in carcinoma of the lung. Am. J. Roentgenol., *57*:339, 1953.

165. McNab, R. F. Jones. The Patterson–Brown–Kelly Syndrome Part II. J. Laryngol. Otol., *75*(6):351, 1961.

166. McNally, E. F., and Katz, I. The roentgen diagnosis of diffuse spasm of the esophagus. Am. J. Roentgenol., *99*(1):218, 1967.

167. Medellin, H., and Wallace, S. Angiography in neoplasms of larynx and hypopharynx. Radiol. Clin. N.A., *8*(3):361, 1970.

168. Meschan, I., Martin, J. F., and Rogers, L. F. *Head and Neck Disorders Syllabus.* Chicago, Ill., Am. Coll. of Radiol., 1974. Vol. 5.

169. Musher, D. R., and Lindner, A. E. Primary melanoma of the esophagus. Am. J. Dig. Dis., *19*(9):855, 1974.

170. Nachlerio, E. D. Surgery of the esophagus. N.Y. State J. Med., *68*:3991, 1968.

171. Nardi, G. L. Colon transplant for artificial esophagus. N. Eng. J. Med., *256*:777, 1957.

172. Nathan, M. H. Radiologic diagnosis of esophageal varices. Radiology, *73*:725, 1959.

173. Nebesar, R. A., and Pollard, J. J. Portal venography by selective arterial catherization. Am. J. Roentgenol., *97*:477, 1966.

174. Netter, F. H. *The CIBA Collection of Medical Illustrations.* Vol. 3, Upper Digestive Tract. CIBA, 1966.

175. Neuhauser, E. B. D. Tracheo-esophageal constriction produced by right aortic arch and left ligamentum arteriosum. Am. J. Roentgenol., *62*(4):493, 1949.

176. Nora, P. F. *Operative Surgery—Principles and Technique.* Philadelphia, Lea-Febiger, 1972.

177. Nasher, J. I., Campbell, L. W., and Seaman, W. B. The clinical significance of cervical esophageal and hypopharyngeal webs. Radiology, *117*(1):45, 1975.

178. Oliphant, W. D., Hills, T. H., Stanford, R. W., and Moore, R. D. Xeroradiology. Br. J. Radiol., *28*:543, 1958.

179. Palmer, E. D. An attempt to localize the normal esophagogastric junction. Radiology, *60*:825, 1953.

180. Palmer, E. D. Dysphagia in Parkinsonism. JAMA, *229*(10):1340, 1974.

181. Palmer, E. D. The fate of esophageal varices in cirrhosis following surgical portal decompression. Gastroenterology, *32*:861, 1957.

182. Pava, S., Pickren, J. W., and Adler, R. H. Ectopic gastric mucosa of the esophagus. N.Y. State J. Med., *64*:1836, 1964.

183. Payne, S. W., and Olsen, A. M. *The Esophagus.* Philadelphia, Lea and Febiger, 1974.

184. Pecora, D. V. The balloon tube as an aid in the roentgenologic examination of the esophagogastric region. Am. J. Roentgenol., *79*:768, 1958.

185. Pernkopf, E. *Atlas of Topographic and Applied Human Anatomy.* Philadelphia, Saunders, 1963. Vol. 1.

186. Pesev, I., and Elenkov, P. Dermatomyositis (translated from Russian). Exc. Med., *23*(8):376, 1969. Abstr. 2261.

187. Peters, P. M. The congenital short esophagus. Thorax, *13*(1):1, 1958.

188. Pitman, R. G., and Fraser, G. M. The post cricoid impression of the esophagus. Clin. Radiol., *16*(1):35, 1968.

189. Polonsky, L., and Girth, P. H. Familial achalasia. Am. J. Dig. Dis., 15(3):291, 1970.

190. Portnoy, L. M., and Sazonov, A. M. Pneumo-esophagotomography. Vestin, Roentgenol., Radial (Russia), 48(2):3, 1973.

191. Porubsky, E. S., Murray, P. J., and Lindsay, L. P. Cricopharyngeal achalasia in dermatomyositis. Arch. Otolaryngol., 98:428, 1973.

192. Preger, L., Maddison, R. E., Won, G., and Brandborg, L. The erection and detumescence of esophageal varices. Am. J. Roentgenol., 107:77, 1969.

193. Babiah, F. A., and Elliott, H. B. Intramural hematoma of the esophagus. Am. J. Dig. Dis., 13(10):925, 1968.

194. Ramirez-Mata, M., Reyes, A. P., Alareon-Segovia, D., and Gorza, R. Esophageal motility in systemic lupus erythematosus. Am. J. Dig. Dis., 19(2):132, 1974.

195. Raphaeal, R. L., Schnabel, T. G., and Leopold, S. S. A new method for demonstrating an aberrant right subclavian artery. Am. J. Roentgenol., 58:89, 1952.

196. Reed, L. J., and Sobonya, M. R. Morphologic analysis of foregut cysts in the thorax. Am. J. Roentgenol., 120(4):851, 1974.

197. Reeder, M. A., and Hamilton, L. C. Radiologic diagnosis of tropical diseases of the gastrointestinal tract. Radiol. Clin. N.A., 7(1):65, 1965.

198. Reuter, R. S., and Atkins, W. T. High dose left gastric angiography for demonstration of esophageal varices. Radiology, 105(3):573, 1972.

199. Rodriques, H. O musculo crico-farmigico e suas relacoes com o musculo farmigo-esofagico e con o esfincter esofagicio superior. Bull. Inst. Cien. Biol. Giocien., University of De Juiz DeFora, Brazil, Bull. 9, Sept., 1974.

200. Rosenkranz, W., and Bryk, D. Pseudo-tumors in large hiatus hernias. Am. J. Roentgenol., 116(2): 289, 1972.

201. Rossetti, M. Die Reflux Krankheit des Oesophagus. Stuttgart, Hippokrates Verlag, 1966.

202. Roswit, B. Complications of radiation therapy: The alimentary tract. Sem. Roentgenol., 9(1):51, 1974.

203. Rubenstein, B. M., Postrana, T., and Jacobson, H. G. Tuberculosis of the esophagus. Radiology, 70(3): 401, 1958.

204. Rubin, P. Cancer of the gastrointestinal tract (esophagus. JAMA, 226(13):1564, 1973.

205. Rudnick, J. P., Ferrucci, J. T., Jr., Eaton, B. S., and Dreyfuss, J. R. Esophageal pseudo-tumor; retrograde prolapse of gastric mucosa into the esophagus. Am. J. Roentgenol., 115(2):253, 1972.

206. Rudolph, I., Herrera, A. F., Stein, G. N., and Roth, J. L. A. Mechanism of Pyrosis. Am. J. Dig. Dis., 16(7):577, 1071.

207. Russell, E., Shapiro, R., and Wilson, G. L. Radiologic aspects of celestin tube intubation for incurable obstructive esophageal carcinoma. Radiology, 102:531, 1972.

208. Saladin, T., French, A. B., Zarafonitis, C. J., and Pollard, M. H. Esophageal motor abnormalities in scleroderma and related diseases. Am. J. Dig. Dis., 11(7):522, 1966.

209. Sandmark, S. Hiatal incompetence. Acta Radiol. Supp. 219, 1963.

210. Sanowski, R. A., and Riegel, N. Pneumatic dilatation of the lower esophageal ring. Am. J. Dig. Dis., 15(5):407, 1970.

211. Schatzki, R., and Gray, J. E. The lower esophageal ring. Am. J. Roentgenol., 75:246, 1956.

212. Schuman, B. M., and Arciniegas, E. The management of esophageal complications of epidermolysis bullosa. Am. J. Dig. Dis., 17(10):875, 1972.

213. Schwedel, J. B. Clinical Roentgenology of the Heart. New York, Haeber, 1946.

214. Seaman, W. B. Functional disorders of the pharyngoesophageal junction. Radiol. Clin. N.A., 7(1): 113, 1969.

215. Seamen, W. B. The significance of webs in the hypopharynx and upper esophagus. Radiology, 89:32, 1967.

216. Shanon, E., and Plaschkes, J. Reconstruction of the pharynx using penile skin graft. Arch. Otolaryngol., 86:119, 1967.

217. Shapiro, J. H., Jacobson, H. G., Stern, W. E., and Poppel, M. H. Posterior mediastinal goiter. Radiology, 71(1):79, 1958.

218. Sheinmel, A., Priviteri, C. A., and Poppel, M. H. A study of the effects of certain drugs on curling of the esophagus. Am. J. Roentgenol., 62(6):807, 1949.

219. Sheppard, I. M., Jacobson, H. G., Zaino, C., and Poppel, M. H. Dynamics of occlusion. J. Am. Dent. Assoc., 58:77, 1959.

220. Sheft, D. J., and Shrago, G. Esophageal moniliasis. JAMA, 213(11):1859, 1970.

221. Shuford, W. H., Sybers, R. G., and Schlant, F. K. Right aortic arch with isolation of the left subclavian artery. Am. J. Roentgenol., 109(1):75, 1970.

222. Singleton, E. B. X-ray diagnosis of the alimentary tract in infants and children. Year Book—1959.

223. Sisson, G. A. The surgical treatment of carcinoma of the cervical esophagus. N.Y. State J. Med., 55:201, 1955.

224. Smith, P. C., Swischuck, L. E., and Eagan, C. J. An elusive and often unsuspected cause of stridor or pneumonia (the esophageal foreign body). Am. J. Roentgenol., 122(1):80, 1974.

225. Smulewicz, J. J., and Dorfman, J. Esophageal intramural diverticulosis. Radiology, 101(3):527, 1971.

226. Som, M. I., and Wolf, B. S. Peptic ulcer of the esophagus and esophagitis in gastric lined esophagus. JAMA, 162(7):641, 1956.

227. Somer, H., Donner, M., Marros, J., and Konttiner, A. Serum lysozyme study in muscular dystrophy. Arch. Neurol., 29:343, 1973.

228. Sperling, H. V., and D'Altario, R. A. Intramural diverticulosis of the esophagus. Am. J. Dig. Dis., 18 (11):978, 1973.

229. Stancin, C., and Bennett, J. R. Smoking and gastroe-

sophageal reflux. Brit. Med. J., *3*:793, 1972. Abstr.: Am. J. Roentgenol., *117*(2):476, 1973.

230. Stein, G. N., and Finkelstein, A. K. *The Esophagus and Stomach—An Atlas of Tumor Radiology.* Chicago, Ill., Year Book Med. Publ., Inc., 1973.

231. Steinberg, I., Esigle, M. A., Halawade, G. R., and Hagstrom, J. W. C. Pseudo-coarctation of the aorta associated with congenital heart disease. Am. J. Roentgenol., *106*(1):1, 1969.

232. Stevens, A. C., and Jackson, C. E. Localization of parathyroid adenomas. Am. J. Roentgenol., *99*(1): 233, 1967.

233. Stewart, J. R., Kincaid, V. W., and Edwards, J. E. *An Atlas of Vascular Rings and Related Malformations of the Aortic Arch System.* Springfield, Ill., Thomas, 1964.

234. Stiennon, A. O. The "captive bolus" test and the pinchcock at the diaphragm. Am. J. Roentgenol., *99*(1):223, 1967.

235. Stout, A. P., and Latters, R. *Tumors of the Esophagus.* Washington, D.C., Armed Forces Institute of Pathology, 1957.

236. Sulway, J. J., Baume, P. E., and Davis, E. Stiff-man syndrome presenting with complete esophageal obstruction. Am. J. Dig. Dis., *15*(1):79, 1970.

237. Sussman, H. M., Weingarten, B., and Massberg, S. M. Localized gastric mucosa hypertrophy simulated tumor. Am. J. Dig. Dis., *10*(1):710, 1965.

238. Sweet, R. H. Esophageal hiatal hernia of the diaphragm. Am. J. Surg., *52*:135, 1952.

239. Swischuck, L. E., Smith, P. C., and Fagan, C. J. Abnormalities of the pharynx and larynx in childhood. Sem. Roentgenol., *9*(1):283, 1974.

240. Takita, H. Endoesophageal intubation. N.Y. State J. Med., *71*:2526, 1971.

241. Texidor, H. S., and Evans, J. A. Roentgenographic appearance of the distal esophagus and stomach after hiatal hernia repair. Am. J. Roentgenol., *119*(2): 245, 1973.

242. Templeton, R. E. *X-ray Examination of the Stomach.* Chicago, University of Chicago Press, 1944.

243. Tento, L. T., and Lattimer, H. F. Congenital H-type TE fistula in young adult. Arch. Otolaryngol., *85*:675, 1967.

244. Terracol, J., and Sweet, R. H. *Diseases of the Esophagus.* Philadelphia and London, Saunders, 1958.

245. Thomas, G. I., and Marendino, A. Jejunal interposition operations. JAMA, *168*(13):176, 1958.

246. Totten, R. S. Tumors of the oral cavity, pharynx and larynx. JAMA, *215*(3):455, 1971.

247. Troupin, R. H. Intramural esophageal diverticulosis and moniliasis. Am. J. Roentgenol., *104*(3):613, 1968.

248. Unger, A. S., and Poppel, M. H. Congenital absence of the middle of the esophagus. Am. J. Roentgenol., *40*(2):240, 1938.

249. Vanasin, B., Wright, J. R., and Shuster, M. M. Pneumotosis cysoides esophagi. JAMA, *217*(1):76, 1971.

250. Victorica, B. E., Van Mierop, L. H. S., and Elliott, L. P. Right aortic arch associated with contra-lateral congenital subclavian steal syndrome. Am. J. Roentgenol., *108*(3):582, 1970.

251. Watson, W., and Bancroft, E. W. Hypertrophic cricopharyngeal stenosis. Surg., Gynecol., Obstet., *62*:621, 1936.

252. Webb, H. E., and Sutcliffe, J. Neurological basis for the abnormal movements in Sandifer's syndrome. Lancet, *2*:818, 1975.

253. Weber, H. L., Kooh Sang, and Watts, B. F. Radiographic examination of gastrointestinal tract in infants and children. Radiol. Clin. N.A., *9*(1):5, 1971.

254. Weitzner, S. Changes in the pharyngeal and esophageal musculature in oculopharyngeal muscular dystrophy. Am. J. Dig. Dis., *14*:11, 1969.

255. Weller, M. H. Intramural diverticulosis of the esophagus. Report of a case in a child. J. Pediatr., *80*:286, 1972. Abstra: Radiology, *104*(2):484, 1972.

256. Weller, M. H., and Lutzker, S. A. Intramural diverticulosis of the esophagus. Radiology, *98*(2):373, 1971.

257. Wells, J. Herniation of gastric mucosa into the esophagus. Am. J. Roentgenol., *58*(2):194, 1947.

258. Whalen, J. P., and Woodruff, L. C. The cervical prevertebral fat strip. Am. J. Roentgenol., *109*(3):445, 1970.

259. Wiesner, P. J., Kleinman, M. S., Contemi, J. J., Resnicoff, S. A., and Schwartz, S. I. Sarcoidosis of the esophagus. Am. J. Dig. Dis., *16*(10):943, 1971.

260. Wilkins, E. W., Jr. Current consideration of esophageal physiology, normal and abnormal. N. Eng. J. Med., *257*(1):24, 1957.

261. Wilson, C. P. Diverticula of the pharynx. J. Roy. Coll. Surg., Edinburg, *4*:236, 1959.

262. Winslip, D. H., Carlton, R., Caflesch, F., Zboroloske, F., and Hogan, W. J. Determination of esophageal peristalsis in patients with alcoholic neuropathy. Gastroenterology, *55*:173, 1968.

263a. Wolf, B. S. Roentgen examination of the esophagus. Gastroenterology, *27*:443, 1957.

263b. Westley, C. R., Herbst, J. J., Goldman, S., and Wiser, W. C. Infantile achalasia inherited as an autosomal recessive disorder. J. Pediatr., *87*(2):243, 1975.

264. Wolf, B. S., Marshak, R. H., Som. M. L., and Winkelstein, A. Peptic esophagitis, peptic ulcer of the esophagus and marginal esophageal ulceration. Gastroenterology, *29*(5):744, 1955.

265. Wright, J. T. Allison and Johnstone's anomaly. Am. J. Roentgenol., *94*(2):308, 1965.

266. Zaino, C. Oil contrast study of the lower esophagus. Am. J. Roentgenol., *67*:942, 1952.

267. Zaino, C., Jacobson, H. G., Lepow, H., and Ozturk, C. H. *The Pharyngoesophageal Sphincter.* Springfield, Ill., Thomas, 1970.

268. Zaino, C., and Poppel, M. H. Acquired hiatal hernia. Dig. Dis. (new series), *5*:215, 1956.

269. Zaino, C., and Poppel, M. H. The lower esophagus. CIBA Symp., 8(1):31, 1956.
270. Zaino, C., Poppel, M. H., and Blazik, C. Roentgenologic study of the abdominal segment of the esophagus in the presence of pneumoperitoneum. Am. J. Dig. Dis., 22:121, 1955.
271. Zaino, C., Poppel, N. H., Jacobson, H. G., and Lepow, H. The Lower Esophageal Vestibular Complex. Springfield, Ill., Thomas, 1963.
272. Zamel, N., Austin, J. H. M., Frof, P. D., Dedo, H. H., Malcolm, D. J., and Nadel, J. A. Powdered tantalium as a medium for human laryngography. Radiology, 94:547, 1970.
273. Zboralske, F. F. The esophagus in the geriatric patient. Radiol. Clin. N.A., 3:321, 1965.
274. Zimmerman, J. M., and King, T. C. Use of Souttar tube in the management of advanced esophageal cancer. Ann. Surg., 169:867, 1969.

INDEX

T

Tantalum, as contrast media, 2–3
Tetanus, effects on swallowing, 182
Thermal trauma, esophagitis from, 217
Thoracic aorta, diseases of, effects on upper alimentary canal, 120–125
Thoracic esophagus
  checklist for barium exam of, 70
  gross anatomy of, 32
  neoplasms of, 256–262
  radiologic anatomy of, 57–61
Thoracic spine
  changes in, affecting upper alimentary canal, 113
  effects on upper alimentary canal, 113–116
Thoracocentesis, effects on esophagus, 297
Thorocoplasty, effects on esophagus, 296
Thoracotomy, effects on esophagus, 296
Thrush, effects on oral cavity and esophagus, 189
Thyroglossal cysts, description of, 75–76
Thyroid gland, enlargement of, 109–112
Thyrotoxicosis, effects on esophagus, 109, 110
Tobacco, excessive use of, esophagitis from, 213
Tomography, description of, 13
Tongue, gross anatomy of, 29, 31
Tonsilitis, acute, 185
Topographic anatomy, of oropharynx and esophagus, 37–38
Toxic myopathics, effects on upper alimentary canal, 182
Trachea, fistulae of, effects on upper alimentary tract, 125–127
Tracheoesophageal fistula, 92
  H-type, 94–96
  repair of, 278, 280
Trauma
  effects on upper alimentary tract, 131
  esophagitis from, 210
Trendelenburg position, description of, 20
Truncus arteriosus, description and diagnosis of, 89
Tubercular granulomas, effects on upper alimentary tract, 128–129
Tuberculosis, of esophagus, 193
Tumors, of thyroid, 111–112

U

Ulcers of esophagus, 188, 217–222
Upper sphincter, checklist for barium exam of, 70
Uvula, gross anatomy of, 31

V

Vagotomy, radiologic changes following, 288–291
Vallecula, neoplasms of, 254
Valsalva maneuver
  description of, 22
  fluoroscopy during, 11

Varices
  esophageal, 4, 23, 24–26, 103, 203–207
  surgery for, 295–296
Vascular rings
  description of, 76–80
  diagnosis of, 78–79, 82, 83
Videotapes, use in radiology, 9
Vigorous achalasia, description of, 146, 148
Volvulus, of esophagus, 165, 168–169
Vomiting, functional, 142

W

Water siphonage test, description of, 23
Web(s)
  congenital, of esophagus, 101–102
  description of, 224–225
  diagnosis of, 28
Wolf's position, description of, 20
"Wooden shoe" cardiac silhouette, in Fallot's tetrad, 88

X

Xeroradiography, description of, 20

Z

Zenker's diverticula, 76
Zollinger–Ellison syndrome, 291